"Dr. Rachel McRoberts has done a masterful job at integrating Jungian concepts into the world of play therapy and counseling. The book is rich with information covering a broad base of Jung's influence over many disciplines, from cognitive-behavioral to the evolving world of neuroscience. This book is a pleasure because she wraps her mind around some very complicated and delicate theoretical concepts and manages to hold onto her sense of humor and wonder about it all."

John Paul "JP" Lilly, MS, LCSW, RPT-S,
Chief Mechanic, Jungian Analytical Play Therapy

"This work is exactly what is needed at this time. We are struggling, as a profession, with cohesive and accessible texts that assist with our understanding of ourselves, as counselors".

Jenna Epstein, PhD, NCC, LPC, ACS,
CTRS, NREMT, *Assistant Professor and*
Programs Coordinator at Frostburg State University

"An insightful journey through the realms of personal and professional growth, this book delves deep into aesthetics of existence, navigating the complexities of post-modernism and the therapeutic alliance. With a focus on ethics, identity, and the influence of Jungian counseling, it offers a profound exploration of the psyche's structure, language, and the transformative power of creative techniques. A must-read for anyone seeking a Jungian-centered approach to counseling and play therapy".

LoriAnn Stretch, PhD, LCMHC-S (NC),
LPC (VA), NCC, ACS, *Professor at University*
of the Cumberlands and President of the Association
for Creativity in Counseling

Jungian Counseling and Play Therapy

Jungian Counseling and Play Therapy is both an introduction to Jung's theory and a practical guide to Jungian-informed practice.

Readers journey through the development of the mental health crisis of the digital age (which Jung foresaw) and are presented with solutions he suggested that are still being met with resistance, despite compelling facts. This book not only advocates for a more widespread integration of Jungian ideas into clinical practice, but also for greater acknowledgement of the integrity, creativity, and intersecting identities of clients, professional counselors, and play therapists. Integrating historical theory with contemporary research, this book helps students to weave creative techniques into their online and in-person clinical work.

This is an ideal text for a psychodynamic theory or methods class, or to support counseling students and supervisors becoming interested in, or familiar with, the work of Carl Jung.

Rachel McRoberts, PhD, LPC-MHSP, ACS, RPT-S, is an award-winning, Jungian-oriented counselor, play therapist, supervisor, and researcher. She is also a Professor at University of the Cumberlands and maintains an atelier private practice.

Jungian Counseling and Play Therapy

Classical Theory for the Digital Age

Rachel McRoberts

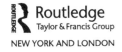
Routledge
Taylor & Francis Group
NEW YORK AND LONDON

Designed cover image: The Tree of Psyche © Rachel McRoberts

First published 2025
by Routledge
605 Third Avenue, New York, NY 10158

and by Routledge
4 Park Square, Milton Park, Abingdon, Oxon, OX14 4RN

Routledge is an imprint of the Taylor & Francis Group, an informa business

ISBN: 978-1-032-55988-9 (hbk)
ISBN: 978-1-032-55983-4 (pbk)
ISBN: 978-1-003-43373-6 (ebk)

DOI: 10.4324/9781003433736

Typeset in Goudy
by Apex CoVantage, LLC

This book is dedicated to
Zo Newell
(1950–2022)
&
"Chief" JP Lilly
(1957–2024)

Contents

Acknowledgements

To my parents; thank you for a childhood cradled in libraries, the Church, Victorian sensibilities, and the arts.

To my husband, Scott, for co-creating in all areas of life with me, endlessly listening, and picking up a ton of slack.

To our sons, Arbor and Xanon, for simply being yourselves. Every moment is a gift.

To Dahlia, for being my best girl.

To Mr. Shevalier for being my first creative writing teacher all those years ago, and continuing to root for me.

To the brilliant artists at Visionary Design Group: Colette Lanham-Stoffel, Michael Stoffel, Taylor Bratcher, and especially Curtis Davidson for helping me bring these images to print.

To Dr. Jenna Epstein, Dr. Dalena Dillman Taylor, and Dr. Linda Homeyer, for your expert feedback in the early stages of this project.

To my teachers in the sandplay community, especially Ellen Saul, Gretchen Watts, Brenda Jacklin, Dr. Lorraine Freedle, and Dr. Jacque Wiersma.

To Dr. Tom Sweeney for your continued advocacy for the counseling profession, your consultation in reference to this book, and bestowing your blessing to highlight the Wheel of Wellness.

To Dr. Gary Landreth, for your steady inspiration and challenge to justify why we might deviate from the child-centered model. I can't imagine what our field would be without your work.

To JP Lilly, for being the official Chief Mechanic of Jungian Analytical Play Therapy. Thank you for sharing your wisdom with humor and humbleness. It's an honor to be your student.

To Lene Rasmussen and Samuel Adler, for witnessing and encouraging me through this process.

To Rinda Skaggs for your mentorship through EFM.

To Dr. "Matt" Lyons and The University of the Cumberlands for supporting this project through the Summer Immersion Grant.

To Princeton University Press for continuing to publish and attempting to make the Collected Works more accessible.

To the editorial team at Routledge, especially Anna Moore, Alison Macfarlane, and Tom Bedford. Your kindness, patience, and expertise are unmatched.

To all those interested in Jungian-oriented scholarship and practice: past, present, and future.

Peace be with you.

Notes

The Collected Works (CW) of C. G. Jung as Referenced Throughout the Book

Throughout the text, while other references will be listed at the end of each chapter, I will reference the Collected Works as CW with the volume, page, and paragraph (i.e., CW#, p. #, § #) for direct quotes, so as to not confuse those who may be searching for a quote in a digital or print copy of different editions. While it is not officially APA style, it is common in the field, as it is more direct and saves space. It is a pet peeve of mine to see Jung's quotes on the internet without a citation to easily go and find them.

For those in the market, I recommend the newest, digital edition of the CW, as it is convenient to search by keyword and a compact addition to any library. Each of the volumes of the CW are thick: several hundred to over 1,000 pages long. Quotes are reprinted here with permission from Princeton University Press (copyright 2014). I will cite the following at the end of each chapter:

Jung, C. G. (2023). *The collected works of C. G. Jung: Revised and expanded complete digital edition.* (CW 1–20). G. Adler, W. McGuire, & H. Read (Eds.), R. F. C. Hull (Trans.). Princeton University Press. https://press.prince ton.edu/books/ebook/9780691255194/the-collected-works-of-c-g-jung

While there are several supplemental volumes to Jung's CW, for a quick reference by subject, I am including here a list of volumes 1–20 with their titles, and publication/copyright date as listed by Princeton University Press at the time this is written. Note that the publication date of the CW does not necessarily reflect the date of Jung's original work; most volumes bridge several decades and are organized roughly by topic. Jung's career spanned from 1900, when he was 25, until his death in 1961 at age 85. He spent a great deal of the last decade of his life retired from clinical practice, devoted to writing (CW 18); some of his last thoughts, though, are contained in CW 14.

CW 1 *Psychiatric Studies* 1970
CW 2 *Experimental Researches* 1973
CW 3 *The Psychogenesis of Mental Disease* 1960/1961
CW 4 *Freud and Psychoanalysis* 1962
CW 5 *Symbols of Transformation 1977/1967*
CW 6 *Psychological Types* 1976/1971
CW 7 *Two Essays on Analytical Psychology* 1972/1967
CW 8 *The Structure and Dynamics of the Psyche* 1970
CW 9i *The Archetypes and the Collective Unconscious 1981/1969*
CW 9ii *Aion: Researches into the Phenomenology of the Self 1979/1969*
CW 10 *Civilization in Transition* 1970
CW 11 *Psychology and Religion: West and East* 1970
CW 12 *Psychology and Alchemy* 1980/1968
CW 13 *Alchemical Studies* 1983/1968
CW 14 *Mysterium Coniunctionis* 1977/1970
CW 15 *Spirit in Man, Art and Literature* 1971/1966
CW 16 *The Practice of Psychotherapy* 1985/1966
CW 17 *The Development of Personality* 1981/1954
CW 18 *The Symbolic Life: Miscellaneous Writings* 1977
CW 19 *General Bibliography of C. G. Jung's Writings* 1979
CW 20 *General Index* 1979

1

An Ongoing Journey

Personal & Professional

. . . if you have nothing at all to create, then perhaps you create yourself.
Jung, CW 8, p. 557, § 906

Jung pioneered the importance of science studying the mind with the body and the spirit, and encouraged his students to refrain from becoming dogmatic with his theories in further developing advancements in practice as evidence emerged (Samuels, 2017; Wilkinson, 2005, 2016). Today, Jungian theory straddles across expressive arts, play, and mind-body therapies that are validated by neuroscience, attachment theory, and the values of the counseling profession. I agree with Sedgwick (2015) that a post-modern study of Jung is prudent, despite what the Jungian celebrity Jordan B. Peterson might think about the term (Peterson & Hicks, 2017; Woien, 2022). I advocate for a balance between classical teachings, richly filled with metaphor and imagery, and adapting to ever-emerging research. While the Jungian model in and of itself may be elusive to many and therefore lack the "evidence-based practice" (EBP) stamp of approval, my aim with this text is to provide ample theory and evidence of why Jungian-oriented counseling may be a more relational, creative, spiritually based approach, and a better fit than many manualized treatments with the EBP gold star. It has been for me and my clients and may be for you and yours.

THE AESTHETICS OF EXISTENCE

It is not I who create myself, rather I happen to myself.

CW 11, p. 259, § 391

DOI: 10.4324/9781003433736-1

I often say that I came to the field of counseling through the backdoor, which is why I may have a slightly different perspective on the field. My mother loves telling the story of how I told her I wanted to be a priest when I was four. While my religious and spiritual practices were, and are, very important to me, I remember realizing, when I was still quite young, that while I found it fascinating and beautiful that there were other religions in the world, others, even within my own parish, didn't feel the same. I could not believe that my way was the only way. I didn't know at the time how to reckon with this (or that I was sensing the idea of the Self, the religious function, and various other Jungian concepts we'll discuss), so I ran away to art school. There, I fully immersed myself in creative expression and found new levels of joy and connection with myself, others, and the divine.

Art making felt deeply personal to me, an intimate conversation, so much so that I wasn't drawn to selling my work professionally. In an attempt to find a career utilizing art, I earned a degree in art education but quickly realized that I didn't feel the need to teach children how to make art at all. I simply had a deep appreciation for what they wanted to say through their symbolic and expressive language. I wanted to see them, hear them, and encourage them. I later learned that this is known as "art as therapy" (Kramer, 2000), which I then pursued graduate studies in. Margarette Lowenfeld, who influenced the development of Jungian sandplay therapy, believed that art education and therapy were inseparable (Allan, 1988). This training, which began my training in Jung and later my adoption by the counseling and play therapy communities, builds upon this sense of knowing: that the act of creation is sacred and an expression of our connection to the Self.

I also learned of the interconnectedness of the fields of aesthetics, ethics, and the history of the power dynamics involved in diagnosing and treating mental illness from the notorious French philosopher Michelle Foucault (1984); he coined the term *aesthetics of existence*, the ethical viewpoint that each person's life is a work of art unto themselves, outside of any other authority. The word "aesthetic", often used to describe an artistic style or symbolic language, has its root in the Greek "aisthitikos" referring to a perceived sense or impression (Macneill, 2017). To live one's life as a work of art, to be a work of one's own creation for the sake of the Self, is an ancient one, but is something that deserves greater consideration in the digital age, where identity politics and mental health diagnoses are significant players in the zeitgeist.

Post-Modernism & the Digital Age

"When I use a word", Humpty Dumpty said, in a rather scornful tone, "it means just what I choose it to mean – neither more nor less".

"The question is", said Alice, "whether you can make words mean so many different things".

"The question is", said Humpty Dumpty, "which is to be master – that's all".

Carroll (1896), *Through the Looking-Glass*

Foucault was one of the first philosophers to talk about power, specifically biopower. Biopower refers to the discourse of surveilling and governing bodies, which today includes the ethics of not only counseling but also medicine, research, education, and the prison-industrial complex, which I will discuss more below. He did not self-identify as a post-modernist but is nonetheless considered one of the most iconic post-modernists (how's that for power influencing the labels we give people?).

Post-modernism, in its broadest sense, is both a time period and a social movement, as well as a method of discourse. As a movement, it is said to have begun in earnest in the mid-20th century (though the term was coined much earlier), after the "modern" age (from after the middle-ages to about the 1960s), in response to the unrest with the changes that occurred with modernity. "Post" modern being "after" the modern age. This is when and where traditional ideas and systems of power began to be openly critiqued, deconstructed, and re-interpreted by intellectuals, artists, and the culture at large.

The discourse around the deconstruction of the meaning of words themselves may be considered the start of the post-modern movement, thanks to literary critics, linguists, and philosophers, perhaps most famously, Jacques Derrida. How words come to have meaning, are understood, and are used all occur in systems of power. Like Humpty Dumpty, we may change a word's meaning by how we use it at any time; if that meaning is accepted and used by others, speaks of the influence of power, be that the editors of a peer-reviewed academic journal, or if the post goes viral. Post-modern artists were the first to deliberately push the boundaries of what was considered "fine art" by splashing paint around onto canvas non-representationally (Jackson Pollock), displaying printed images of commercial products and celebrities (Andy Warhol), and brandishing political ideals (the Guerilla Girls, who were also feminists). Second-wave feminism, too, in the post-modern era, overtly challenged traditional gender roles, as women began to take birth control pills, go to college, and attempt to redefine "femininity", regardless of previously established norms.

While the age we are in at the time this book is being written is commonly called "modern", technically, it is not since that time period is over. By dictionary definition, it would be more accurate to call any time we live in together "contemporary". However, we are also well into the "digital age". The digital age, sometimes called "the information age", can arguably be considered to have started with the widespread use of electricity and the printing press. Nevertheless, what is commonly referred to as the "digital age" is a transition that occurred within my adult life: computers in nearly every home, let alone pocket, have become a societal norm in America. And we're not even all the way in yet. While Americans have been spending most of their waking hours on some kind of digital platform for several years, it was only after the COVID-19 pandemic that I even came to imagine that art and play therapy could be facilitated online, let alone be practiced . . . by me. Online counseling is becoming increasingly popular.

Perhaps confusingly, "modernity", or wanting to continually improve and advance society with capitalism, industrialization, and staunch individualism, is still a thing. Post-modernism, too, is still a methodology used formally in qualitative research, which continues to deconstruct ideas and power systems to amplify the voices of its participants so we can better understand their lived experiences. Regarding counseling in America today, specifically, I think a post-modern approach is wise, especially today, because there is so much that is up for interpretation.

It is interesting to me that one of the most famous Jungians (admittedly also one of the most infamous educators, mental health providers, and social commentators), Jordan Peterson, is so vocal in speaking out against "the post-modernists", often combining that label with "Marxist". Foucault was adamant that he was not a Marxist (Wade, 2019). It seems to me and others that he's frustrated with people thinking that they can make up their own version of reality, attempt to change the meaning of words, attempt to impose new beliefs and practices upon others, and calling society's complacency with, or overt perpetuation of, that type of behavior post-modernism (Woien, 2022). However, I would argue that it is the post-modernists who would question all the power structures involved, the words themselves, as well as the thoughts and feelings expressed by all groups, both "in" and "out". Also, I believe that we can critique through a post-modern lens, while still holding on to personal and professional values, even if those fall under "traditional". Maybe Jordan and I can have a clinical debate about this someday. That would be fun! And terrifying.

Speaking of "in" and "out" groups, it may be helpful to note that there is discourse in the field about what/who is "Jungian" and what/who is "post-Jungian". I won't get into it too much here. However, I will discuss a bit more about the historical hierarchies that stem from valuing the ability to trace one's training lineage directly back to Jung himself. Some argue that everything thought or written after Jung's death is post-Jungian. I like to call myself a Jungian because I am reading Jung and applying his work to mine; it's more straightforward, and I am not a fan of the excessive use of hyphens; I already have one in post-modernism.

As a self-identifying Jungian-oriented counselor and post-modernist in the digital age, I am skeptical of all systems of power: the government, the media, and the mental health system. I think it is my ethical duty as a white woman, mother, person of faith, counselor, educator, supervisor, and researcher to take responsibility for my role within systems of power that have historically and continue to oppress people. Sitting in my positions of power, I agree with Peterson that I have a great deal of responsibility to clean up my own messes (Peterson et al., 2018), but I respectfully disagree that I need to perfect anything before critiquing various systems of power that influence and intersect with our collective identity as counselors.

Foucault discusses the idea of *the Panopticon* at length in his book *Discipline & Punish: The Birth of the Prison* (1977). I highly recommend this reading (. . . it makes me quite unpopular at parties), especially for those working in rehabilitation, corrections, schools, and really any type of institution. The Panopticon, referring to the Greek for "all seeing", was an efficient, circular prison structure designed in the 1700s; one guard could see into every cell, but because prisoners cannot know if they are being watched or not, they internalize that sense of being watched and begin to act as if they always actually are.

The idea of the "all seeing" can be considered an archetype, known across time and cultures from the "eye of Providence" (on the back of the US Dollar), to the third eye of Shiva, to the concept of an authority being able to assess the state of an internal process such as mental health. The Panopticon, then, is also a metaphor for any type of surveillance system, the discourse of the power dynamics between the watched and the watcher (Foucault, 1977).

The Panopticon is like Big Brother (Orwell, 2021), or the Eye of Sauron (Tolkien, 2020), but more inside our heads, like in *Brave New World* (Huxley, 2006), where it is "normal" to take anesthetizing pills to stay happy; where the word "mother" is taboo; where children are thought to be better raised by the State; where culture is homogenized. This is probably not good, right? Or maybe even wrong (Huijer, 1999; Koenderink, 2014). It is science fiction from the 30s. Or is it? Look around. Many well-meaning State agencies, schools, scientists, and mental health counselors sing variations of this panoptic tune and call it "objectivity", "anti-bias", "established best practice", "evidence-based", and even "good". That is beyond an ethical dilemma for me, and why I also need the aesthetics of existence in order to keep me grounded in this identity and work.

The Panopticon, from my Jungian framework, is the shadow of our profession.

While I do believe that we need standards in the field to make sure we do not go completely off the rails, I, like ACA (2014), value people's autonomy and see it as my duty to continue to help them if they ask for it, to continue to be, and feel, free. I have to continually wrangle with the paradox of being an authority and giving that power back to the people it rightfully belongs to. And I'm here to help others do the same.

It is one of my "unpopular feminist opinions" (which is a book in the making) that the pop culture fascination, or, as we say, *archetypal possession*, with self-diagnosis, trauma, "girl-bosses", and "toxic masculinity" is part of the Panopticon of the digital age, perpetuating the biopower of the prison-industrial complex, to the benefit of the mental health system (see also This Jungian Life, 2021). The Panopticon is already inside our heads, invited in by the tiny computers on our wrists and in our pockets, and we aren't really talking about or taking responsibility for this. The answer to what exactly is driving this, if there is an ultimate authority, I have to leave to the theologians and the conspiracy theorists. I just know that identifying with powerful archetypes such as The Victim, The Addict, The Fool, The Rebel, and The Judge are on trend. The Healer, The Priest, The Teacher, The Mother, The Father . . . not so much. But I'm delighted you're here. As we will discuss, all of these archetypes have value, as well as light and dark sides that, if we aim to cultivate aspects of both the Seeker and Servant Leader, I think we'll be all right.

ACA (2014) says it is our ethical duty to be aware of the "historical and social prejudices in the diagnosis of pathology" (E.5.c.). Know this: when men were primarily diagnosing mental illness at the dawn of psychology, many "difficult women" were targeted and imprisoned in mental institutions. Jung helped fight against that system and worked to lift women up by training them as analysts (Kirsch, 2000). Today, the mental health counseling field is over 70% white women and growing in demand (DATA USA, 2024; US Bureau of Labor and Statistics, 2022b). You would think we'd know better and use that power wisely. But the US has a long history of enslaving people simply for who they are, what they think, what they believe, and how they behave, even in private, and white women have a long history of being complicit. And it's not over. We counselors are still part of the problem.

Slavery is still legal in American prisons, and it is a billion dollar industry (ACLU, 2023; Berkeley Law, 2023). The "War on Drugs" increased the rate of incarceration in the US and the consumption of mental health services exponentially after decades of deinstitutionalization (Vera Institute for Justice, 2023). It is not a secret that about half of the people who are incarcerated also meet criteria for a mental health and a substance use disorder (SAMHSA, 2023). Despite increased discourse about restorative justice, we are still locking people up faster than any other civilized nation, often because they are caught using drugs or failed to pay court costs; at the same time, more children are placed in charge of the State for more hours a day than they see their parents (National Center on Early Childhood Quality Assurance, 2019; Prison Policy Initiative, 2023; US Bureau of Labor and Statistics, 2022a; Vera Institute for Justice, 2023).

Despite our knowledge about the importance of play in a child's development, that it can prevent and cure mental illness, recess and the arts are still continually cut in public schools. Being removed from the classroom, which happens to boys more often, especially if they are poor or part of a minority group, exponentially increases the risk of being funneled into the juvenile justice system (GAO, 2018; Institute for Policy Studies, 2019); 50% of young people report symptoms of depression (The White House, 2022). What is happening? More counselors are being brought into schools as an attempt to "help", but are we?

How are we, as counselors, combating the everyday use of the term "behavioral health" in the field that directly points to a panoptic control of one's behavior and not our professional value of wellness and empowerment? How are we assisting the government and its "behavioral risk factor surveillance system", which includes collecting data on children's mental health and funneling them deeper into additional systems of power (CDC, 2019)? How are we experiencing ourselves within these power relations? How do we know and determine what is true? What about our rights to live freely?

In short: The professional codes of ethics I choose to abide by as a counselor and play therapist serve a critical, authoritative role: to hold us accountable to collective standards. However, they are insufficient for me, my clients, students, and the profession. I did not get into this work in order to conform to a perpetuating system that devalues the rights of children, families, and communities over the will of the State. The honest answer will not be found telling or otherwise trying to teach people that their thinking or behavior is somehow wrong. I must thereby ascribe to an additional ethic, the aesthetics of existence.

I still have my old paperback of *Madness & Civilization* (Foucault, 1965), which I also highly recommend. It sits next to the copy of Jung's *Psyche & Symbol* (de Laszlo, 1958) that I, admittedly, stole from my dad when I was in high school.

Ethics & Identity

Both Jung and Foucault critiqued the rapid changes of the modern age and the increasing popularity of mental health treatment. They valued the pursuit of finding deeper, spiritual truths through our personal and collective identities. Both challenged an ongoing discourse regarding who has the power to change lives and to dictate that change and suggested we adopt a new ethic. The ongoing call is to learn to read, decipher, and critique subtexts, be that unconscious content or unspoken agendas underlying the power structures that influence us all. Both men revered the subjectivity of personal and collective creative experience within a larger contextual framework of power relations. Where Foucault often talks about systems of governance, Jung talks about the collective. The question of how a society may be structured around the aesthetics of existence continues to be explored not only as a personal challenge, psychological theory, political agenda, or a bridge between disciples but also as an ethical duty (Cochrane et al., 2014; Foucault, 1984; Guilfoyle, 2016; Macneill, 2017; Peters, 2005). It is a sentiment that I read between the lines while reading Jung and bring into my work as a counselor, educator, and supervisor. We might ask ourselves:

What is the role of the individual in society? Are we the creators of our own lives, and to what degree? To what degree are we subject to powerful forces within or outside ourselves, be they unconscious, metaphysical, or governmental? What is "normal", and who decides who is a "deviant" from that "norm", for how long, to what degree, and to what end?

It is an ancient, honorable duty for leaders, and thereby mental health professionals, to live by the Socratic principles to know and care for oneself. Through these ongoing practices, along with our responsible relationship with the power dynamics involved in our roles, we become useful and ethical as practitioners (ACA, 2014). Jung (CW 16) was clear that we need to do our own work as Wounded Healers, including embracing our creativity, in order to help others; this is a sentiment gaining some traction, especially as we talk about ideas such as the parallel process and gatekeeping (Rønnestad & Skovholt, 2003; St. Arnaud, 2017). Playfulness, an aspect of creativity (Glynn & Webster, 1992), is also described as a virtue in leadership, as it can put people at ease and assist in building relationships, encouraging creative problem solving and stress management (Mullen et al., 2007).

The question of ethics in the West used to be primarily governed by the Church. I would like to acknowledge Spinoza's early, albeit controversial, efforts to marry the ideas of science and spirituality in his controversial work, *Ethics* (1677/1993). While Jung did not openly address Spinoza in the lineage of dual-aspect philosophers, the influence is incontrovertible. Pervasive mental health discourse, including the mind-body connection, the value and reality of the subjective experience, intergenerational trauma, mode-shifting, and multiple aspects of modern humanism, can all be traced back to Spinoza (Den Uyl, 2008). Specific to Jungian theory, ideas about the collective unconscious, the dual nature of archetypes, the nature and function of the psyche, and even individuation might not exist without Spinoza (Atmanspacher & Fach, 2015; Langan, 2019). With modernity and the increased value of science and reason, faith and religion eventually fell out of fashion, a trend that continues today. Jung (CW 11) observed and predicted a correlation that we now know: that with the decrease in religious and spiritual practices comes the fractioning of communities as well as the psyche. How are people forging their identities in the digital age?

Some suggest that while we are more connected in some ways through the internet, we are less connected physically, socially, and spiritually. There remains a hunger for connection to something larger than ourselves. While most people still believe in God, they identify with specific religions less, attend church less, and suffer more (Pew Research Center, 2019, 2022; Saad & Hrynowski, 2022). Higher levels of religious and spiritual engagement as positive coping have been associated with improved mental health (Lucchetti et al., 2021). Many people, especially racial, ethnic, and cultural minorities in America, still prefer spiritual guidance over mental health treatment (Blogger & Prickett, 2021). There is a call to help bridge the gap between religion and mental health; the field of counseling has been heeding it (Epstein et al., in submission; Lucchetti et al., 2021; Oxhandler & Parrish, 2018). We need to really HEAR people, though, and not simply push our secular, panoptic agenda onto folks who do not want it. THEY know BETTER than US, right? Isn't that what our "theory" says? What if we offered a more numinous, culturally flexible approach to mental health treatment (Lönneker & Maercker, 2021)?

Being a Jungian-oriented counselor is about embracing creative and empowered transformation, both for the practitioner and the client. We hold a great deal of power in our positions as counselors. People who are suffering come to us for answers. Like it or not, we also work within an extensive government surveillance system, which includes schools, mental health providers, insurance companies, and prisons (Center for Disease Control, 2019; Institute for Policy Studies, 2019). While we may only work with one person at a time, we are encouraged to look both deep within and to the world around us to find collaborative and healing solutions.

COUNSELING INFLUENCERS

> The important thing is not the neurosis, but the man who has the neurosis. We have to set to work on the human being, and we must be able to do him justice as a human being.
>
> CW 16, p. 83, § 190

Counseling might be traced back to ancient times, but to this day, we are still struggling to agree on a unified definition of our professional identity both worldwide and within the US. In the UK, counseling is still kind of a snot-nosed-little-kid compared to psychotherapy (McLeold, 2013), while in the US, psychotherapy is the more elusive term. Psychotherapy emerged first in the UK during the Industrial Revolution when society's values shifted considerably as industry moved people out of their communities and away from their families. As machines increasingly replaced humans, science began to replace religion. There was little room anymore for those who could not perform like a machine or with dwindling community support. Medical doctors became experts in "lunacy", hypnosis, psychiatry, and later, psychotherapy; Freud and his school, which includes Jung, were influential in that transition, as well as the idea that a theory of mind might be relevant to everyone, not just those with mental illness. However, the Victorian sensibilities of psychotherapy did not sit well with Americans for long. The concrete thinking of behaviorism made a big splash and still saturates the mental health market today.

"Therapy" is now short for "psychotherapy", but there is no license to be a "psychotherapist" in the US. Psychotherapist organizations tend to welcome therapists from all mental health disciplines. While that may be heartwarming, it also does not provide for distinction in our disciplines that may be fundamental. For example, in the UK, in contrast to most states in the US, counselors often do not have standardized training requirements, and their services are often not acknowledged as proper mental health services by the government. Similarly, counselors on both sides of the Atlantic tend to take a less pathologizing, whole-person, strength-based approach to providing support, and many work toward bridging the gap between counseling and psychotherapy. In the US, while licensed psychiatrists, psychologists, social workers, and counselors can all engage in counseling, counselors are the experts in counseling. Most states now license counselors with the ability to diagnose and treat mental health conditions, but some still have additional or optional requirements to do so. Counselors are trained in many manualized therapies, though, including the widely government- and insurance-funded cognitive behavioral therapy (CBT) and dialectical behavioral therapy (DBT); manualized treatments tend to be shorter, and government funding often has a limited number of sessions as well, so there is still a stigma in the field that a counselor does not, or should not, "keep" a client in treatment as long as a psychotherapist would, nor go as deep. While there are many definitions of counseling, I will share my favorite, and the working definition in this book, taken from the American Counseling Association (ACA) Code of Ethics (2014, p. 20). Please note that the bolding is mine:

> Counseling is: a professional **relationship** that **empowers** diverse individuals, families, and groups to accomplish mental health, wellness, education, and career goals.

There are also three common characteristics of all counseling (ACA, 2023), and I have to bold them all because they are just that important:

1. A client-centered approach
2. A wellness-based philosophy
3. A commitment to ethical & culturally inclusive practices.

We will be circumambulating around all those ideas throughout this book, but I wish I could repeat them for emphasis. There are a few counseling influencers that I feel obliged to highlight here, beyond mere acknowledgments, who have guided me on this journey, none of whom happen to be Jungians, namely Doctors Carl Rogers, Gary Landreth, and Thomas Sweeney.

I see Carl Rogers, father of the client- or person-centered movement, as a bridge between psychotherapy and counseling, mental health and power discourse (like Foucault), experience and transformation, the spiritual and scientific (like Jung), and between counseling and Jung. While he was an advocate and model for the counseling field, he also criticized the social sciences for clamoring for power within larger governing bodies. Rogers was a psychologist but is also acknowledged as developing the foundation of counseling with a more egalitarian approach and utilizing client-centered ways of relating through empathy, listening, and reflecting. In the 1940s, he began to use the terms "counseling" and "psychotherapy" interchangeably (Rogers, 1942, 1951). Both Rogers and Jung, as well as their followers, have historically, and continue to be, accused of being "unscientific", accused of "playing doctor", and practicing outside of their scope. Some, though not many, credit Jung with influencing the client-centered movement (Douglas, 2005). Rogers (1977) himself spoke of the Jungian analysts Dr. John W. Perry and Dr. Howard Levine as examples of developing a person-centered Jungian approach at Diabasis (Greek for "crossing over"), a center for young people with schizophrenia. Rogers admits that the model was challenging for the general establishment, even Jungians. At Diabasis, the focus was on, and power was distributed between, each person, regardless of their credentials or diagnosis. Even the word "patient" was dropped in favor of "person" (hence the favor for the term person-centered, as well as the common practice of counselors preferring the word "client" over "patient"). I thank Rogers and these Jungians for their efforts in speaking up and out about how it is the experience of the process that is important, both the therapeutic relationship and the spontaneity of manifestations of the unconscious within a safe and protected space.

Gary Landreth is a Licensed Professional Counselor and Registered Play Therapist-Supervisor who has transformed how we view and treat children in the play therapy community. I will reference his work frequently throughout this book. His humanistic approach to counseling children, child-centered play therapy (CCPT), is clearly outlined in his book *Play Therapy: The Art of the Relationship* (2024), which is now in its fourth printing. CCPT not only extends ACA counseling values toward children more than any theory (IMHO) and is one of the most heavily researched and evidenced-based practices (Evidence-Based Child Therapy, 2023) but fills some gaps between Jungian analysis, sandplay therapy, and counseling. For example, while there is a growing body of evidence that Jungian psychotherapy is effective, the field cannot agree on a set of procedures that defines Jungian "psychotherapy" or "analysis" enough to conduct randomized control trials to dispel the burden of proof (Roesler, 2018). Jungian analysts have criticized sandplay therapy for not addressing, nor seemingly valuing, the importance of ongoing, relational, verbal interactions (Kirsch, 2000). While sandplay therapists may ultimately integrate other interventions, including verbal ones, with children, it is traditionally taught as a silent process with a minimal, scripted verbal protocol. The Sandplay Therapist of America's (STA, 2012) current procedure manual does indicate, though, that if a response by the therapist is deemed necessary, it should be person-centered (STA, 2012), or as Landreth calls it when working with children, *child-centered*. Landreth provides us with clear, developmentally appropriate, nurturing guidelines for how to speak with children therapeutically in a way no other resource, Jungian or otherwise, has provided to date. His philosophical explanations for being non-directive, especially if we are going to call ourselves "person", "client", or "child" centered, extends all the way to avoiding the use of questions.

Tom Sweeney and his brilliant, beloved late wife, Jane Myers, are legends in the American counseling field. They influenced the development of the ACA, Chi Sigma Iota (CSI, the counselor honor society), early CACREP programs, and the establishment of the counselor ethics of cultural responsiveness, servant leadership, and wellness (Ivey & Ivey, 2020). Tom (whom he insisted I call him when I reached out about this book) has boldly advocated for counselor licensure and professional identity distinction since the 70s (Sweeney & Sturdevant, 1974). Tom, like Carl Rogers, uses both the terms "counseling" and "psychotherapy" in his Adlerian book, now in its sixth printing (Sweeney, 2019). I'll give it to him that Adlerians tend to be more pragmatic and cooperative (. . . I will get to Jungians' reputation in a bit). Tom recognizes that we live and work in a pluralistic world and wants to reach a broad audience. He advocates for a non-pathologizing approach but also recognizes that we need to adapt to work within the structures that allow us to serve others affordably. I truly appreciate how he advocates for Adler to be acknowledged for his influential work, which parallels my passion for doing so with Jung.

These folks, in particular, have directly inspired me to be able to integrate Jung into my identity as a mental health counselor in profound ways. Without them, I could not have cohesively brought it together. There are simply too many elements between contemporary counseling and Jungian theory that seem discordant. This is part of why I think there aren't many people hanging their shingles out this way. I do think, though, that there is a hunger in the collective to go deeper. Underneath, we are very much the same.

Only after this circumambulation around my intersecting personal and professional identities did I discover Purton's (1989) article on the

"Person-Centered Jungian". He identifies several sentiments that Rogers and Jung shared:

1. Clients Know Best. Therapists Are to Serve & Not Impose.
2. The Person-of-the Therapist & Their Attitudes Trump Technique. We Can't Hide.
3. We Try to Adapt by Wearing Masks When We Sense a Misalignment Between the Self and the World.

There's the most succinct description of how this all makes sense to me. If you want to stop reading right here, you got the gist of what this book is about.

WRITING JUNG BACK IN

> . . . the constant flow of life again and again demands fresh adaptation. Adaptation is never achieved once and for all.
>
> CW 8, p. 108, § 143

Carl Gustav Jung was an Edwardian who lived from 1875–1961. His father was a pastor, and his aunt was a spiritualist. Spiritualism was quite in vogue at the time when psychotherapy was being developed. Historically, scientists have had to contend with the spiritual as an authority; it is only quite recently in human history that this has shifted. Many are aware that Jung was Freud's star pupil for a time, at the dawn of the psychoanalytic movement, and that they had a falling out that ultimately led to the development of Jung's own theory: analytic psychology. Jung was hesitant to discuss the fallout with Freud in-depth, but we speculate it had much to do with Jung's acknowledgment of the importance of the symbolic, the unconscious, and spiritual life. Jung can be credited with bringing psychology to the spiritual movement in America in the 1920s, though some criticize him for it (Noll, 1994), as well as increasing women's role in mental health (Kirsch, 2000). It seems that with the trend to write religious and spiritual education and research out of the discourse between the 1920s and the 1980s (Oxhandler & Parrish, 2018), Jung was written out, too, just as counseling was developing as a unique mental health field.

I like to think of Jung as our long-lost Grandpa. Let's trace our roots back.

Cultural Responsiveness

As an American counselor in the digital age, I am ever more aware that we need to be on our toes, ready for anything. The discourse about "cultural competencies" has been around for a while but still struggles to gain traction (Ratts et al., 2015). While "multicultural" training is continuing to increase in frequency, it still has an air of "othering" and a bad habit of perpetuating stereotypes. Placing people into demographic boxes, then putting together a list of statistics, generalizations, and suggested adaptations for what counselors might do to "help them" is often not, I'm afraid, promoting its aim. I, for one, cannot ever hope to be "competent" in any culture other than my own, unless perhaps I was adopted by or otherwise lived within another culture for a significant period of time. Why and how I would do that is also an area of question. For this reason, I prefer the idea of "cultural humility" (Tervalon & Murray-García, 1998) to keep me humble. I cannot, and will not, assume to know what it is like for any person to identify with, or live within a particular culture, nor what I think is best for them, especially as a white woman, an "expert" in counseling with a terminal degree. As Jung suggested, this collaborative process of becoming and knowing is lifelong, and when it comes to treatment, it matters much less what I think than what my client does. To this end, I ultimately hold myself to the charge of attempting to remain "culturally alert" and an active participant in cultural discourse (McAuliffe & Associates, 2013).

I am, in fact, hyper-alert to the fact that we are giving anti-racism a lot of lip service but continue to hold colonialist ideals to our breast, including imposing our diagnostics (especially pathologization), demographics, quantitative research practices without disclosing our positionality, and presenting manualized treatment practices onto marginalized peoples. I am also hyper-alert that the cultural discourse in the digital age is continuing to be divisive and expects us to "take sides" when I know that the ability to see things from both or many sides is a gift, a virtue, and a skill I call mode-shifting (inspired by Jung). Jung's concept of archetypes and the Self, now being validated by affective neuroscience (Alcaro et al., 2017), directly addresses the fundamental importance and interconnectedness of the personal and collective psyche. So many people in America have been stripped of their culture, family, land, religion, language, multigenerational livelihood, and overall freedom in favor of industrialized capitalism. What would be the "normal" response here?

Folks, something much bigger is going on, and I don't hear us talking about it directly. Counseling is a culture, too – a powerful one. But we are selling out. We are appeasing social media inspired talking points, self-diagnosis, insurance companies, and our FOMO with pre-packaged treatment modalities and techniques. It's a great disservice to our history, professional identity, and humanity. It is also chipping away at our attention span and self-efficacy. We need a robust theoretical foundation. For some of us, like our traumatized clients, there is no "going back to a previous level of functioning". We have to start anew with hope and vision for the future.

Jung gives me that. If you get to know him a little better, he might give it to you, too.

Theoretical Foundation

We know from attachment theory that having a secure base is psychically necessary to make sense of the world, organize our thoughts about it, and see ourselves safely in it (Bowlby, 1988). Jung's theory of the mind, personally and collectively, is vast. While he knew he did not have all the answers, and was sometimes contradictory, he wrote prolifically about his ideas. In this way, I find his theory strong yet flexible, not unlike how a tree must be rooted, yet free to grow, and bend in the wind. If we are not securely rooted, and know to a degree where we stand, we are at risk of being blown away by any gust of influence. There are hundreds of theories, and new ones emerging all the time, resulting in most counselors identifying or at least practicing in an integrative or eclectic way. However, proper theoretical integration requires competence in multiple theories (Peabody & Schaefer, 2016). I find that student and experienced counselors alike do not dig deep enough into one theory to really get to know it, let alone embody it, before they start cherry picking. I agree that cherries ARE delicious, but if we aren't careful, we can find ourselves uprooted, disoriented, and not, frankly, practicing ethically.

Counselors may feel pressure to keep up and adapt not only to the latest thing, but also to predominating "evidence-based practices", as dictated by their sites, supervisors, or insurance companies. I need to give this some serious attention, y'all, because this topic grinds my gears. For one, there is no universal definition of EBP. Some people try to say that one generally accepted theory is more evidence-based than others, but I challenge that on several levels. For one thing, identifying with a theory is not necessarily a practice protocol. I can identify as a Jungian-oriented counselor and run a DBT workbook group; it doesn't identify who I am. Second of all, "EBP" seems to have come to mean "manualized treatment protocol", but I rarely see people doing CBT by the book anymore; in fact, they kind of promote not doing it like that anymore (Beck Institute, 2023; TF-CBT Therapist Certification Program, 2023), but they sure did back in the day.

However, EBP is not a single, manualized treatment protocol (not that I would talk through a manual and try to call that counseling, anyway) but a process involving being informed about the existing research surrounding knowledge of the mind, the population we are working with, specific treatment interventions, and more, COMBINED with our codes of ethics, level of training in that area, clinical judgment, and most of all, the client's preferences (Shedler, 2018). There are certification programs for all the so called EBP, but they are generally acquired at post-graduate level. They are all specialty areas, and, therefore, optional, so not foundational to who we are as counselors. Jungian, and psychodynamic therapies in general, are, indeed, based on evidence (Roesler, 2018; Wiersma et al., 2022), as are the other established therapies and theories that we teach in university, for that matter. Counselors (. . . not therapists . . . COUNSELORS), though, value and focus the clinical portion of our training on the slightly more intangible relational-based factors that are tougher to manualize (CACREP, 2024; Lambie et al., 2018; Sommers-Flanagan, 2015). Maybe those Jungian analysts have a point.

While we may need to adapt our practices to meet specific requirements, authorities do not have the right to change what we believe. To identify as a counselor means to be client-centered, wellness-focused (not disease-focused, like the medical model is based on), and culturally humble, right? While we are bound to our ACA Code of Ethics (2014), we still need to decide for ourselves how we conceptualize the human experience, what causes suffering, and how we see our role as assisting in the healing process. While it is true that no one theory has been proven to treat everyone effectively, research also shows (Holland, 1997; Prescod & Zeligman, 2018; Rønnestad & Skovholt, 2003) that we may suffer personally and professionally if our theoretical orientation does not:

- match our personality, values, or goals
- normalize or encourage ongoing reflective practices
- encourage holistic growth and adaptability
- discourage pathologizing people.

Jung does this for me.

Professional Identity

With so many theories and interventions to choose from, and so many pressures to be what our clients need us to be, it is easy to see how a counselor may become overwhelmed, and not have a strong sense of professional identity. Who we are as counselors is a developmental process. It is not only the step-by-step process of our completion of courses, tests, and various governmental forms that we become counselors. We "become" counselors through relationship: with our teachers, supervisors, peers, and clients. Through these relationships, we develop a sense of belonging and self-efficacy needed for fulfilling and sustainable careers. Where I feel like I belong, and where others might, too, is in the Jungian community. Our identities, like our psyches, are rooted in both the personal and the collective. Having a grasp of Jungian concepts gives me the clarity, confidence, and satisfaction that helps me feel rooted and flexible enough to utilize my creativity.

My research recently has been around professional identity and creativity, both quantitatively and qualitatively. At first I thought that maybe there was something about Jungian training that increased creativity, but it looks like I may have been mistaken (though I think further research is warranted); creatives may be drawn to Jung, especially so at midlife (CW 17; McRoberts, 2022, 2023). Counselors, in general, though, seem to be creative people, even though they may not realize it . . . and also subject to experiencing a high level of stress (McRoberts & Epstein, 2023). This is another reason why writing Jung back in is essential. Jung highly valued creativity and recognized its innate healing power, made artwork, and encouraged his patients to do so. In this way, he can be seen as the founder of the expressive therapies, especially art and play therapy, though I don't see him cited enough, which I think, frankly, is unethical. It also ties back to professional identity and our sense of belonging. You might currently or one day identify as an art or play therapist as well. Creativity, though, encompasses a much broader expanse, as we will explore in this book. Creative thinking is involved in curiosity and perspective taking, which is at the heart of what we do as counselors. The legend is that Jung's theory grew from his love of anthropology. This seems to naturally fit in with our ever increasing global landscape, as well as counselor preparation for cultural humility, and spiritually informed practices (Kondili et al., 2022; Ratts et al., 2015).

Identifying as a Jungian may help with finding community support. By having a term to identify ourselves with, we can more easily look for resources in our local communities and online. While this may be for continuing education of interest, it might also be reaching out to ask for our own spiritual or mental health support. Even though our training stresses that we practice from a wellness model, promoted in our professional organizations and accrediting boards (CACREP, 2024; CSI, n.d.), and we have an ethical obligation to do our own work (ACA, 2014). I still see a stigma in the counseling community at large around mental health treatment. This may stem, in large part, from the larger culture of managed care, which requires a diagnosis, or pathology, in order to use insurance to pay for counseling. I understand that in many places in Europe, insurance pays for Jungian analysis, but counseling has a dodgy reputation. In the US, it is the Jungians who are often considered elitist, elusive, and, as I often jokingly admit, considered "woo woo" for their spiritual and artistic approach.

THE CULT OF JUNG

> . . . psychology without the psyche . . . suits people who think they have no spiritual needs or aspirations . . . it is only meaning that liberates.
>
> CW 11, p. 330, § 496

There are real barriers to identifying as a Jungian in the US. Some people are freaked out by the spiritual aspect of it. I hear counselors talking more about "bracketing out" their spirituality much more than I hear about integration. Some might get around this by working for a faith-based counseling agency, where they can hang their shingle out freely, leaving out many folks who might want services. Others say they fear being perceived as forcing their beliefs on people so they don't bring it up. I think there's something in between. You guessed it: a Jungian-oriented approach.

But what does it mean to be "Jungian"? Where do I find one? Do I have to join a cult?

While there are unique mentorship opportunities, creative practices, and encouragement, or rather, requirements, to engage in personal processes, there is an extensive financial and time commitment, not to mention limited access to classical Jungian training. To some, being a Jungian means being trained as a Jungian Analyst, with a post-master's degree in analytic psychology from the Inter-Regional Society of Jungian Analysts (IRSJA). To others, it means being certified as a Sandplay Therapist through the Sandplay Therapists of America. Still others say that no one, and no one organization, owns Jung, his ideas (or ANY ideas), art therapy, or play therapy. Jung himself reportedly said he was thankful he was not a Jungian, and if there was such a thing, he was the only one (Casement, 2018; Fordham, 1988; Hannah, 1976).

Politics are involved in the Jungian world, like in other systems we work in. Some have gone so far as to call the Jungian community a "cult" and liken Jungian training to a pyramid scheme, with only a few at the top holding power to gatekeep the tight-knit community (Noll, 1994; Slater, 2012). While I do value standards, and have collected various letters next to my name, as is customary in our field, part of my work, and the writing of this book, is to help level the playing field a bit more. I believe that we can identify as Jungian, or embrace Jungian theory, without being required to jump through endless hoops, especially if they are ultimately inaccessible or unnecessary. Perhaps it is the American Protestant in me, but it seems that Jung's work is out there for anyone to read and adapt as they see fit, within their own ethical codes. Yes, there needs to be a balance between mentorship and idealization of our teachers, and yes, I think some folks hang onto the idea of being a Jungian so tightly that they become out of touch with the general practice of mental health counseling. And, yes, some groups of Jungians seem a bit cult-y.

Sometimes, attempts to organize ideas and people can lose sight of the forest for the trees. Jung is cited widely for his resistance to standardizing and training others in his method, partly because he was humble, wanted the field to grow in ways he could not envision, and was aware of how an institution's power can corrupt. I have heard many Jungians take an elitist position that training is difficult because Jung and the processes he inspired are not for everyone, sometimes referencing Jung saying that the "experience of the unconscious is a personal secret communicable only to very few, and that with difficulty; hence the isolating effect . . ." (CW 12, p. 52, § 61). While I agree that not everyone may seek out experiences with the unconscious, as a trainee or a client, and that it definitely can be hard (for many reasons that we'll discuss in this book), I do not believe that means training should be inaccessible or unreasonably accessible. I think that Jung also recognized that all people do experience the unconscious in one way or another: through dreams, synchronistic events, relationships, and emotions that may seem to bubble up from nowhere and carry us away. Yes, not everyone will be able to decode the "secret" symbolic language of their own psyche, but I think that it is the human condition that we are driven to try. I do not think Jung would disagree with me on that.

I have trained extensively over my 20+ year career with many Jungian teachers in various Jungian organizations, have done, and continue to do my own work, and still do not hold the titles and certifications that some think I need to identify as a Jungian. I am here because I can finally say that I don't care about that anymore. I'm not definitively writing off any possibilities, or suggesting we all go rogue, but there is work to be done, and I'm called to do it. Maybe you are, too. So here I am, with you, gentle reader. Let's do this.

WHO THIS BOOK IS FOR

> In elfin nature wisdom and folly appear as one and the same . . . Life is crazy and meaningful at once. And when we do not laugh over the one aspect and speculate about the other, life is exceedingly drab, and everything is reduced to the littlest scale. There is then little sense and little nonsense either.
>
> CW 9i, p. 31, § 65

This book is for the rest of us. I specifically wrote it for counselors because there isn't one. To paraphrase Muncey (2005), the expert voices have not been telling my version of the story. Many other texts out there will talk about Jungian "analysis", "psychotherapy", or "psychology", or present Jungian play therapy from a social worker's perspective, but, again, I'm a counselor, and so are my students. I wanted to see a book that integrates counseling language, both for them, and so it can simply exist in the world. Using a common language can help break barriers and make education and services more accessible. I am passionate about that. It's why I chose and have stayed with this field, and heeded the call to earn my PhD in counselor education and supervision, and enter academia.

You may identify with one of these labels, or you may be a student, for the first time, again, or still. You might be licensed in another mental health discipline, curious about Jung for personal or professional reasons, or practice the art of counseling and would like to learn more about it. I often tell my students that many professions incorporate counseling into their practice, such as psychologists, psychiatrists, and social workers, but counselors are the specialists in counseling. I want to help develop the identity of a "Jungian Counselor". Jung says we get to create ourselves, right?

In addition to identifying as a counselor, I am also a play therapist, currently holding the Registered Play Therapist-Supervisor credential with the Association for Play Therapy (APT). The APT encourages members to obtain training in a variety of theoretical orientations. We have a very small community of Jungians. Some of us identify as "Jungian Play Therapists". Others say "Jungian Analytic Play Therapist". Even here, we have our own distinctive styles: various levels of how we use directives, how much and often we reference Jung; how we interpret, reframe, and integrate his work; how much we use case examples to illustrate our points; how interested we are in research or publishing in general; how collaborative we are, and more (Allan, 1988; Allan & Bertoia, 2003; Green, 2014; Lilly, 2015). There are several books on sandplay therapy, which is Jungian-oriented, but there is some disagreement in the community about if sandplay therapy is play therapy. While STA as an organization is an APT Approved Provider at the time this book is being written, most STA trainings, save for the conference, simply don't bother to meet the minimum requirements to do so.

Contemporary post-modern philosophers are leading an important discussion about biopower and the mental health system (Macneill, 2017). They promote a shift toward the active practice of the aesthetics of existence as an ethical practice. This requires us to challenge the idea of, and bias toward, objective truth as dictated by any book or authority (hey, little "O" on our SOAP notes), including ourselves as those who, like it or not, sit in a position of power over our clients. No matter how hard we try to promote an egalitarian relationship, the fact remains that someone who is vulnerable and wounded has come to us for help. We must be vigilant to that dialectic.

We all, as healthcare providers, are accused of only giving lip service to our value of emotions and the subjective, lived experience of our clients. Counselors are creative, but we continue to be complacent in utilizing dry, manualized treatments, or at least touting to funders, supervisors, and colleagues that we do. I propose that we continue to deny our own creativity, associative processes in general, and distrust our client's natural creative ability to heal inside a therapeutic relationship (despite the gobs of evidence) in part, at least, because we're scared. We have cast our creativity into Shadow. We are afraid of accusations that we're trying to be secular priests (like Jung experienced) or imposing our values onto others (like students of faith have admitted when I asked why they never talked about spiritual issues in supervision). While we may be called to be Servant Leaders, we remain Wounded Healers. We have a responsibility to do as Jung (1973) asks us, to stop projecting, take a good, hard look inside ourselves, and awaken: for the sake of ourselves, our clients, and the world. The

Panopticon is here, in the digital age, and as those licensed by the State, we are a part of its all seeing eye. Be mindful.

The culture of the digital age bombards us with imagery but robs us of our symbolic function. It presents us with contradicting messages to do it all, while at the same time, be present and relax. It attempts to control our minds and bodies by convincing us to keep scrolling, because even though we're not good enough the way we are, the next new "clinically proven" pill, cream, or method is right around the corner. Don't buy it.

Identifying as a Jungian-oriented counselor inspires me to be the Servant Leader I am called to be. I now know that my relationship with, and value of, the spiritual, creative expression, and working with people is part of my individuation process. Embracing Jungian ideas allows me to practice the Art of the Self and assist others in doing so as well. While I practice from the ACA and the APT codes of ethics, I also value aesthetics as a form of ethics, especially concerning the biopower involved in the mental health system. While counseling has fought to be legitimized as a science, it is also an art. We are not only allowed, but obliged to learn and utilize the language of the unconscious.

I hope that you feel comfortable enough to stay for a spell, safe to explore, and become uncomfortable enough to grow. Take what you need, and leave the rest. Jung knew that this work will change us in mysterious ways if we allow it to.

Reflections

1. What drew you to this book?
2. Do you know a Jungian? Do you identify as one? Why or why not?
3. What professional identities do you currently embrace? Are you working on one? How? Do you have an end in mind?
4. In what ways do art, creativity, and/or religious and spiritual practices influence you personally? How about professionally?

REFERENCES

Alcaro, A., Carta, S., & Panksepp, J. (2017). The affective core of the Self: A neuro-archetypical perspective on the foundations of human (and animal) subjectivity. *Frontiers in Psychology*, 8(1424), 1–13. https://doi.org/10.3389/fpsyg.2017.01424

Allan, J. (1988). *Inscapes of the child's world: Jungian counseling in schools and clinics.* Spring Publications.

Allan, J., & Bertoia, J. (2003). *Written paths to healing: Education and Jungian child counseling.* Spring Publications. (Original work published 1992).

American Civil Liberties Union (ACLU). (2023). *Captive labor: Exploitation of incarcerated workers.* www.aclu.org/news/human-rights/captive-labor-exploitation-of-incarcerated-workers

American Counseling Association (ACA). (2014). *ACA code of ethics.* www.counseling.org/resources/aca-code-of-ethics.pdf

American Counseling Association (ACA). (2023). *What is a counselor?* www.counseling.org/about-us/what-is-a-counselor#:~:text=1%3A%20A%20Client%2DCentered%20Approach%20That%20Focuses%20on%20You&text=A%20professional%20counselor%20is%20likely,your%20relationships%20or%20self%2Desteem

Atmanspacher, H., & Fach, W. (2015). Mind-matter correlations in dual-aspect monism according to Pauli and Jung. In E. F. Kelly, A. Crabtree, & P. Marshall (Eds.), *Beyond physicalism: Toward reconciliation of science and spirituality* (pp. 195–226). Rowman & Littlefield.

Beck Institute. (2023). *Understanding CBT.* https://beckinstitute.org/about/understanding-cbt/

Berkeley Law. (2023). *Corporations use of prison labor.* https://sites.law.berkeley.edu/sustainability-compliance/corporations-use-of-prison-labor/

Blogger, D., & Prickett, P. J. (2021). Where would you go? Race, religion, and the limits of pastor mental health care in black and latino congregations. *Religions, 12*(12), 1062. https://doi.org/10.3390/rel12121062

Bowlby, J. (1988). *A secure base: Clinical applications of attachment theory.* Brunner-Routledge.

Carroll, L. (1896). *Through the looking-glass.* (Public domain in the USA).

Casement, A. (2018). *Who owns Jung?* Routledge.

Center for Disease Control (CDC). (2019). *Behavioral risk factor surveillance system ACE data* [Violence prevention]. www.cdc.gov/violenceprevention/childabuseandneglect/acestudy/ace-brfss.html

Chi Sigma Iota (CSI). (n.d.). *Wellness in counseling.* www.csi-net.org/group/wellness

Cochrane, M., Flower, S., Mackenna, C., & Morgan, H. (2014). A Jungian approach to analytic work in the twenty-first century. *British Journal of Psychotherapy, 30*(1), 33–50. https://doi.org/10.1111/bjp.12060

Council for Accreditation of Counseling and Related Programs (CACREP). (2024). *2024 CACREP standards*. www.cacrep.org/wp-content/uploads/2023/06/2024-Standards-Combined-Version-6.27.23.pdf

DATA USA. (2024). *Mental health counselors*. https://datausa.io/profile/soc/mental-health-counselors#:~:text=In%202021%2C%2066.1%25%20of%20the,or%20More%20Races%20(7.1%25)

de Laszlo, V. (1958). *Psyche & symbol: A selection from the writings of C. G. Jung*. Doubleday Anchor Books.

Den Uyl, D. (2008). *God, man, and well-being: Spinoza's modern humanism*. Peter Lang.

Douglas, C. (2005). Analytical psychotherapy. In R. J. Corsini & Q. Wedding (Eds.), *Current psychotherapies* (pp. 96–129). Thomson Learning.

Epstein, J., McRoberts, R., & Todd, S. (in submission). Engaging the numinous: Predictors & perceptions of religious and spiritual integrated practice (RSIP) among Licensed Counselors. [Unpublished manuscript].

Evidence-Based Child Therapy. (2023). Home page. http://evidencebasedchildtherapy.com/

Fordham, M. (1988). Michael Fordham in discussion with Karl Figlio. *Free Association, 1*, 7–38.

Foucault, M. (1965). *Madness & civilization: A history of insanity in the age of reason*. Vintage Books.

Foucault, M. (1977). *Discipline & punish: The birth of the prison*. Vintage Books.

Foucault, M. (1984). *The Foucault reader*. P. Rainbow (Ed.). Pantheon Books.

Glynn, M. A., & Webster, J. (1992). The Adult Playfulness Scale: An initial assessment. *Psychological Reports, 71*, 83–103.

Government Accountability Office (GAO). (2018). *K-12 education: Discipline disparities for black students, boys, and students with disabilities*. US Government Accountability Office. www.gao.gov/assets/700/690827.pdf

Green, E. (2014). *The handbook of Jungian play therapy with children & adolescents*. Johns Hopkins University Press.

Guilfoyle, M. (2016). Therapy and the aesthetics of the self. *British Journal of Guidance & Counseling, 44*(1), 1–11. http://dx.doi.org/10.1080/03069885.2014.1002075

Hannah, B. (1976). *Jung, his life and work: A biographical memoir*. Putnam Adult.

Holland, J. L. (1997). *Making vocational choices: A theory of vocation-personalities and work environments* (3rd ed.). Psychological Assessment Resources.

Huijer, M. (1999). The aesthetics of existence in the work of Michel Foucault. *Philosophy & Social Criticism*, *25*(2), 61–85. https://doi.org/10.1177/01914537990 2500204

Huxley, A. (2006). *Brave new world*. Harper Perennial. (Original work published 1932).

Institute for Policy Studies. (2019). *Report: Students under siege*. https://ips-dc.org/ report-students-under-siege/

Ivey, A., & Ivey, M. B. (2020, April 30). *Jane Myers and Tom Sweeney: Servant leaders and advocates for the counseling profession*. https://ct.counseling.org/2020/04/ jane-myers-and-tom-sweeney-servant-leaders-and-advocates-for-the-coun seling-profession/

Jung, C. G. (1973). C. G. *Jung Letters: Volume 1, 1906–1950*. G. Adler, A. Jaffe et al. (Eds.), R. F. C. Hull (Trans.). Routledge.

Jung, C. G. (2023). *The collected works of C. G. Jung: Revised and expanded complete digital edition*. (CW 1–20). G. Adler, W. McGuire, & H. Read (Eds.), R. F. C. Hull (Trans.). Princeton University Press. https://press.princeton.edu/books/ ebook/9780691255194/the-collected-works-of-c-g-jung

Kirsch, T. B. (2000). *The Jungians: A comparative and historical perspective*. Routledge.

Koenderink, J. (2014). The all seeing eye? *Perception*, *43*, 1–6. https://journals.sage pub.com/doi/pdf/10.1068/p4301ed

Kondili, E., Isawi, D., Interiano-Shiverdecker, C., & Maleckas, O. (2022). Predictors of cultural humility in counselors-in-training. *Counselor Preparation*, *61*, 129–140. doi:10.1002/ceas.12230.

Kramer, E. (2000). *Art as therapy: Collected papers*. Jessica Kingsley Publishers.

Lambie, G. W., Mullen, P. R., Swank, J. M., & Blount, A. (2018). The Counseling Competencies Scale: Validation and refinement. *Measurement and Evaluation in Counseling and Development*, *51*(1), 1–15. doi:10.1080/07481756.2017.1358964.

Landreth, G. (2024). *Play therapy: The art of the relationship* (4th ed.). Routledge. (Original work published 1991).

Langan, R. (2019). Jung, Spinoza, Deleuze: A move towards realism. In *Holism: Possibilities and problems*. Routledge. doi:10.4324/9780367824389-11.

Lilly, J. P. (2015). Jungian analytical play therapy. In D. A. Crenshaw & A. L. Stewart (Eds.), *Play therapy: A comprehensive guide to theory and practice* (pp. 48–65). Guilford Press.

Lönneker, C., & Maercker, A. (2021). The numinous experience in the context of psychopathology and traumatic stress studies. *Culture & Psychology*, *27*(3), 392–416. https://doi.org/10.1177/1354067X20922139

Lucchetti, G., Koenig, H. G., & Lucchetti, A. L. G. (2021). Spirituality, religiousness, and mental health: A review of the current scientific evidence. *World Journal of Clinical Cases, 9*(26), 7620–7631. doi:10.12998/wjcc.v9.i26.7620.

Macneill, P. (2017). Balancing bioethics by sensing the aesthetic. *Bioethics, 31,* 631–643. doi:10.1111/bioe.12390. PMID: 28901599.

McAuliffe, G. J. & Associates (Eds.) (2013). *Culturally alert counseling: A comprehensive introduction.* Sage Publications.

McLeold, J. (2013). *An introduction to counselling* (5th ed.). Open University Press. (Original work published 1993).

McRoberts, R. (2022). Addressing the creativity crisis: Sandplay therapists' mode-shifting and professional identity development. *Journal of Sandplay Therapy, 31*(2), 129–142. www.sandplay.org/journal/research-articles/addressing-the-creativity-crisis-sandplay-therapists-mode-shifting-and-professional-identity-development/

McRoberts, R. (2023). The white rabbit: Sacred & subversive. *ARAS Connections: Image and Archetype, 2,* 1–32. https://aras.org/newsletters/aras-connections-image-and-archetype-2023-issue-2

McRoberts, R., & Epstein, J. (2023). Creative self-concept, post-traumatic growth, and professional identity resilience in counselors with traumatic experiences: A conical correlation analysis. *Journal of Creativity in Mental Health,* 1–15. doi:10.1080/15401383.2023.2232730.

Mullen, J. A., Luke, M., & Drewes, A. A. (2007). Supervision can be playful, too: Play therapy techniques that enhance supervision. *International Journal of Play Therapy, 16,* 69–85. http://dx.doi.org/10.1037/1555-6824.16.1.69

Muncey, T. (2005). Doing autoethnography. *International Journal of Qualitative Methods, 4*(3), 5. www.ualberta.ca/~iiqm/backissues/4_1/pdf/muncey.pdf

National Center on Early Childhood Quality Assurance. (2019). *Addressing the decreasing number of family child care providers in the United States.* https://childcareta.acf.hhs.gov/sites/default/files/addressing_decreasing_fcc_providers_revised_final.pdf

Noll, R. (1994). *The Jung cult: Origins of a charismatic movement.* Free Press Paperpacks.

Orwell, G. (2021). *Nineteen eighty-four.* Penguin Classics. (Original work published 1949).

Oxhandler, H. K., & Parrish, D. E. (2018). Integrating clients' religion/spirituality in clinical practice: A comparison among social workers, psychologists, counselors, marriage and family therapists, and nurses. *Journal of Clinical Psychology, 74,* 680–694. doi:10.1002/jclp. 22539.

Peabody, M. A., & Schaefer, C. E. (2016). Towards semantic clarity in play therapy. *International Journal of Play Therapy, 25*(4), 197–202. http://dx.doi.org/10.1037/pla0000025

Peters, M. A. (2005). Foucault, counseling and the aesthetics of existence. *British Journal of Guidance & Counseling, 33*(3), 383–396. doi:10.1080/03069880500179616.

Peterson, J. B., & Hicks, S. R. C. (2017). *Postmodernism: History and diagnosis.* www.jordanbpeterson.com/transcripts/postmodernism-history-and-diagnosis/

Peterson, J. B., Doidge, N., & Van Sciver, E. (2018). *12 rules for life: An antidote to chaos.* Random House Canada.

Pew Research Center. (2019). *Religion's relationship to happiness, civic engagement and health around the world.* www.pewresearch.org/religion/2019/01/31/religions-relationship-to-happiness-civic-engagement-and-health-around-the-world/

Pew Research Center. (2022). *How US religious composition has changed in recent decades.* www.pewresearch.org/religion/2022/09/13/how-u-s-religious-composition-has-changed-in-recent-decades/

Prescod, D. J., & Zeligman, M. (2018). Career adaptability of trauma survivors: The moderating role of posttraumatic growth. *The Career Development Quarterly, 66,* 107–120. doi:10.1002/cdq.12126.

Prison Policy Initiative. (2023). *Mass incarceration: The whole pie.* www.prisonpolicy.org/reports/pie2023.html

Purton, C. (1989). The person-centered Jungian. *Person-Centered Review, 4*(4), 403–419. www.dwelling.me.uk/PCJUngian.htm

Ratts, M. J., Singh, A. A., Nassar-McMillan, S., Butler, S. K., & McCullough, J. R. (2015). *Multicultural and social justice counseling competencies.* www.counseling.org/docs/default-source/competencies/multicultural-and-social-justice-counseling-competencies.pdf?sfvrsn=20

Roesler, C. (2018). *Research in analytical psychology: Empirical research.* Routledge.

Rogers, C. R. (1942). *Counseling and psychotherapy; newer concepts in practice.* Houghton Mifflin

Rogers, C. (1951). *Client-centered therapy: Its current practice, implications, and theory.* Houghton Mifflin.

Rogers, C. (1977). *On personal power: Inner strength and its revolutionary impact.* Dell Publishing, Co.

Rønnestad, M. H., & Skovholt, T. M. (2003). The journey of the counselor and therapist: Research findings and perspectives on professional development. *Journal of Career Development, 30*(1), 5–44. doi:10.1023/A:1025173508081.

Saad, L., & Hrynowski, Z. (2022). *How many Americans believe in God?* Gallup. https://news.gallup.com/poll/268205/americans-believe-god.aspx

Samuels, A. (2017). The future of Jungian analysis: Strengths, weaknesses, opportunities, threats ("SWOT"). *The Journal of Analytical Psychology, 62*(5), 636–649. https://doi.org/10.1111/1468-5922.12351

Sandplay Therapists of America (STA). (2012). *Procedure manual for research using sandplay therapy as originated by Dora Kalff.* www.sandplay.org/wp-content/uploads/2012/11/Procedure-Manual-for-Sandplay-Research.pdf

Sedgwick, D. (2015). On integrating Jungian and other theories. *The Journal of Analytical Psychology, 60*(4), 540–558. https://doi.org/10.1111/1468-5922.12169

Shedler, J. (2018). Where is the evidence for "evidence-based" therapy? *Psychiatric Clinics of North America, 41*(2), 319–329. https://doi.org/10.1016/j.psc.2018.02.001

Slater, G. (2012). Between Jung and Hilman. *Quadrant, 4*(2), 14–37. www.cgjungny.org/q-vol42-2-summer-2012/

Sommers-Flanagan, J. (2015). Evidence-based relationship factors. *Journal of Mental Health Counseling, 37*(2), 95–108. https://doi.org/10.17744/mehc.37.2.g13472044600588r

Spinoza, B. (1993). *Ethics.* G. H. R. Parkinson (Ed.). Everyman. (Original work published 1677).

St. Arnaud, K. O. S. (2017). Encountering the wounded healer: Parallel process and supervision. *Canadian Journal of Counselling and Psychotherapy, 51*(2), 131–144. https://cjc-rcc.ucalgary.ca/article/view/61147

Substance Abuse and Mental Health Services Administration (SAMHSA). (2023). *About criminal and juvenile justice.* www.samhsa.gov/criminal-juvenile-justice/about

Sweeney, T. J. (2019). *Adlerian counseling & psychotherapy: A practitioner's wellness approach* (6th ed.). Routledge.

Sweeney, T. J., & Sturdevant, A. D. (1974). Licensure in the helping professions: Anatomy of an issue. *The Personnel and Guidance Journal, 52,* 575–581. https://doi.org/10.1002/j.2164-4918.1974.tb04056.x

Tervalon, M., & Murray-García, J. (1998). Cultural humility versus cultural competence: A critical distinction in defining physician training outcomes in multicultural education. *Journal of Health Care for the Poor and Underserved, 9*(2), 117–125. doi:10.1353/hpu.2010.0233.

TF-CBT Therapist Certification Program. (2023). *TF-CBT implementation resources.* https://tfcbt.org/resources/implementation/

This Jungian Life. (2021, January 14). *Inflation: The challenge of archetypal possession.* https://thisjungianlife.com/episode-146-inflation-the-challenge-of-archetypal-possession/

Tolkien, J. R. R. (2020). *The fellowship of the ring.* Clarion Books. (Original work published 1954).

US Bureau of Labor and Statistics. (2022a). *Average hours per day parents spent caring for and helping household children as their main activity.* www.bls.gov/charts/american-time-use/activity-by-parent.htm

US Bureau of Labor and Statistics. (2022b). *Substance abuse, behavioral disorder, and mental health counselors.* www.bls.gov/ooh/community-and-social-service/substance-abuse-behavioral-disorder-and-mental-health-counselors.htm

Vera Institute for Justice. (2023). *Incarceration statistics.* www.vera.org/ending-mass-incarceration/causes-of-mass-incarceration/incarceration-statistics

Wade, S. (2019). *Foucault in California [A true story – wherein the great French philosopher drops acid in the Valley of Death].* Heyday.

The White House. (2022). *Reducing the economic burden of unmet mental health needs.* www.whitehouse.gov/cea/written-materials/2022/05/31/reducing-the-economic-burden-of-unmet-mental-health-needs/

Wiersma, J. K., Freedle, L. R., McRoberts, R., & Solberg, K. B. (2022). A meta-analysis of sandplay therapy treatment outcomes. *International Journal of Play Therapy, 31*(4), 197–215. https://doi.org/10.1037/pla0000180

Wilkinson, M. (2005). Undoing dissociation: Affective neuroscience: A contemporary Jungian clinical perspective. *The Journal of Analytical Psychology, 50*(4), 483–501. https://doi.org/10.1111/j.0021-8774.2005.00550.x

Wilkinson, M. (2016). Review of The body keeps the score: Mind, brain and body in the transformation of trauma. *The Journal of Analytical Psychology, 61*(2), 239–244. doi:10.1111/1468-5922.12213.

Woien, S. (Ed.). (2022). *Jordan Peterson: Critical responses.* Open Universe.

2
Why Jung?

Freedom is not a mere abstraction, it is also an emotion. Reason becomes unreason when separated from the heart, and a psychic life void of universal ideas sickens from undernourishment.

Jung, CW 18, pp. 310–311, § 745

- Why Jung?
- Didn't Freud kick him out cuz he was so weird?
- Aren't his ideas outdated?
- He sounds cool but I have to use EBP . . .
- Yeah, but he's too hard to read . . .
- What book of Jung's would you recommend I read first?

I am naturally skeptical when I hear of the latest and greatest developments in mental health. This may be due to my post-modern sensibilities, but I also have the uncanny ability to find a thread that leads back to Jung. Over 300 counseling theories are recognized by the counseling field (Neukrug, 2015); there are infinite ways to integrate them with various techniques, and more are being developed, combined, re-packaged, and sold every day. So why Jung? In short, he said a lot of it first. I also find him infinitely inspiring, freeing, and see his influence everywhere. That's why I'm compelled to write this book. You're welcome.

I know it's getting worse as I get older, but I've always been skeptical, especially of groupthink and the logical fallacy of appealing to authority. Remember, the word "skeptic" comes from Greek philosophy. While it tends to have negative connotations, it embraces the notion that while we may be out in search of truth, we can't know everything, even those who have the power to say they do. I certainly don't know everything about anything. I certainly don't know anything definitively about my clients; I can IMAGINE and gather information,

DOI: 10.4324/9781003433736-2

but I can't know what it is actually like to be someone else. In fact, I think it is dangerous to say we can or do, and pre-package a one-size-fits-all approach to treatment. I stop counselors when they postulate that a client "is" something, especially without consulting with them, or "will" or "should" do this or that, especially without asking what the client thinks. Jung often quotes Kant, who was a philosopher in his own right, but with a big dollop of skepticism.

I'll admit that I fall into the camp that thinks Jung was also a philosopher, though he didn't overtly identify as one. He identified as a scientist, and I agree he was. But more than forming questions, developing a method, and coming up with conclusions, he encouraged his students, (and still does to this day) to continue to seek, use their unique talents and perspectives, and to find their own path to wholeness, whatever that might look like for them. He combined many aspects of truth-knowing (Claugh, 2013), all of which we look to in the counseling world: rationalism (does it make logical sense), empirical research (is it observable, measurable, and "scientific"), subjectivity (which is also "scientific" when we study the phenomenon properly; it is also a part of our counselor ethics to respect our clients' lived experience), and pragmatism (is it do-able?). I often say that Jung invites me to wonder with my clients, and know my history and the research well enough to back that up. I find that creative, ethical, trauma-informed, and intelligent. In this chapter, I will share some things that might give perspective to how a counselor might construct an argument that being Jungian is rooted in history, evidence, and counselor values. I do this because I want to empower others to embrace their weirdness, too.

Jung was a child of the Industrial Revolution, both immersed in and fearful for the growing Westernized culture, which was beginning to reject spiritual traditions in favor of new scientific findings. Jung (CW 16) asked long ago if the churches were adapting to meet the changing zeitgeist, and it seems they're still trying to catch up. Witnessing humanity's growing detachment from the earth, our creative instincts, and cultural practices, he predicted the mental health crisis that we're experiencing today. Not only was he a prolific writer and lecturer, but he was a deep thinker and developed a working theory which is also a worldview.

Jung developed a model for conceptualizing both our individual and collective psyches, and laid a strong foundation on which we can continue to build for culturally humble counseling practices. At the same time, his ideas can seem wide open, like playing in the key of C. This can be very frustrating for new counselors and researchers alike because they want a concrete method. However, increasing our *tolerance for ambiguity* is a specific counseling skill (Professional Dispositions Competency Assessment, PDCA-R; Garner et al., 2016).

Today, Jungian theory straddles across expressive arts, mind-body, and traditional talk therapies that are culturally humble, trauma-informed, and validated by affective neuroscience and attachment theory. It just mostly lives in relative obscurity. Jungians tend to cluster in small circles, hang back, and in America, primarily publish (mostly case studies and theory) in their own journals, with a few notable exceptions (Kirsch, 2000; Roesler, 2013, 2019; Wiersma et al., 2022). They have a reputation for not liking having their methods pinned down and seem not to mind being the weird kids of the psych world. We could all learn to embrace our weirdness a little more.

I think it's important to remember that counseling is based on philosophy, not just prescriptive interventions, and Jung constantly reminds me of that and holds me accountable. He called it years ago, somewhere around 1934, that it was more to do with the personalities of the client and the therapist than it was about any technique (CW 10, p. 159). Without a well-constellated philosophy of humanity, we risk, at best, sailing adrift, and at worst, being vulnerable consumers of the trendiest, most highly marketed interventions and exploitation of our client's suffering. JP Lilly (2015), the self-proclaimed "mechanic" of Jungian Analytical Play Therapy, taught me that it's beyond irresponsible not to have a solid theoretical foundation. It's dangerous.

I'd like to add a little chart here (see Figure 2.1) to highlight some common misconceptions and counter-arguments I plan to make throughout this book.

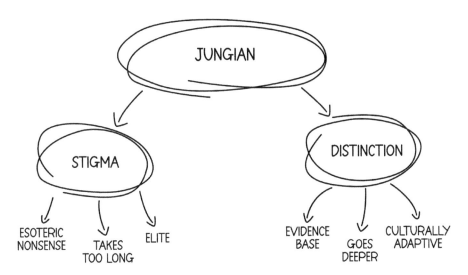

Figure 2.1 A Jungian Approach. (Reprinted with permission. Further reproduction is prohibited without the author's written authorization. All rights reserved. Copyright © 2023 by author, Rachel McRoberts.)

GIVING CREDIT WHERE CREDIT IS DUE

> There are in fact many different methods, standpoints, views, and beliefs which are all at war with one another, chiefly because they all misunderstand one another and refuse to give one another their due. The many-sidedness, the diversity, of psychological opinions in our day is nothing less than astonishing, not to say confusing.
>
> CW 16, p. 54, § 116

Let's give Jung credit where credit is due. Perhaps it is because humans are naturally meaning-making creatures, or I have a Jungian bias, but I can see Jung's influence all over the mental health world. The more I read his work, too, the more I see. Rarely, though, even when reading and teaching in the psychodynamic field, do I see or hear his name. Perhaps folks are unaware that Jung may have said it first. Maybe Jung's been pushed into Shadow so the egos of the age can shine.

While Jungians are a distinct population, since Jung was a student of Freud, and Jung's theory is acknowledged under the psychodynamic umbrella, along with Freud, Adler, Klein, and others (Jacobs, 2017), I would like to see more depth of focus on his work in the field. It seems he's been all but written out, even by theoretical kin. Jung helped to pioneer the importance of science, studying the mind with the body, co-regulation in the therapeutic relationship, and encouraged his students not to become dogmatic with his theories in further developing advancements in practice as evidence emerged. While he wrote and lectured prolifically, he said several times that he didn't claim to have it all together and was resistant to having a cult following (Bulkeley & Weldon, 2011).

Sorry, man.

Jung was one of the first to recognize that psychic material, left unprocessed, tended to manifest, both within the individual and collective; this concept is now being validated by neuroscientific developments: unspoken or unconscious processing may connect in deeper ways than previously realized (Leader, 2015; Wilkinson, 2005). It's also a cultural competency to see individuals as having various intersecting identities that may impact our mental health (Ratts et al., 2015). This "both/and" dialectic is becoming increasingly popular in the fields of counseling, creativity, problem solving, and leadership. This often paradoxical concept of "both/and" helps to challenge "either/or" thinking, that which may be found beyond the binary and the assumptions and expectations therein, both individually and collectively (Heracleous & Robson, 2020; Moradi & DeBlaere, 2010; Reid, 2022). This even includes the counselor, and our ability to integrate various evidence and practices within a theoretical framework. I used to have a little tag hanging up in my office that said "both/and" as a reminder to myself and clients. Jung's work itself reflects that life is a paradox, including the therapeutic process. And as counselors, that process begins and exists within the relationship.

THE THERAPEUTIC RELATIONSHIP

> For two personalities to meet is like mixing two different chemical substances: if there is any combination at all, both are transformed. In any effective psychological treatment, the doctor is bound to influence the patient; but this influence can only take place if the patient has a reciprocal influence on the doctor . . .
>
> CW 16, p. 71, § 163

Jung (CW 16) also postulated that the therapeutic relationship is dynamic, impacting both the client and the therapist. Instead of having his clients lay on a couch to be examined, he had more of a conversational, egalitarian, client-centered approach. This concept of engaging co-regulation in a dyad (Bradway & McCoard, 1997) has been witnessed in brain imaging studies and is recognized as the foundation for building safety, attachment, and transformation in treatment, including sandplay therapy (Wiersma et al., 2022).

Treating from a Jungian perspective, integrating play therapy and expressive arts techniques, is ideal for several reasons, including the therapeutic relationship itself. Beginning with the conceptualization of the mind, through valuing and understanding how symbols arise from the unconscious (possibly as symptoms but also as wisdom) to speaking indirectly, often less threatening, through play and artmaking, the Jungian counselor creates a safe container for clients to explore and express themselves (Allan, 1988; Turner, 2005; Winnicott, 1971); Jung (CW13, CW16) called this container of the transformational relationship the "*vas Hermeticum*", commonly referred to just as "the vas", which may be symbolized by a basin, a bath, a mother's womb, or, even more basically, a circle; the waters contained within the vas represent the unconscious. This is the place where things begin to form, are nurtured, washed, healed, and made anew, sometimes by heating up, or "cooking" items that have been brought together. Like the phrase "cooking something up" suggests, various conditions and processes often interact in the mind, and between minds, and may take time to develop. Acknowledging the importance of nature, nurture, and co-regulation in healthy psychic development comes from a century of scientific studies, especially attachment and neurobiology, providing a framework for understanding the impact of trauma on empathy and creativity in a relational model of Jungian psychology.

According to Fordham (1994), a prominent student of Jung himself, the quality of the therapeutic relationship, and maintenance of the analytic attitude is the primary technique in Jungian treatment, as discussed above. Allan (1988) identified a framework for a Jungian way of being in a counseling relationship with children, which focuses on the relationship itself, valuing the client, their means of expression, symbolic content, and limiting the use of directives. Compared with child-centered play therapy (CCPT; Landreth, 2024), this is quite similar; primarily, the selective use of questions and the carefully timed analysis distinguishes Jungian play therapy from CCPT.

I often emphasize with those I supervise, especially when they are struggling with theory or which interventions they "should" choose, that counseling is first and foremost a relationship. The American Counseling Association (ACA, 2014) says so . . . right in our Code of Ethics (full quote in Chapter 1): Counseling is a *relationship*. I would like us all to remember that every time we walk into a session with a client. This is about developing a relationship that empowers people to meet their goals. How do we truly assess and navigate that type of relationship, in all its complexities?

ASSESSMENTS, PARTS, & NEURO

> In considering the problem of typical attitudes, and in presenting them in outline, I have endeavoured to direct the eye of my readers to this picture of the many possible ways of viewing life, in the hope that I may have contributed my small share to the knowledge of the almost infinite variations and gradations of individual psychology.
> CW p. 673, § 848

Jung can be credited with developing some of the first assessments that continue to be used today, and influenced others in the areas of personality and creativity. He may be most unsung for his influence on pop psychology and the use of personality tests. Personality tests are all over the internet and used for everything from entertainment, to diagnosing mental health issues, and pre-determining job placements. A funny YouTube video exemplifies just how popular personality tests are these days (It's a Southern Thing, 2023). There is even an article attempting to analyze Jung's typology on a website called Personality Junky (2023).

Jung's most notable and direct influence is the Myers-Briggs (The Myers-Briggs Foundation, 2023). Jung identified the concept of personality types

(CW 6) based on three groups of characteristics on a continuum: extroversion/introversion, sensing/intuition, and thinking/feeling; Myers & Briggs added one more dichotomy, judging/perceiving, to Jung's existing model (remember these dual processes when we get to mode-shifting). However, Jung eventually conceptualized that "typology" was merely a symbolic way of talking about tendencies, not a firm diagnostic classification system for people. He thought about types, in the end, more like a continuum, which could also be situationally dependent. In this way, he began the conversation about the ethical dilemmas of making concrete decisions about people.

Jung's influence, though, can also be seen in the growing popularity of the enneagram (The Enneagram Institute, 2021), and Internal Family Systems (IFS Institute, 2023). Both utilize ideas of typology and symbolic representations of parts, or characteristics of self, which mimic ideas of persona and archetypal influence, which we will discuss later in this book.

His Word Association Test (WAT) (CW 2), though, really helped introduce him to the world, as he was recognized at the time for significantly contributing to the study of diagnosing psychopathology. In the WAT, the interviewer says a word and the client says the first word that comes to mind; the interviewer then looks for atypical or delayed responses, suggesting "complexes" or "trigger" words, then analyzing the associations for meaning. The WAT is one of the first examples of Jung's use of "associative" and "analytic" processes, which is now foundational to how we understand the bi-lateral neuro-processing in the brain that informs our counseling techniques, and mode-shifting theory. I believe that this includes not only creative techniques, which we will discuss further, but also, if we give credit where it is due, an overall contemporary neuropsychological focus on the right and left hemispheres, the two poles of which may be considered the creation of soothing, understanding, or effective action when they harmonize, as well as the explanation of how eye movement desensitization and reprocessing (EMDR) works (McGilchrist, 2010; Pettigrew, 2001; Shapiro, 1995, 2014).

Let's get geeky. We all love a little neuroscience, right?

The right hemisphere of the brain develops first in humans and is primarily in charge of body data as well as symbolic attachment and threat patterning; the left hemisphere is mainly responsible for symbolic mastery, including language and logic-curiosity, and "danger-denying" (McGilchrist, 2010; Petchkovsky et al., 2013). Resonance circuitry has been observed in both hemispheres, though, suggesting that both symbolic and verbal interactions stimulate brain activity of internal awareness and empathetic responses very quickly. Jung's suggestion that being over-analytic, or left brain dominant, may be considered a complex; the neural exploration of suppressing deep emotional resonance can lead to additional disconnection, more popularly known as "negativity bias", and, if left to run amuck, can impact our perceptions of ourselves, our performance, and our mental health (Müller-Pinzler et al., 2019; Petchkovsky et al., 2013). Jung (CW 16) suggested that the function of mental health treatment was to draw people out of their well-worn paths of thinking, which is a metaphor still used today in neuroscience.

The WAT has recently been studied under fMRI conditions showing that complexed responses can be witnessed in the brain, giving further evidence that psychological stressors can impact limbic system regulation, attachment, cognition, attention, emotional regulation, and meaning making, including symbolically (Escamilla et al., 2018; Petchkovsky et al., 2013). It was discovered that not only does the left hemisphere override the right within seconds when triggered, but that activation patterns of complexed responses can be witnessed in the brain: mirror neurons, anterior insula, and cingulated gyrus, thought to be responsible for empathy, self-awareness, and conflict resolution, respectively. Triggering words from the WAS has been seen to activate 2 brain circuits: (1) Those responsible for episodic memory responses below the level of consciousness, including episodic memory (superior parietal cortex), anticipation (frontal lobe), mirror neuron activation (frontal lobe and postcentral gyrus), body and sensory information (parietal lobe), and motor movement (primary motor cortex), (2) Subcortical structures involving attachment, attention, learning, memory, emotions, sensory associations, and meaning making were bi-laterally activated (Escamilla et al., 2018). We will discuss this finding later as the symbolic function.

In other words, while both hemispheres of the brain, right and left, have their own jobs, they are also interconnected. This jostling of ideas from an associative or affective state to a more analytic or logical one is how we make both emotional and cognitive sense of the world, and is influenced by our early childhood experiences, including our exposure to trauma (where we many develop complexes). Contemporary attachment theory reinforces that affective patterning and symbol development occurs early in life and can have lifelong influence referred to neurologically as resonance circuitry (Siegel, 2007), or shared circuitry (Keysers, 2011), which is important for empathy and mindfulness. It also explains why archetypes come in pairs (Panksepp & Biven, 2012). Jung's influence may have cast a much wider net across theories than he's given credit for. This also illustrates his influence on the concept of mode-shifting as an assessment for personal and professional creativity (McRoberts, 2022; Pringle & Sowden, 2017).

Jung (CW 6 & 8) said that creativity is a literal basic human instinct, a figurative doorway to the unconscious, and a state where happiness is experienced. In my search for creativity assessments I found the Mode Shifting Index (Pringle & Sowden, 2017), which immediately looked Jungian to me. It measures not only one's ability to shift back and forth, but also our awareness of shifting in both personal and professional contexts. Looking into the history of the development of the measure, Epstein (2003) is credited with first describing associative-experiential & analytic-rational processes of creative thought, developing the REI (Pacini & Epstein, 1999) to measure trait creativity. Gabora and Ranjan (2013) were the first to distill and use the terms associative and analytic to describe these modes. The MSI differs from the REI in that it focuses on "state" rather than "trait" creativity (Pringle & Sowden, 2017), which may provide more growth models of creativity research in the future. I find this hopeful when talking to people who say they're not creative (as a trait); Jung said we all are, and I like believing that. It inspires me to help people develop at least a creative state. Creative thinking involves all kinds of processing, including making clinical diagnoses (Durning et al., 2016), especially relevant for counselors. In fact, we have a whole branch of ACA called the Association for Creativity in Counseling (ACC, n.d.). I used the Mode-Shifting Index to measure Sandplay Therapists' creativity (McRoberts, 2022). However, as I have taught the model, it seems like this is how we can more easily illustrate how play, art, and expressive therapies work, and makes a case for integrating them more frequently into mental health counseling.

It is important to remember, too, that in counseling, even if we don't use *formal assessments*, or measures, with our clients, we are using *informal assessments* all the time. Through our attunement with our client, we imagine what it might be like in our client's shoes while applying what we have learned in our training. We might not be directly asking ourselves, but may be intuiting (or using our intuition to imagine) how our client feels, what they might be thinking, how their decisions may have made perfect sense at the time, and even what to say or do with our clients next. To me, that is all part of assessment. I also think of it as an aspect of mode-shifting.

MODE-SHIFTING

> We have, therefore, two kinds of thinking: directed thinking, and dreaming or fantasy-thinking.
>
> CW 5, p. 18, § 20

I like to think about this back and forth, right and left hemisphere, thinking and feeling, but more-than-dual-processing way of looking at and working with the psyche as "mode-shifting" (see Figure 2.2). Jung said we have "two main tendencies. One is the way of creative formulation, the other the way of understanding" (CW 8, p. 119, § 172), but we need both to be well balanced. These two modes are what we now call *associative* (more right-brained) and *analytic* (more left-brained) modes. We know that being aware and able to shift between modes can lead to creative and therapeutic outcomes. In Jungian-oriented counseling and play therapy, we don't expect this process to be linear, and we see it as more interconnected. Ideas are observed, nurtured, explored, and expanded on in a process we call *circumambulation*. Circumambulation is an ancient term that means creating a sacred circle.

Jung theorized years ago that some disturbances of the mind can lead to one-sided, rigid, ego-centric, over-analytical thinking (CW 8). You may have heard this called "black or white thinking" in CBT circles. I prefer to call this "getting stuck in analytic mode" and it affects counselors-in-training as well. Sometimes, even if we are trying our best to be "non-judgmental" in our counseling relationships, the reality is that we are trained to analyze. That is what assessments, diagnoses, and clinical impressions are. I am still curious why Jung chose the term *analytic psychology* to describe his method, when he seemed to want to distinguish his value of the unconscious, and associative processes as well; he actually says that "analytical" DOES mean that to him

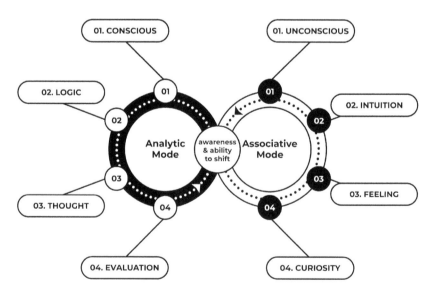

Figure 2.2 Mode-Shifting. (Reprinted with permission. Further reproduction is prohibited without the author's written authorization. All rights reserved. Copyright © 2023 by author, Rachel McRoberts.)

(CW 9i). While I call out his Humpty Dumpty nonsense here, I give him credit for the concept of mode-shifting anyway.

Contemporaries have also begun to use this language, differentiating between more unconscious/associative processes and conscious/analytical ones, as well as how they interact and work together (Macchi & Bagassi, 2015). Nobel laureate Daniel Kahneman's research (2011) identified two major modes in his book *Thinking Fast and Slow*: the automatic experiential-intuitive system, and the rational-analytic system; this both supports the mode-shifting theory of creative cognition, as well as describes the role of Jungian, and other psychodynamically oriented counselors working as translators between the modes and assisting with making the unconscious more conscious. Research also demonstrates Jung's theory that over-reliance on either mode can cause difficulties (Shapiro & Marks-Tarlow, 2021), from repetition-compulsion (anxiety) to rigid thinking (referred to as thought-distortions in the CBT world), to psychosis (or a flooding from the unconscious).

Both we and our clients experience this *tension of the opposites*, as Jung called it (Hannah, 1976), which frequently arises in our work, and is especially relevant to those who have been abused by those they love, as the vast majority of children who have been abused are (National Children's Alliance, 2023). Clients may be of "two minds" about many aspects of themselves, their abuser, and the situation they find themselves in. Kalashed (1996), a Jungian therapist, recognized that trauma interrupts the internalized balance, the transitional space between the real and imaginary, the conscious and unconscious, where people interpret and express their perceptions of the world; the Jungian concept of *conjunction oppositorum*, or a joining of the opposites, must be acknowledged and worked through symbolically, in a recovered or discovered transitional space for integration to occur (CW 8. This being of two minds is an issue that Jung addressed in his time, and is being further studied in neurobiological effects on the brain, as well as neuro-inspired mental health treatments, such as EMDR (EMDRIA, 2023; Parnell, 2013; Shapiro, 1995; Silverstein, 2014).

We have a wealth of worldwide research (like, literally from the World Health Organization) suggesting that the arts are good for promoting wellness, as well as preventing and treating various illnesses (Fancourt & Finn, 2019). Working on our creative cognition must include actively engaging in creative or experiential activities, including playing, mark making, and experimenting, suspending our judgment for a significant period of time while we make. Popular neuroscientist Dan Siegel (2007) identifies that the ability to imagine, or conceptualize a mental image of experience, supports healthy structural brain development; this supports Jung's ideas about the creative instinct (CW 8), what we now call the symbolic function (Boukhabza, 2023), the skill of *active imagination* (CW 18; CW 7), and the neurobiological benefits of sandplay therapy (Akimoto et al., 2018; Foo & Pratiwi, 2021; Freedle, 2019) all of which we will cover later in this book.

Suppose we practice being curious, playing with ideas, and imagining various possibilities, staying with the metaphors and feelings. In that case, we open ourselves and the relationship, and provide room for our clients to explore more freely. If we mode-shift, we'll likely encourage more mode-shifting. It is more difficult to judge if we are aware and able to balance associative and analytic processes. We may be less inclined to jump to conclusions or pathologize others in our counseling relationships.

A NON-PATHOLOGIZING, SPIRIT-CENTERED APPROACH

> Tears, sorrow, and disappointment are bitter, but wisdom is the comforter in all psychic suffering.
>
> CW 14, p. 247, § 330

Jung noticed a shift in our mental health as the symbolic and religious interaction declined; he even lamented that there were "as yet no statistics with actual figures to prove this" (CW 11, p. 336, § 514). The Jungian-oriented counselor is especially likely to be drawn to a non-pathologizing approach. Counseling values a strength-based wellness model, with spirituality at the hub (CSI, 2023). The Wheel of Wellness is often cited as an infographic illustrating the interactive and interconnected aspects of life that impact our overall wellness, both personal and collective. It is based on the work of Jung's contemporary, Alfred Adler, and his theory of the importance of a sense of wholeness, otherwise known as *holism*, and the *indivisibility of the self*, as well as the completion of life tasks within a social context (Sweeney, 2019). Both Adler and Jung were students of Freud who broke away to develop their own theories, both with a focus on the somewhat intangible, philosophical, spiritual core grounding one's sense of self as one moves through and is impacted by the world, as well as a high value for creativity. (Alder's "individual psychology" seems as much of a misnomer as Jung's "analytical psychology", though.) The brilliant minds that developed the Wheel of Wellness were also staunch counseling advocates before and after.

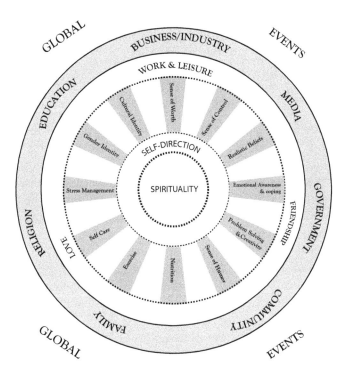

Figure 2.3 The Wheel of Wellness. (Reproduction by special permission of the Publisher, Mind Garden, Inc. www.mindgarden.com from the Wellness Evaluation of Lifestyle by Jane E. Myers, Thomas J. Sweeney, & Melvin Witmer. Copyright © 2001 by Jane E. Myers. Further reproduction is prohibited without the Publisher's written consent.)

Wellness is a complex concept, and determining the higher-order factors conclusively across populations remains elusive. Where we end and the world begins, and how much of each goes into each conscious decision, cannot be accurately quantified, especially day-to-day or in the counseling relationship. Through it all, though, the Wheel of Wellness (Myers et al., 2002; see Figure 2.3) remains influential and helpful to counselors and clients alike as an illustration of what forces may impact our sense of self.

In recent years, many counselors have adopted more medicalized models being sold as "evidence-based" practice, in part to "legitimize" the profession in competition with other healthcare providers, often within the same workplace. Jung (CW 10) was wary way back in the day about therapies whose idealized protocol attempted to predict what might be best for a particular individual; there are too many variables to consider and what matters is the client's Self-knowledge. What sets one free is another's prison; it is the same with "normality and adaptation" (CW 16, p. 70, § 163). As a population, we have already begun to forget who we are, pushing our values, the definition of evidence-based, and the actual evidence for a holistic, creative, relational way of working into Shadow.

Jung struggled with assisting the field in attempting to understand and find a balance between science and spirituality; it was a big part of why he broke with Freud. Jung took a more Eastern philosophical approach to viewing suffering: it is inevitable, but we are designed to seek balance. The Jungian idea of the Self, or the wise inner guide, can be traced back to ancient Eastern concepts of *brahman, atman,* and the *Tao,* and to contemporary mindfulness trends in the mental health field (though Jung and Eastern religions/philosophies are rarely cited). The Tao is closely linked with the idea of flow, like that of one being in and of the water. "Flow" is both an ancient aspect of mindfulness and a contemporary measure of creativity (Kelly, 2006). Jung brought the two together 100 years ago. He said that the "steady flow of life manifests itself" in undisturbed thinking and "has a progressive creative quality"; should this process become interrupted, one may be:

> . . . plagued by afterthoughts, contenting itself with constant broodings on things past and gone, chewing them over in an effort to analyze and digest them. Since the creative element is now lodged in another function, thinking no longer progresses, it stagnates.
>
> CW 6, p. 495, § 592

Clients often describe this stagnation as feeling or being "stuck". One of the ways people try to escape their feeling of stuckness is through the use of substances. While I do not usually hear about Jung's influence in alcohol and drug treatment circles, Jung had a direct influence on the development of Alcoholics Anonymous (AA) in the 1930s. A comprehensive overview is outlined in McCabe's (2015) book on the subject. However, in short, Jung saw addiction as a spiritual problem, inspired one of AA's founders, Bill W., and corresponded with him as he developed the 12 Steps, an immersive spiritual program. AA is unique because it is a member-led fellowship, blending the spiritual and scientific, the individual and the collective. All are welcome. Members self-identify as alcoholics; while other providers may refer clients to meetings, and they might even be court-ordered, no one gets formally diagnosed in the program. Notably, AA has recently been found to be as effective as, or even more effective than, other manualized mental health treatments such as CBT (Kelly et al., 2020). And it's free!

Counselors often joke that we are trying to work ourselves out of a job. But the need is so great, and ever growing. What is going on? Both Jung and his student, Neumann (1959), criticized growing modernity for separating us from our developmental, relational, creative, and spiritual processes. Even then, they recognized that both professionals, and the masses, were downright defensive of the conscious, ego-centric, "rational" mind and continued attempts to dismantle the power of historical cultures. The idea of culture, our collective history, our drives, and our connection to the Self, are all thought to reside in the unconscious. We may be seeing a revolt from the unconscious: wisdom rearing up, being "socially unacceptable" in service of the Self and the greater good. Jung was curious about how what we might call symptoms, neurosis, or complexes may be messages from the unconscious that a change is needed, and even how to go about making that change (CW 4; CW 14). Like the Humanists after him, Jung trusted that people know themselves the best and can find their own solutions. He said:

> We should not try to "get rid" of a neurosis, but rather to experience what it means, what it has to teach, what its purpose is. We should even learn to be thankful for it, otherwise we pass it by and miss the opportunity of getting to know ourselves as we really are. A neurosis is truly removed only when it has removed the false attitude of the ego. We do not cure it – it cures us. A man is ill, but the illness is nature's attempt to heal him. From the illness itself we can learn so much for our recovery, and what the neurotic flings away as absolutely worthless contains the true gold we should never have found elsewhere.
>
> CW 10, p. 170, § 361

Every time I teach a Play Therapy course, and talk about Gary Landreth's development of child-centered play therapy (CCPT), I hear Jung's message amplified. Gary says that focusing on the problem makes us lose sight of the person and refers to "the playing cure" as a complementary alternative to "the talking cure" introduced by the psychoanalysts in the early 1900s (Landreth, 2024). However, Jung takes us a step further by asking us to consider what the disturbance means. Here, we practice interpretation, but in collaboration with our clients. Jung suggests that the unconscious manifests disturbances in the ego because it is trying to get our attention. The unconscious holds the answer to problems the ego can't solve. When worrying about our next move, frozen in our despair, or reliving past traumas, we may want to run away from, control, and "get rid" of them.

Counselors across theoretical orientations intuitively know that what is really needed is to sit down, unpack, and then process these phenomena more deeply.

I was trained in art therapy before I was trained in counseling. There, we valued "art as therapy". The art making, or associative process, is considered the therapy itself, no matter the diagnosis, or if there is one or not. In this way, CCPT also resonated with me. For generations, the art therapist Edith Kramer (2000) advocated against the use of therapist-predetermined, banal, art-based interventions, as they do not spring from and resonate within the client, and fail to accept them as they are; Jungian sandplay therapists have traditionally also taken a non-directive stance, as have child-centered play therapists. While some clinicians have expressed a desire or perceived need to intervene if a child seems stuck behaviorally, emotionally, or in a symbolic stereotype, or replaying, that may be considered symptomatic of the trauma experience (Gil, 2006; Green, 2008; Shelby & Felix, 2006), others advise against it in service of self-determination and trusting the process (Fordham, 1994; Lowenfeld, 1939; Turner, 2005), or encourage elaboration on the theme to expand the client's awareness (Michael, 1982; Robertson, 1982). A less directive approach has been shown to positively affect self-esteem, emotional regulation, and social skills (Scott et al., 2003).

When a child has a history with a symbol or play theme that has appeared over time, the therapist may intervene through wondering aloud about the work, which is considered partially directive, and when well attuned and timed, can lead a client deeper into their process; when a client appears to be overly anxious about engaging in the process, directly inviting them toward activities or materials that may soothe, resonate with, or activate salient feelings may be helpful (Allan, 1988). This process should be harmonious, in that the highly skilled and attuned therapist can resonate with and riff off the client to create a transformational experience based on presented needs and themes (Schmidt, 2014).

Counseling continues to expand the idea of wellness, encouraging us to advocate for the legitimacy of feelings that clients may be pressured to cut off because of a collective fear, anxiety, or rejection. Counselors are also encouraged to develop our knowledge of and humility regarding the cultures of the world, which we now recognize comes from knowing ourselves more deeply (Ratts et al., 2015). However, Jung (CW 10) observed that what many people may call "self-knowledge" is merely ego-awareness and does not delve deep enough into the unconscious to evoke real insight.

Jung was one of the first to de-medicalize and de-pathologize his method, analytic psychology, and focus on empowerment, especially for women. While it is now a requirement in many Jungian professional organizations to hold a mental health license, before credentialing that was not the case (Kirsch, 2000); for many years, a graduate degree in any field (not necessarily medicine, which was the norm), personal process, and specialized Jungian training was the norm. To become an analyst, one had to be a patient first. Many Jungians today hold such a non-pathologizing approach that they refuse to diagnose, much like strict humanistic counselors. This may be a challenge for those who want to work in an agency setting or bill insurance. However, it can be done more easily in private practice and in faith-based or other non-profit organizations.

One of the reasons that I advocate for my counseling supervisees to delve deeply into a theory of practice, and not to become prescriptive too early, is so they can confront themselves more deeply. If we are too quick to bounce away from an uncomfortable concept or situation while working, this might speak of our own anxieties, and distrust of the process. Jung knew that it was important for those who wanted to be helpers first to do their own work because if we grow to maturity, we inevitably have wounds, unprocessed unconscious material (we'll talk more about the Wounded Healer later . . .), and even if everything has been rosy, we are still walking own path on our way to becoming who we are. In the counseling literature we see this topical referred to as "the person of the therapist".

THE PERSON OF THE THERAPIST

> The cure works best when the doctor himself believes in his own formulae otherwise he may be overcome by scientific doubt and lose the proper convincing tone.
>
> CW 4, p. 353, § 578

While some therapists may be looking for a theory of practice that involves purely reason, and adherence to a medical model, others may feel called to this work on a deeper level. Jung acknowledges, throughout his work, not only that his theory attempts to build a bridge, understanding that there is a psychological function for spiritual connection, but also that the person of the therapist, and their belief in their method, matters. We now have evidence that the therapeutic relationship itself may be the most determining factor of successful treatment outcomes across theories (Wampold &

Imel, 2015). That means we have to buy what we're selling, or, even better, embody it. Who we are is more important than what we do. This discourse is cited in the literature as the *person of the therapist*.

Though reflective practices are a big part of counselor training assessments, requiring counselors to go to counseling themselves is an ethical considera-tion being discussed in America and abroad which we'll discuss further in this book. It goes without saying, though, that in general, contemporary cultur-ally informed and anti-racist policies require us all to take a good hard look. And in order to exude and inspire creative cognition and expression, we must value creativity, believe ourselves to be creative, and act creatively, embracing the aesthetics of existence (Foucault, 1984). This involves ethical self-care for one's life and profession, to become a living work of art. We have to actively engage in life and the creative process. Not doing our own work but attempt-ing to help others do theirs is as ridiculous as trying to teach someone to cook when we've never cooked in our lives (Ammann, 1991). Jung himself humbly claimed that his entire body of work was entirely subjective (CW 18).

If there is one thing that a Jungian counselor must ascribe to, it is the val-uing of the unconscious and the creative process it engages in. That's the thing that really divided Jung from Freud. Jung said that Freud thought of the unconscious as the garbage can of consciousness (Jung, 2023), "just a receptacle for all unclean spirits and other odious legacies from the dead past" (CW 4, p. 448, § 760). Jung's message that resonates across time is that the unconscious is a vital half of our psyche so much so that we can't have consciousness without it.

We have known for a while that counselors-in-training, and especially those who do not trust their supervisors for a variety of reasons, may be afraid of openly engaging in reflective practices, which can do a great disservice to themselves and, ultimately, their clients (Bernard & Goodyear, 2014; Eryılmaz & Mutlu, 2017; Nissen-Lie et al., 2017; Rønnestad & Skovholt, 2003). Jung called this holding back "concealment", and identified it as characteristic of the isolation and "irritability of the over-virtuous" (CW 16, p. 58, § 130). We don't want to be like that! "True education can only start from naked reality, not from a delusive ideal" (CW 7, p. 62, § 93). This is why I urge all counselors-in-training to seek out supervision that is sup-portive and validating, if not downright theoretically aligned (McRoberts, 2019). We need mentors. And not just any mentors. It needs to be a good fit, just like in counseling.

There is gobs of research on how supervisor's modeling is important and can impact creativity, intrinsic motivation, sense of belonging, as well as client care outcomes (it's called a parallel process); here are a few references just to get you started if you want to go see for yourself: (Bernard & Goodyear, 2014; Chong & Ma, 2010; Deci, 1972; Grant & Berry, 2011; Inman & Soheilian, 2010; Mullen et al., 2007; Reisetter et al., 2004; Smith-Adcock et al., 2015; VanderGast & Hinkle, 2015; Zellars et al., 2002). Our supervisors are like mirrors. And like Jung said in 1931:

> If we do not fashion for ourselves a picture of the world, we do not see ourselves either, who are the faithful reflections of that world. Only when mirrored in our picture of the world can we see ourselves in the round. Only in our creative acts do we step forth into the light and see ourselves whole and complete.
>
> CW 8, p. 491, § 737

Remember how counseling is a relationship? Counselor education and supervision is a relationship, too. That makes me, as a counselor, educator, and supervisor, want to explicitly say that if you aren't getting the kind of supervision you want from your boss (because I know sometimes that's the reality of our work), I hope that you are empowered to ask for what you want from them, or to seek supervision elsewhere. There are several assessments, but one of my favorites is currently available online and is called What I Want from Supervision (Heartland Health Outreach, n.d.). I encourage my supervisees to fill it out at the beginning and end of semesters, and any time they want to reassess how things are going.

Like the *individuation process*, Jung's phrase for becoming who we are, our counselor identity can be a long, winding road with many shifts in awareness and prioritization of personal and professional development (Rønnestad & Skovholt, 2003). That also sounds a lot like mode-shifting to me. They say it takes a lifetime. I kind of hope it does.

SO WHY JUNG?

> . . .life is a disease with a very bad prognosis: it lingers on for years, only to end with death.
>
> CW 11, p. 105, § 167

After over 20 years in the field of counseling and play therapy, even though I can see Jung's influence everywhere, I still get significant side-eye from other professionals. I often joke about the "woo woo" of being Jungian, because I can be playful with the idea of how serious this all is. I am writing this book to explain how Jung helps me provide this freedom and responsibility to help empower myself and others: my students, supervisees, their other supervisors, our clients, and maybe others who know, hear, and love us. Jung said years ago that we were on a slippery slope to a mental health crisis, and folks, we're there. As counselors we are called to do something about that. For me, it starts with me and my relationship to the Self. What do I believe about life, what's meaningful, what the mind is, and how to conceptualize how I might be helpful to myself, my clients, and the world? No other theorist makes me question all of this, gives me a map, and inspires me to keep searching, like Jung. I am glad you are here and can be a part of this phenomenon of amplifying Jung's work. I hear it's catching on (Cheslaw, 2023).

Reflections

1. What is your current primary theoretical orientation? Does it fit perfectly or have you had to make little adjustments along the way? If so, describe them.
2. Where does the personal and professional intersect for you? How does one feed the other? What is the boundary?
3. Where do you find yourself mirrored in the World?
4. Why are you drawn to learning more about a Jungian approach? What aspects?

REFERENCES

Akimoto, M., Furukawa, K., & Ito, J. (2018). Exploring the sandplayer's brain: A single case study. *Archives of Sandplay Therapy, 30*(3), 73–84. https://doi.org/10.11377/sandplay.30.373

Allan, J. (1988). *Inscapes of the child's world: Jungian counseling in schools and clinics.* Spring Publications.

American Counseling Association. (2014). *2014 ACA code of ethics.* www.counseling.org/resources/aca-code-of-ethics.pdf

Ammann, R. (1991). *Healing and transformation in sandplay: Creative processes become visible.* Open Court Publishing Company.

Association for Creativity in Counseling (ACC). (n.d.). Home page. The American Counseling Association. www.creativecounselor.org/home-1

Bernard, J. M., & Goodyear, R. K. (2014). *Fundamentals of clinical supervision* (5th ed.). Pearson Allyn & Bacon.

Boukhabza, D. (2023). *A Jungian understanding of symbolic function and forms: The dream series.* Routledge.

Bradway, K., & McCoard, B. (1997). *Sandplay: Silent workshop of the psyche.* Routledge.

Bulkeley, K., & Weldon, C. (2011). *Teaching Jung.* Oxford Press.

Cheslaw, L. (2023, September 13). *How This Jungian Life made Carl Jung Cool Again.* Vulture. www.vulture.com/2023/09/this-jungian-life-podcast-psychoanalysis-carl-jung.html

Chi Sigma Iota (CSI). (2023). *Wheel of wellness.* www.csi-net.org/members/group_content_view.asp?group=162835&id=573587

Chong, E., & Ma, X. (2010). The influence of individual factors, supervision and work environment on creative self-efficacy. *Creativity and Innovation Management, 19*(3), 233–247. https://doi.org/10.1111/j.1467-8691.2010.00557.x

Claugh, W. R. (2013, October 27). *Jung and philosophy.* The Jung Page. https://jungpage.org/learn/articles/analytical-psychology/89-jung-and-philosophy. (Original work published 1997).

Deci, E. L. (1972). Intrinsic motivation, extrinsic reinforcement, and inequity. *Journal of Personality and Social Psychology, 22*(1), 113–120. https://doi.org/10.1037/h0032355

Durning, S. J., Costanzo, M. E., Beckman, T. J., Artino, A. R., Roy, M. J., van der Vleuten, C., Holmboe, E. S., Lipner, R. S., & Schuwirth, L. (2016). Functional neuroimaging correlates of thinking flexibility and knowledge structure in memory: Exploring the relationships between clinical reasoning and diagnostic thinking. *Medical Teacher, 38,* 570–577. doi:10.3109/0142159X.2015.1047755.

EMDR International Association (EMDRIA). (2023). Home page. www.emdria.org

The Enneagram Institute. (2021). *Type descriptions.* www.enneagraminstitute.com/type-descriptions

Epstein, S. (2003). Cognitive-experiential self-theory of personality. In T. Millon & M. J. Lerner (Eds.), *Handbook of psychology: Personality and social psychology,* Vol. 5 (pp. 159–184). John Wiley & Sons.

Eryılmaz, A., & Mutlu, T. (2017). Developing the four-stage supervision model for counselor trainees. *Educational Sciences: Theory & Practice, 17,* 597–629. http://dx.doi.org/10.12738/estp. 2017.2.2253

Escamilla, M., Sandoval, H., Calhoun, V., & Ramirez, M. (2018). Brain activation patterns in response to complex triggers in the Word Association Test: Results from a new study in the United States. *The Journal of Analytical Psychology, 63*(4), 484–509. https://doi.org/10.1111/1468-5922.12430

Fancourt, D., & Finn, S. (2019). *What is the evidence on the role of the arts in improving health and well-being? A scoping review.* WHO Regional Office for Europe. (Health Evidence Network (HEN) synthesis report 67).

Foo, M., & Pratiwi, A. (2021). The effectiveness of sandplay therapy in treating patients with generalized anxiety disorder and childhood trauma using magnetic resonance spectroscopy to examine choline level in the dorsolateral prefrontal cortex and centrum semiovale. *International Journal of Play Therapy, 30*(3), 177–186. doi:10.1037/pla0000162.

Fordham, M. (1994). *Children as individuals.* Free Association Books.

Foucault, M. (1984). *The Foucault reader.* P. Rainbow (Ed.). Pantheon Books.

Freedle, L. R. (2019). Making connections: Sandplay therapy and the Neurosequential Model of Therapeutics. *Journal of Sandplay Therapy, 28*(1), 91–109.

Gabora, L., & Ranjan, A. (2013). How insight emerges in a distributed, content addressable memory. In O. Vartanian, A. S. Bristol, & J. C. Kaufman (Eds.), *The neuroscience of creativity* (pp. 19–44). Oxford University Press.

Garner, C. M., Freeman, B. J., & Lee, L. E. (2016). Assessment of student dispositions: The development and psychometric properties of the professional disposition competence assessment (PDCA). *Vistas, 52,* 1–14. www.researchgate.net/publication/346119851_Assessment_of_Dispositions_in_Program_Admissions_The_Professional_Disposition_Competence_Assessment-Revised_Admission_PDCA-RA

Gil, E. (2006). *Helping abused and traumatized children: Integrating directive and nondirective approaches.* Guilford Press.

Grant, A. M., & Berry, J. W. (2011). The necessity of others is the mother of invention: Intrinsic and prosocial motivations, perspective taking, and creativity. *Academy of Management Journal, 54*(1), 73–96. https://doi.org/10.5465/AMJ.2011.59215085

Green, E. J. (2008). Reenvisioning Jungian analytical play therapy with child sexual assault survivors. *International Journal of Play Therapy, 17*(2), 102–121. http://dx.doi.org/10.1037/a0012770

Hannah, B. (1976). *Jung: His life and work.* Chiron Publications.

Heartland Health Outreach. (n.d.). *What I want from supervision.* https://nhchc.org/wp-content/uploads/2019/08/What-I-Want-From-Supervision.pdf

Heracleous, L., & Robson, D. (2020, November 11). *Why the "paradox mindset" is the key to success.* Worklife. www.bbc.com/worklife/article/20201109-why-the-paradox-mindset-is-the-key-to-success

IFS Institute. (2023). Home page. https://ifs-institute.com/

Inman, A. G., & Soheilian, S. S. (2010). Training supervisors: A core competency. In N. Ladany & L. J. Bradley (Eds.), *Counselor supervision* (4th ed., pp. 413–436). Routledge.

It's a Southern Thing. (2023). *Personality tests are out of control.* [YouTube video]. https://youtu.be/2q4q_CBdoFs

Jacobs, M. (2017). *Psychodynamic counselling in action* (5th ed.). Sage.

Jung, C. G. (2023). *The collected works of C. G. Jung: Revised and expanded complete digital edition.* (CW 1–20). G. Adler, W. McGuire, & H. Read (Eds.), R. F. C. Hull (Trans.). Princeton University Press. https://press.princeton.edu/books/ebook/9780691255194/the-collected-works-of-c-g-jung

Kahneman, D. (2011). *Thinking, fast and slow.* Farrar, Strauss and Giroux.

Kalashed, D. E. (1996). *The inner world of trauma: Archetypal defenses of the personal spirit.* Routledge.

Kelly, J. F., Humphreys, K., & Ferri, M. (2020). Alcoholics Anonymous and other 12-step programs for alcohol use disorder. *Cochrane Database of Systematic Reviews, 3,* CD012880. https://doi.org/10.1002/14651858.CD012880.pub2

Kelly, K. E. (2006). Relationship between the Five-Factor Model of Personality and the Scale of Creative Attributes and Behavior: A validational study. *Individual Differences Research, 4*(5), 299–305.

Keysers, C. (2011). *The empathic brain: How the discovery of mirror neurons changes our understanding of human nature.* Social Brain Press.

Kirsch, T. B. (2000). *The Jungians: A comparative and historical perspective.* Routledge.

Kramer, E. (2000). *Art as therapy: Collected papers.* L. A. Gerity (Ed.). Kingsley Publishers.

Landreth, G. (2024). *Play therapy: The art of the relationship* (3rd ed.). Routledge. (Original work published 1991).

Leader, C. (2015). Supervising the uncanny: The play within the play. *Journal of Analytical Psychology, 60*(5), 657–678. doi:10.1111/1468-5922.12178.

Lilly, JP (2015). Jungian analytical play therapy. In D. A. Crenshaw & A. L. Stewart (Eds.), *Play therapy: A comprehensive guide to theory and practice* (pp. 48–65). Guilford Press.

Lowenfeld, M. (1939). The world pictures of children. *British Journal of Medical Psychology, 18,* 65–73.

Macchi, L., & Bagassi, M. (2015). When analytic thought is challenged by a misunderstanding. *Thinking & Reasoning, 21*(1), 147–164. http://dx.doi.org/10.1080/13546783.2014.964315

McCabe, I. (2015). *Carl Jung and Alcoholics Anonymous: The Twelve Steps as a spiritual journey of individuation.* Routledge.

McGilchrist, I. (2010). *The Master and his emissary: The divided brain and the making of the Western world*. Yale University Press.

McRoberts, R. (2019). The middle ground: Theoretically matched play therapy supervision: community considerations. *Play Therapy Magazine, 14*(3), 28–29.

McRoberts, R. (2022). Addressing the creativity crisis: Sandplay therapists' mode-shifting and professional identity development. *Journal of Sandplay Therapy, 31*(2), 129–142. www.sandplay.org/journal/research-articles/addressing-the-creativity-crisis-sandplay-therapists-mode-shifting-and-professional-identity-development/

Michael, J. (Ed.). (1982). *The Lowenfeld lectures*. Pennsylvania State University Press.

Moradi, B., & DeBlaere, C. (2010). Replacing either/or with both/and: Illustrations of perspective alternation. *The Counseling Psychologist, 38*(3). https://doi.org/10.1177/0011000009356460

Mullen, J. A., Luke, M., & Drewes, A. A. (2007). Supervision can be playful, too: Play therapy techniques that enhance supervision. *International Journal of Play Therapy, 16*, 69–85. http://dx.doi.org/10.1037/1555-6824.16.1.69

Müller-Pinzler, L., Czekalla, N., Mayer, A. V., et al. (2019). Negativity-bias in forming beliefs about own abilities. *Scientific Reports, 9*, 14416. www.nature.com/articles/s41598-019-50821-w

The Myers-Briggs Foundation. (2023). *MBTI basics*. www.myersbriggs.org/my-mbti-personality-type/mbti-basics/home.htm?bhcp=1

National Children's Alliance. (2023). *National statistics on child abuse*. www.nationalchildrensalliance.org/media-room/national-statistics-on-child-abuse/

Neukrug, E. S. (Ed.). (2015). *The SAGE Encyclopedia of Theory in Counseling and Psychotherapy*. Sage Publications.

Neumann, E. (1959). *Art and the creative unconscious*. Princeton University Press.

Nissen-Lie, H. A., Rønnestad, M. H., Høglend, P. A., Havik, O. E., Solbakken, O. A., Stiles, T. C., & Monsen, J. T. (2017). Love yourself as a person, doubt yourself as a therapist? *Clinical Psychology and Psychotherapy, 24*, 48–60. doi:10.1002/cpp. 1977.

Pacini, R., & Epstein, S. (1999). The relation of rational and experiential information processing styles to personality, basic beliefs, and the ratio-bias phenomenon. *Journal of Personality and Social Psychology, 76*(6), 972–987. https://doi.org/10.1037/0022-3514.76.6.972

Panksepp, J., & Biven, L. (2012). *The archaeology of mind: Neuroevolutionary origins of human emotion*. W. W. Norton & Company.

Parnell, L. (2013). *Attachment-focused EMDR: Healing relational trauma.* W. W. Norton & Co.

Personality Junky. (2023). *Enneagram 4, 5, or 9? Insights from analyzing Jung's personality type.* https://personalityjunkie.com/08/enneagram-4-5-9-jung-personality-type/

Petchkovsky, L., Petchkovsky, M., Morris, P., Dickson, P., Montgomery, D., Dwyer, J., & Burnett, P. (2013). fMRI responses to Jung's Word Association Test: Implications for theory, treatment and research. *The Journal of Analytical Psychology, 58*(3), 409–431. https://doi.org/10.1111/1468-5922.12021

Pettigrew, J. D. (2001). Searching for the switch: Neural bases of perceptual rivalry alternations. *Brain and Mind, 2,* 84–115.

Pringle, A., & Sowden, P. T. (2017). The Mode Shifting Index (MSI): A new measure of the creative thinking skill of shifting between associative and analytic thinking. *Thinking Skills and Creativity, 23,* 17–28. https://dx.doi.org/10.1016/j.tsc.2016.10.010

Ratts, M. J., Singh, A. A., Nassar-McMillan, S., Butler, K., & McCullough, R. (2015). *Multicultural and social justice counseling competencies.* American Counseling Association. www.counseling.org/docs/default-source/competencies/multicultural-and-social-justice-counseling-competencies.pdf?sfvrsn=20

Reid, K. (2022, February 22). Is a "both/and" approach to integration possible? A practice reflection on working with children in out-of-home care and their caregivers. *Australian & New Zealand Journal of Family Therapy.* https://doi.org/10.1002/anzf.1476

Reisetter, M., Korcuska, J. S., Yexley, M., Bonds, D., Nikels, H., & McHenry, W. (2004). Counselor educators and qualitative research: Affirming a research identity. *Counselor Education and Supervision, 44,* 2–16. http://dx.doi.org/10.1002/j.15566978.2004.tb01856.x

Robertson, S. M. (1982). *Rosegarden and labyrinth: A study in art education.* Spring Publications.

Roesler, C. (2013). Evidence for the effectiveness of Jungian psychotherapy: A review of empirical studies. *Behavioral Sciences, 3,* 562–575. doi:10.3390/bs3040562.

Roesler, C. (2019). Sandplay therapy: An overview of theory, applications and evidence base. *The Arts in Psychotherapy, 64,* 84–94. https://doi.org/10.1016/j.aip.2019.04.001

Rønnestad, M. H., & Skovholt, T. M. (2003). The journey of the counselor and therapist: Research findings and perspectives on professional development. *Journal of Career Development, 30*(1), 5–44. doi:10.1023/A:1025173508081.

Schmidt, M. (2014). Influences on my clinical practice and identity Jungian analysis on the couch: What and where is the truth of it? *The Journal of Analytical Psychology*, *59*(5), 661–679. http://dx.doi.org/10.1111/1468-5922.12116

Scott, T. A., Burlingame, G., Starling, M., Porter, C., & Lilly, JP (2003). Effects of individual client-centered play therapy on sexually abused children's mood, self-concept, and social competence. *International Journal of Play Therapy*, *12*(1), 7–30. https://doi.org/10.1037/h0088869

Shapiro, F. (1995). *Eye movement desensitization and reprocessing: Basic principles, protocols and procedures* (1st ed.). Guilford Press.

Shapiro, F. (2014). The role of eye movement desensitization and reprocessing (EMDR) therapy in medicine: Addressing the psychological and physical symptoms stemming from adverse life experiences. *The Permanente Journal*, *18*(1), 71–77. doi:10.7812/TPP/13-098.

Shapiro, Y., & Marks-Tarlow, T. (2021). Varieties of clinical intuition: Explicit, implicit, and nonlocal neurodynamics. *Psychoanalytic Dialogues*, *31*(3), 262–281. https://doi.org/10.1080/10481885.2021.1902744

Shelby, J. S., & Felix, E. D. (2006). Posttraumatic play therapy: The need for an integrated model of directive and nondirective approaches. In L. A. Reddy, T. M., Files-Hall, & C. E. Schaefer (Eds.), *Empirically based play interventions for children* (pp. 79–104). American Psychological Association.

Siegel, D. J. (2007). *The mindful brain: Reflection and attunement in the cultivation of well-being*. W. W. Norton.

Silverstein, S. M. (2014). Jung's views on causes and treatments of schizophrenia in light of current trends in cognitive neuroscience and psychotherapy research: Psychological research and treatment. *The Journal of Analytical Psychology*, *59*(2), 263–283. http://dx.doi.org/10.1111/1468-5922.12073

Smith-Adcock, S., Shin, S. M., & Pereira, J. (2015). Critical incidents in learning child-centered play therapy: Implications for teaching and supervision. *International Journal of Play Therapy*, *24*(2), 78–91. https://doi.org/10.1037/a0039122

Sweeney, T. (2019). *Adlerian counseling and psychotherapy* (6th ed.). Routledge.

Turner, B. A. (2005). *The handbook of sandplay therapy*. Temenos Press.

VanderGast, T. S., & Hinkle, M. S. (2015). So happy together? Predictors of satisfaction with supervision for play therapist supervisees. *International Journal of Play Therapy*, *24*(2), 92–102. https://doi.org/10.1037/a0039105

Wampold, B. E., & Imel, Z. E. (2015). *The great psychotherapy debate*. Routledge.

Wiersma, J. K., Freedle, L. R., McRoberts, R., & Solberg, K. B. (2022). A meta-analysis of sandplay therapy treatment outcomes. *International Journal of Play Therapy*, *31*(4), 197–215. https://doi.org/10.1037/pla0000180

Wilkinson, M. (2005). Undoing dissociation: Affective neuroscience: A contemporary Jungian clinical perspective. *The Journal of Analytical Psychology, 50*(4), 483–501. https://doi.org/10.1111/j.0021-8774.2005.00550.x

Winnicott, D. W. (1971). *Playing and reality.* Basic Books.

Zellars, K. L., Tepper, B. J., & Duffy, M. K. (2002). Abusive supervision and subordinates' organizational citizenship behavior. *Journal of Applied Psychology, 86,* 1068–1076. http://dx.doi.org/10.1037/0021-9010.87.6.1068

3
The Structure of the Psyche

Individuation and collectivity are a pair of opposites, two divergent destinies.
They are related to one another by guilt. The individual is obliged by the collective
demands to purchase his individuation at the cost of an equivalent work for the
benefit of society. So far as this is possible, individuation is possible.

Jung, CW 18, p. 452, § 1099

What makes us uniquely human? Where is the line between us and the rest of the world? How do we grow to become the best version of ourselves? These questions have historically been deferred to philosophers and theologians, but the social sciences have recently entered the discourse. What do we mean when we talk about "the mind", or "mental health"? How is it that counseling has become the new norm? When I read the quote above, I think again of mode-shifting and our ability to balance and actively relate with our associative and analytic processing, testing our perceptions both within and without ourselves. Jung taught that we all struggle with life's big questions, and everyone is on their own path to individuation which he said:

> . . . means becoming an "in-dividual", and, in so far as "individuality" embraces our innermost, last, and incomparable uniqueness, it also implies becoming one's own self. We could therefore translate individuation as "coming to selfhood" or "self-realization".
>
> CW 7, p. 238, § 266

The individuation process might also be compared to self-actualization, becoming who we "really are", or as some people say, "walking the path" created for us, or the one we make by walking. However, we are not alone. We are of the world and live in the world.

> Individuation does not shut one out from the world, but gathers the world to oneself.
>
> CW 8, p. 293, § 432

DOI: 10.4324/9781003433736-3

The individuation process may not truly begin until a great conflict is experienced, either within the psyche, or in external life events, in which our egos are forced to give up their illusions of control. We develop and count on our ego-defenses to protect us and make life easier. We'd simply be overwhelmed if we were always aware of everything we could possibly know. But sometimes, we need a wake-up call, so to speak, that it's time to go deeper. It might be when we first realize our childish ways no longer get us what we want; this might happen early on if parenting is not "good enough". It may be a "breakdown" in mid-life that seemingly emerged out of nowhere. More and more, it seems, people are coming to counseling after realizing they've experienced a trauma. Something brings them in. Something rocked their world. And, yes, it hurts.

> There is no birth of consciousness without pain.
>
> CW 17, p. 193, § 331

The individuation process starts a spiritual and psychological rite of passage, leading to confrontation with the Shadow, and ending with a reckoning of duality (integration is arguable among scholars). Along the course of spiritual development, regardless of one's religious affiliation or lack thereof, as one begins to emerge, one is at the highest risk for a variety of psychological disorders; it is unknown if this disturbance is a side effect of the quintessential Dark Night of the Soul (St. John of the Cross, 1908), or if it is because those who are suffering psychologically might seek out spiritual engagement. The good news is that spiritual maturity, or individuation, is a protective factor for our mental health (Choi et al., 2020).

As counselors, we encounter this duality of the "individual", or "personal", and the "collective" within ourselves and with our clients, yet are asked to hold a non-dual stance of suspending judgment and interpretation. Though we are ever more aware that systems impact our clients, we still primarily treat individuals 1:1. How we internalize and balance our desires with the world's expectations, developing patterns of feeling, behaving, and acting, is still quite abstract. Jung gives us a way to concretize these internal structures as part of ourselves and the world.

> The psychological rule says that when an inner situation is not made conscious, it happens outside, as fate. That is to say, when the individual remains undivided and does not become conscious of his inner opposite, the world must perforce act out the conflict and be torn into opposing halves.
>
> CW 9ii, p. 100, § 126

Jung defined the *psyche* (sometimes with a capital P) as "the totality of all psychic processes, conscious as well as unconscious" (CW 6, p. 640, § 797). Psyche attempts to self-regulate and heal, just as our bodies do. Having favorable conditions is ideal, but Jung believed we also have instinctual drives toward getting those needs met, which went far beyond Freud's drive theory (see Chapter 4). Each aspect within the structure of the psyche can be thought both as a part of one person, and an archetype, or a universal idea.

Jung's conceptualization of the psyche makes his theory infinitely richer and deeper than many others. It is also a lens through which we can continue to view new developments, be they personal or collective. Jung's work in this area is some of his earliest, developed around the time of his break with Freud, much of which can be found in Volume 8 of his Collected Works. It is said that Jung's approach to the psyche developed in response to the pervasive ego-centric mindset of the age which he proposed isolates us from the natural world, and therefore our human nature, which he considered to be a major contributor of mental health issues (Samuels et al., 2013). Jung's entire CW 8 is entitled *The Structure and Dynamics of the Psyche*. It is a humbling task to present this brief and vastly incomplete summary. Many of these concepts were initially presented very early in his career, around the time of his break with Freud, but continued to develop throughout his life, and are at times still argued about by Jungians.

There are numerous diagrams of Jung's structure of the psyche, but I have worked with the digital artists at Visionary Design Group (2023) to re-imagine this abstract concept here (see Figure 3.1). It's heavily inspired by Estelle Weinrib's (1983/2004) version (which has been my go-to for years), and the 15th-century image of The Dream of Nebuchadnezzar in Jung's CW 8. Weinrib's version looks to me a bit like a flashlight shining in the darkness: we may not see nor understand the working mechanisms of the flashlight (the unconscious); too close, and we can only see the nose in front of our face, but if we back up, so much more is revealed. In the image of Nebuchadnezzar, a large tree emerges from the sleeping king's body, and it warns that ignoring our history and our dreams, a portal to the Self, can be our downfall. Jung describes Nebuchadnezzar's dreams: first of an angel that instructs that a great fruit tree's branches must be cut off, the roots should be allowed to remain, in order to change the man's heart; in the second dream, the king becomes the tree itself. The Tree is an archetypal symbol, in and of itself (CW 13).

These concepts came together for me when I saw the Tree of Good and Evil Knowledge (Eckhardt, 1785). It was created, in part, to help teach

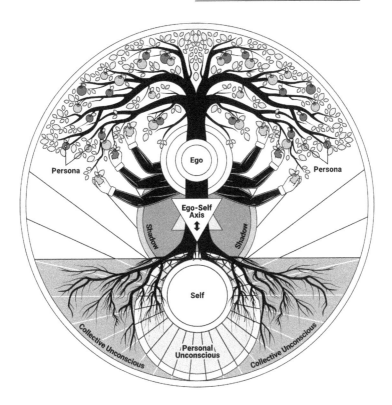

Figure 3.1 The Tree of Psyche. (Reprinted with permission. Further reproduction is prohibited without the author's written authorization. All rights reserved. Copyright © 2023 by author, Rachel McRoberts.)

philosophical and scientific findings to those steeped in the stories, or myths, of the Judeo-Christian tradition; in the book of Genesis, there are two trees in the Garden of Eden: The Tree of the Knowledge of Good and Evil, and the Tree of Life. Jung was fascinated by early scientific pursuits, especially alchemy (early chemistry) and Hermeticism in general, which sought unifying truths about God, humanity, and the natural world. The Tree of Good and Evil Knowledge holds many symbols and metaphors relevant to the structure of the psyche:

The tree is one, but bears two kinds of fruit, and with that, the tension of duality. It is tempting, especially when we feel dis-ease, to attempt to will additional fruit, or franticly try to grasp and own it. What we may not realize is that the fruit buds, blooms, and ripen in its own time. Stealing from a place in our meager will and understanding will not be in alignment with our Self. We may be dis-"armed" if there is a misalignment from the persona to the Self, mediated by the ego-Self axis. Through seeking Wisdom, we have the potential to embody the whole tree. In this way, we both create the fruits and are known by them. The fruit, too, is not truly meant for us, though we could choose to eat it; it holds the seeds of the next generation, and ultimately feeds the earth that holds the tree's roots. Those seeds and their nourishment go underground, sometimes for several seasons. The numinous light perpetuates from the center, and will overcome any darkness if we bring our attention to it. Humanity's task is to come to understand, to remain grounded, and survive the battle.

There is that which is above, and so it is below. That which is conscious or directly interacts with the world is above, and below is the unconscious. It is not as simple as being awake or asleep; the realms are more interactive than that. The tree is firmly rooted in the ground below, but must sprout and grow above to live. It may be difficult to reckon with the unconscious, which we value in Jungian counseling, to be underground, when many religious traditions imagine the divine, or good, above, and the advisory, or evil below. I would ask the reader, though, to remember that we are attempting to illustrate the psychological here, and not the theological. In common American language we often say that things are "rooted" somewhere, and as Jungians, we conceptualize this in the unconscious. We say, too, to "get grounded" in the "reality" of the "here-and-now" which is also frequently symbolized by the earth and actions toward becoming more "in touch" or "earthy". In sandplay therapy, too, which we'll discuss more later, we literally "dig down", "dig up", or "bury" things in the sand, revealing aspects of the unconscious. Also, remember that in counseling we are often presented with client behavior that they are quick to judge as "good" or "evil". While we may or may not be people of faith, we are not there to make that judgment in our counseling role. We seek to be curious about their values and goals, tending to speak more about what might "help or harm", what they "truly" want, to seek and get to know the Self.

Let's go deeper . . .

> No tree, it is said, can grow to heaven unless its roots reach down to hell.
> CW 9ii, p. 69, § 78

PERSONA

> To the degree that the world invites the individual to identify with the mask, he is delivered over to influences from within.
> CW 7, p. 266, § 308

"Persona" and "person" come from the same Latin root word, referring to the masks that the ancient Greeks wore during stage performances to amplify their facial expressions and voices (CW 18); think of the comedy and tragedy masks often used as symbols of the theater. We all have figurative masks we wear, or roles we play in life. Not all of these roles are false, either. They often speak of our identities within our most important relationships, personally and professionally. They may include our intersecting developmental factors, roles, and expression of our various identities, including:

- gender
- age
- familial and social relationships
- religious, spiritual, and cultural practices
- our professional identity
- interests/hobbies.

Our personal expression of these roles is part of our personae, but our perceptions of cultural norms and expectations also influence them. How we act in specific contexts may be very different than others, as is considered appropriate by various sub/culture norms. For example, how we might interact with our pets when they need attention often looks and sounds very different than when we're in a formal work meeting. In this way, personae are considered social archetypes. (Archetypes will be discussed more below as well as in Chapter 5.)

Personae should be flexible, though, not rigid, and be able to be taken off, like masks, or in our fruit metaphor, picked at the right time. We might become stunted or seem one-dimensional if we only serve, or over-identify with, one role all the time, all our lives. We can't just eat one kind of fruit, especially if it doesn't agree with us. We do not want to be "acting" all the time. Jung goes so far as to say that a persona, or mask, "*feigns individuality*, making others and oneself believe that one is individual, whereas one is simply acting a role through which the collective psyche speaks" (CW 7, p. 376, § 245) blocking us from being whole, and *real*. A persona is a type of compromise between us and the world, but is often at least partially unconscious (CW 18). The fruit holds a seed that begins to grow after it falls to the ground.

While we may consciously adapt to a role and do what we must to get by, owning up to being one-dimensional or "phony" can be hard. For example, someone who over-identifies as a businessman might miss out on the fun and relaxing aspects of being a parent. An adult child who never moved out of their parents' house and neglected their dreams to please them may feel unfulfilled and not know why. In this way, personae act as mediators between the outside world and our ego; our psychic branches that reach out to the world and attempt to bring back nourishment, or perhaps nefarious fulfillment, from it. Ideally, though, all of our personae should be able to be well aligned with the ego and the Self, through the *ego-Self axis* (Edinger, 1972). Another way to think about this is that even though our mask is what others in the world may see, it is not our whole Self; it is just a part. If we are always playing one role, we may be impersonating our Self.

During significant transitions, we are often called to adapt or change roles dramatically, including in the therapeutic process. Sometimes we are unmasked, our branches stripped bare. While this stripping can release potential energy that could be channeled into new ways of being, and be more *real*, we must tread lightly. Ego-consciousness may be so intertwined with the persona, we may have difficulty differentiating them from the Self (CW 7). We may have never known any different. For example, a young child who always tried to be The Good Girl in an abusive household may suddenly manifest reactionary "acting out behaviors". Jungians tend to take a different view of "symptoms" in that we value the survival instinct. Our instincts are not just wild, they are also wise. They are part of our ancestral knowledge, the *archetypal self-care system* (Kalsched, 1996). The right brain is especially impacted by trauma, exponentially for children experiencing relational trauma, and therefore may affect the associative mode, and the connection with the unconscious (Schore, 2003; Winnicott, 1971). Instead of trying to deaden instinctive reactions, or "symptoms", we invite a deeper understanding of and compassion for what the Self might be trying to tell us through unconscious manifestations (through play, art making, dreams, or "bizarre" behavior). Is it not adaptive to experience anxiety when one is about to go into an abusive family situation or a soul-sucking job? A contemporary Jungian perspective for mental health includes increasing knowledge, and having compassion for and developing a working relationship with the Self and the archetypal patterns it presents. This is quite akin to Internal Family Systems, but with more complexity and variability. We are not meant to do this alone.

Especially as counselors, we would not want to disarm a client and leave them psychologically bare and vulnerable. Remember, the persona mediates between the us and the world through the ego. We also have no right to pick the fruit from another's tree without permission. Without our personae we may be left confused, wondering who we are, and what we're supposed to do. We commonly call this "flooding" today in trauma work; Jung said it first, though, and suggests that this information may seem to come up suddenly, when in actuality, there have been symbolic signs for some time:

> The moment of irruption can, however, be very sudden, so that consciousness is instantaneously flooded with extremely strange and apparently quite unsuspected contents.
>
> CW 7, p. 241, § 270

This process may be largely unconscious, and is generally thought of as working in service of the ego, though it is painful. It may be part of our work to eventually look back and see if there is increased awareness about a possible catalyst to the disarmament. The ego may be delighted to rule the psyche and resent being dethroned.

THE EGO

> Egoists are called "selfish", but this, naturally, has nothing to do with the concept of "self" as I am using it here.
>
> CW 7, p. 238, § 267

"What an ego!"
"She's so egotistical!"
"He's such an ego maniac!"
"They're all ego!"

The ego gets a really bad wrap. Jung knew this very early on in the budding days of psychology. He admitted that the world of the ego can be "petty, over-sensitive, personal . . . touchy" and can be filled with "personal wishes, fears, hopes, and ambitions which always has to be compensated or corrected by unconscious counter-tendencies" if not kept in check (CW7, § 275, p. 244). Our egos are important, especially for Westerners, in our staunchly individualistic culture, and may need to become inflated sometimes in order to see us through tough times alone.

But the idea of the ego is quite complex. From a Jungian perspective, the ego is the very seat of our consciousness. It encompasses all that we are aware of, including our "somatic and psychic" functioning (CW 9ii, p. 18, § 3), that is, our awareness of what our bodies and minds are doing, how we are feeling, as well as our ability to control those things (though how much we actually control is questionable and a topic of later discussion here). Our ego-functioning allows us to learn about, adapt, and choose to be functioning members of society. It allows us to be aware of conflicts, within us and outside of us, to both tolerate and resolve tension, and to "grow as a person" (Jung calls this process part of the transcendent function, which will be discussed in the next chapter). We need to be "firmly rooted" in this ego-functioning (CW 7, p. 110, § 113), aligned with our sense of Self, in order to be oriented in what most people call "reality", or to feel mentally healthy. From an Eastern perspective, the ego is also an illusion in that it is only our perception of who we are and what is happening around us. What we think we know might not be accurate. Cognitive behaviorists might call misaligned thoughts "cognitive distortions".

However, fellow Westerners, please do not attempt to "kill" your ego, nor anyone else's, as some pop-psychology fake gurus might encourage. Our egos are there to protect us: from the world and the unconscious. We need our egos, or conscious awareness, to focus our attention, to concentrate, to make rational judgments, and generally, be thoughtful (CW 9ii). Killing our egos would mean we would be completely unconscious; this is generally thought of in the field as psychosis. Our unconscious mind, personally and collectively, is the world of myth and dreams, filled with fantastic and imaginal spaces and creatures. Without our egos, we live in a dream world that might not make much sense to us, or anyone else. Paradoxically, though, Jung says (1933), as Landreth (2024) did later, that children naturally begin to develop a sense of identity, or ego-consciousness, through playing out their unconscious life, a language made of symbols, not words.

While our little egos may develop largely without our conscious awareness, as we grow, we can become more aware of it and make more conscious choices. A child who pretends to be a ballerina, even if they have never seen one, or cannot remember seeing one, may pursue the idea in unconscious play, mannerisms, their dress, music, and room color choices, and in more conscious conversations, eventually convincing their parents for lessons, and ultimately become one. However, the little dancer who grows to become tyrannically absorbed by their physical performance, to the detriment of all other aspects of their life, and others', can be said to have an inflated ego.

Ideally, our personas develop in service of the ego. To paraphrase Frank-N-Furter from Rocky Horror Picture Show, it is not good enough to just dream it . . . we gotta be it (O'Brien, 1974). While we might have unconscious urges, or perhaps unrealistic fantasies that well up, our ego-consciousness might choose to take some on, fully or partially. A child who often plays the boss might indeed practice this persona throughout their life, be rewarded, adapt in service of the ego, consciously decide to pursue a career path, and become a successful leader. In addiction recovery, some common phrases are "fake it till you make it", and "act as if"; these can be helpful tools for someone who wants to increase their awareness and the strength of their ego. The message is "I can do this (e.g., call my sponsor instead of use) because I AM this (a person in recovery)". In this case, as counselors or sponsors, we may lend ego strength to others: we may have an awareness of our own empathy, personal experience and knowledge of recovery, and have the confidence to ride the wave with them; that is, our ego is strong enough to take it.

Problems with the ego might emerge in any case. Like with the businessman persona example above, someone might take on too much and say of any characteristic, or symptom, "but this is who I AM", becoming rigid in their ego. Or the ego may "split" and we might find ourselves being "totally different people", feeling like we lead a "double life", or develop a "complex", or symptoms. We may have pushed essential pieces of our ego into Shadow. We can think of this splitting occurring when the flow of the ego-Self axis is off; humanists may call this *incongruence*. While we will discuss the Self more below, simplistically a misaligned ego-Self axis means that how we experience ourselves (our ego) is not congruent with who we feel or sense deep down we are supposed to be . . . who we REALLY are or know we can be. Jung says:

> The ego is, by definition, subordinate to the self and is related to it like a part to the whole.
>
> CW 9ii, p. 20, § 9

It is thought that most people have an innate sense of their Self: their inner voice, moral compose, the feeling when they know something is true even if it is hard to accept. When the ego-Self axis is off it may sound like: "I don't feel like myself", "I don't like/know who I've become", "Something is very wrong but I don't know what it is", "I have no right to be depressed; I'm so successful/loved/etc.". Or it might be posed as a question: "Why am I so anxious?", "What's wrong with me?", "Why now?". Other times, too, it is simply, "Who am I?". On the way to the Self, which we will explore more below, it is thought that we also encounter the anima and animus.

ANIMA/ANIMUS

> We are each "a compound of two mixtures . . . the female and the male".
>
> CW 9ii, p. 83, § 100

Although we might be used to the more open discourse today about distinctions between sex and gender, I urge readers to excuse some of Jung's clunkiness when reading his work on the anima and animus (such as using the term "man" to describe "people" or "humans" . . . which is still commonly heard, especially in science). Please remember that he was revolutionary by presenting these ideas in academia, especially considering psychology was still trying to legitimize itself in medicine. He proposed the idea of *psychifica-tion*, or the intersection of psyche and soma, around 1936 (CW 9ii), though not the word itself; this concept remains a mystery today, but still a topic of scientific inquiry (Fuentes, 2022).

There has been some re-envisioning with revisiting Jung's concepts of the anima and animus over the years, and they continue to evolve with the post-Jungians. While Jung recognized that people are a mixture of mas-culine and feminine characteristics, he initially described these archetypes as the "not-I" or "soul images" of the opposite sex in the psyche (CW 6): the anima as the idealized feminine (traditionally imagined in the man) and the animus as the idealized masculine (traditionally imagined in the woman). He proposed that we fall in love with the person on whom we can project our other side of our psyche, with whom we can then feel more whole; the "mar-riage" occurs not only between people, but within each individual's psyche as well. Jung also proposed that one could become "possessed" by one's anima (if one was a man) or animus (if one was a woman), and take on unconscious emotional characteristics of the opposite sex.

But what if there are more than two genders? What exactly are the distinc-tive characteristics? What is feminine or masculine? What does it mean to be a boy or a girl? A woman or a man? Both? Neither? A mother, father, parent in general, a caregiver, or an adult with no children? Are archetypes gendered? What if or if not? Is sex and/or gender in the body and/or in the mind and/or as a concept in the collective?

You'll forgive me for not putting these archetypes on the Tree of Psyche.

More contemporarily, we might think of the anima and animus as both personal and collective archetypes for what is thought of, perceived, and felt about the feminine and masculine, or even, more broadly, what is "inner" and what is "outer", and how they fit together, like plumbing fixtures (which are often referred to as being male or female). Like all archetypes, these qualities resist literal definitions, but each of us has a felt sense of what this might involve. Contemporary gender theory dis-course presents biological and social distinctions between sex and gender, challenging various aspects of "traditional" gender roles and stereotypes, including archetypal dualism (Nesbitt-Larking, 2022; Peterson, n.d.); however, demonizing any culture's history and values, including around ideas, or ideals, about sex and gender is not exactly culturally aware and may be doing more harm than we realize. We are feeling this tension in personal, political, and social realms. Jung saw it happening in his time, too, though it may have been more covert:

> There are far more people who are afraid of the unconscious than one would expect. They are even afraid of their own shadow. And when it comes to the anima and animus, this fear turns to panic.
>
> CW 9ii, p. 57, § 62

Social media today is full of people talking about the questioning and queering of gender roles, and even developing new archetypes such as The Soyboy and The Trad Wife (short for traditional) as seeming stand-ins for the animus and the anima; I have even actually heard the word "archetype" in some of these conversations (thank you, Mbowe, 2023). Some are excited and feel freed by releasing societal expectations of their gender performance, while others feel safer and more spiritually secure with clearer definitions. This may be considered the anima and animus at work in the collective. Identifying and unpacking individual and collective experiences of sex, gender, and messages about perceived roles may well be part of the personal and professional counseling process, and one we should prepare for and broach. They can impact our self-concept and intimate relationships (Saiz & Grez, 2022). There are real physical and psychological implications for how we assist clients in managing their gender identities that require candid, ongoing interdisciplinary discourse (APA, 2018a, 2018b; Chan Swe et al., 2022; Levine & Abbruzzese, 2023; Pinna et al., 2022; Swe et al., 2022). An open exploration of the anima and animus may assist us on our journey toward the Self.

THE SELF

> The self is not only the centre, but also the whole circumference which embraces both conscious and unconscious; it is the centre of this totality, just as the ego is the centre of consciousness.
>
> CW 12, p. 41, § 44

The Self is a central and yet still disputed concept in the Jungian world, which Jung says "cannot be fully known" (CW 9ii, p. 20, § 9). If the psyche is the entire contents of the conscious and unconscious mind, the Self is that, transcended beyond one to many; from me-ness to we-ness (Watts, 1970). Contemporary Jungians tend to capitalize Self to denote it as an archetypal concept. It is important to note that person-centered approaches also consider "the self" (lower case) to be central to the organizing structure of the personality as well, comprised of the total perceptions of an individual as they interact with their world, in need of unconditional positive regard to obtain a sense of wholeness (Landreth, 2024; Rogers, 1951); they do not tend to talk about the unconscious as much. It is, paradoxically, both a part of and a container for the whole person. Jung said it can't be "localized in an individual ego-consciousness, but acts like a circumambient atmosphere to which no definite limits can be set, either in space or in time" (CW 9ii, p. 208, § 257).

From a Jungian perspective, the Self contains all our concepts of universal truth, everything related to the spiritual as well as our sense of and connections to them (see also the religious function). Jung called the Self, from a psychological perspective, as our concept of the "God-within" (CW 7, p. 325, § 399). This includes our ever-developing, complex, and integrated ideas, images, and practices regarding what is moral, holy, and true (Corbett, 2021; Pew Research Center, 2009). In the West we might call the Self many different things including: our highest potential, the most evolved sense of being, a sense of purpose, our humanity, our moral compass, our heart, or even, in Judeo-Christian or Muslim traditions, the soul. In Indian philosophy, *the atman* is similar to this idea of Self, which is also part of *brahman*, the creative life force for the entire cosmos. From Chinese philosophy, the *tao*, or "the Way", the underlying structure, or flow, that connects everything in the universe, comprised of both yin and yang, and by extension, all of the paradoxes that have been, are, and can ever be, in harmony, understood intuitively, with wisdom.

The Self is non-dual and all inclusive. From research on the Wheel of Wellness (Myers & Sweeney, 2007), we may come to understand the Self to be our indivisible core which also contains the interactive components of our personal and collective being. It acknowledges, holds, values, and plays with the tension of the opposites in the game of life. There is no music without both sound and silence. There is no freedom unless there is more than one choice and the choices are known. The purpose of the dance is the dance itself. Real play is spontaneous, creative, flows freely, and is sacred; this ancient, archetypal concept extends beyond philosophy and religion to developmental theory, to CCPT and sandplay therapy. I love the sound of the Sanskrit word for divine play: "lila". The Self may be conceptualized both as playing the game for us, or the part of us that inherently knows what is and what must be.

How often, though, do we reference the Self without considering all of what it entails? You might reflect on a few of the phrases represented in Figure 3.2.

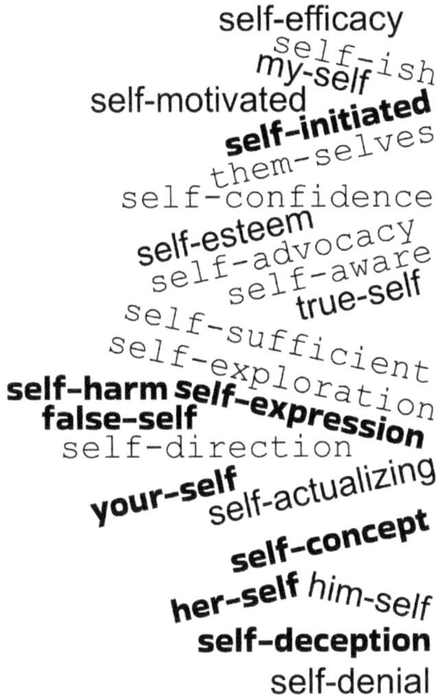

self-efficacy
self-ish
my-self
self-motivated
self-initiated
them-selves
self-confidence
self-esteem
self-advocacy
self-aware
self-true-self
self-sufficient
self-exploration
self-harm self-expression
false-self
self-direction
your-self
self-actualizing
self-concept
her-self him-self
self-deception
self-denial

Figure 3.2 Self-Phrases. (Reprinted with permission. Further reproduction is prohibited without the author's written authorization. All rights reserved. Copyright © 2023 by author, Rachel McRoberts.)

While the ego might crave, strive, and sometimes think it is in control, the Self knows there is no control; there is simply the flow of life. Nonetheless, aligning the ego-Self axis can be seen as the process and ultimate goal of individuation, which can be compared to Maslow's idea of "self-actualization" or finding one's "true self" (Maslow, 1943). An integrative perspective of disruption of the ego-Self axis might suggest that if the ego does not receive enough validation, or positive regard, even through the development of various persona, the ego-Self axis may become misaligned. An individual may feel like they fundamentally do not belong, are "broken", "bad", or even "abandoned by God". The Hindu myth of the Ramayana illustrates this idea of the ego-Self axis: Rama, the personification of the Self, and Sita, the intelligence of the ego, are separated when Sita is kidnapped by Ravana (a demon disguised as brahman); they are reunited through Rama's collaborative efforts, and Sita's practice of yoga and meditation (Newell, 2021).

Jung considered the interactions with the Self to be a psychic phenomenon worthy of an entire volume, which he adamantly states is not a "confession of faith" (CW 9ii, p. 14), but one which, nonetheless, cannot be separated from our propensity to form and hold a God-image (see also the religious function). He acknowledges the psychological implications of various perceived interactions with images and concepts of the divine. The Self is thought to spontaneously manifest images of completion, or the closest thing to perfection we can imagine, as well as the ability to hold the tension of the opposites, and is ultimately responsible for healing (CW 7). This can be true for people even if they are atheists; for them, the Self may be an abstract place deep inside themselves, yet still an idealized part: the part of themselves that knows what is true and real, where paradoxes come together and are held with compassion, understanding, and love.

Jung taught that "Self-alienation in favor of the collective" is a paradox: it is both socially sanctioned and can "also be misused for egotistical purposes" (CW 7, p. 238, § 267). There are many times and situations where we must cater to the World and put ourselves aside. Contemporary Jungians have suggested that we are challenged in the digital age with imagining and aligning a World-Self axis in order to become re-enchanted with the new reality of our home (Main, as cited in Casement, 2018). For all of us, interactions with the Self can be how we come to know ourselves fully, including our "dark side", or Shadow.

THE SHADOW

> The shadow is a moral problem that challenges the whole ego-personality, for no one can become conscious of the shadow without considerable moral effort.
>
> CW 9ii, p. 24, § 14

> . . . the perceived or assumed "negative side of the personality".
>
> CW 9ii, p. 27, § 19

When conceptualizing the idea of the Shadow, I imagine it as everything we feel pressured to cut off from ourselves but cannot . . . not fully. While we may think and speak in dualistic or binary terms (good and bad, etc.) many things are not so easily categorized. Parts of us that we might find to be unacceptable, for whatever reason, may still BE; to deny them may be a form of denial, suppression, or repression. For example, if the ego decides that one persona is "too much" for our idea of ourselves, that persona may be pushed into shadow. We may not become a florist, even though it is a lifelong dream, because it seems frivolous at the time, and we choose something more practical like becoming an accountant. It might serve us well to live that lifestyle for a while and we may not even think of flowers or even see them all around us. One day, though, flowers may show up for us in synchronistic events. People may give them to us. We may notice them growing through the cracks in the sidewalk. This may be an invitation to do Shadow work. Perhaps by exploring the aspect of ourselves that we have neglected, we may find new inspiration.

As we know, defense mechanisms are often automatic, powerful, and tend to work for a while. However, Shadow material, especially if it contains unresolved trauma or unfulfilled dreams, may emerge as its own force. We may discover that we are isolating, judging others harshly, or becoming steadfast in our ideas; this may be projecting our shadow onto others. "The psychological rule says that when an inner situation is not made conscious, it happens outside, as fate" (CW 9i, p. 101, § 126). When clients come in talking about feeling "out of control", "completely crazy", or doing things they cannot even imagine, leaving them full of shame, and "not at all" themselves, the Shadow is said to be at play. They might even recognize a pattern on some level, saying things like, "Why does this keep happening to me?", "I never saw it coming, but here I am again!". Jung reminds us that we all contain light and dark aspects; we are not whole or fully human without our Shadow (Jung, 1933). It cannot be done away with. It must be reckoned with.

The Shadow is both an archetype in and of itself, and an element of every archetype: almost anything can cast a Shadow. Every coin has two sides. Shadow can contain material from both the personal and collective unconscious, yes, but I've chosen to place it here, above, on the other side of the ego. I often hear Shadow talked about with more tangible presence than just what is "below the surface" with the rest of the unconscious. I think of Shadow more like the "dark side" of the ego, like "the dark side of the moon", in that it is right there, part of the whole, it just isn't lit. Or, we cast Shadow when light shines upon our egos, especially if we are quite "opaque" and not being "transparent", or open. Talking about our "evil twin" is common with people who experience being out of emotional alignment, like "Jekyll & Hyde", or the involuntary transformation of the werewolf from civilized person to animal, giving in to primal urges. Because the Shadow contains aspects of our ego that we reject, but is not necessarily "bad", such as in our florist metaphor above, Shadows of Light, or Light Shadow is also a concept I have heard spoken of in Jungian circles. We might be unaware that we have rejected parts of ourselves that others may even be able to see, or sense, as radiant. If we look, we may see glimmers of our path from the ego to the Self, like fairy lights in a darkened forest.

One way of viewing the rapid increase of mental health diagnoses in the digital age is that we are so cut off from our-Selves, and the ability to accept who it is we truly are in all our complexity, that our ego is allowed to drive too much into Shadow. Shadow now rears. Paradoxically, what may initially seem like a brutal attack is a revolt against the divided psyche. We must look at both sides and transcend the tension of the opposites. The storm is necessary to bring the rain that makes the flowers bloom.

THE UNCONSCIOUS: PERSONAL & COLLECTIVE

> Hence, "at the bottom" the psyche is simply "the world".
>
> CW 9i, p. 173, § 291

The unconscious may also be known as the Realm of Dreams, but it is more commonly reduced to our *autonomic nervous system*. Jungians, though, acknowledge and value the language of the unconscious, which is symbolic, and may be accessed through our associative processes. It holds a deeper sense of knowing than we can put into words: one of feeling, perception, reaction, and images. It is in control of all of those things we take for granted when we are busy "thinking", or up-in-our-heads: our breathing, our heart beating, our micro-expressions, our sense of direction, our bias, and other seemingly automatic responses (Bargh & Morsella, 2008). While it may seem that calling the unconscious a "lower level" of functioning is insulting it, Jung and others who appreciate the unconscious prefer to think of it as "deeper" (hence the term "depth psychology", or suggestive induction to "go deeper"). While many of us would like to think we have the power to consciously steer our life on course to the Good Life (hi there, CBT!), there are compelling arguments that it is the unconscious who is the actual captain of the ship (Lahav & Neemeh, 2022; Morsella et al., 2016; Pollard-Wright, 2021).

Jung's idea of the unconscious consists of two layers: the personal unconscious and the collective unconscious. The personal unconscious sits closer to our conscious mind, is based on our personal life experiences, and contains our most private thoughts, and our "feeling-toned complexes" (CW 9i, p. 4, § 4). The personal unconscious can be thought of as the scrapbook, or memory keeper, of our individual life. Neuroscientists are still studying the nuances of memory (Takehara, 2021), such as how experiences become memories, how associations are tied to memory, and why sometimes memories are not formed or may degenerate over time, but any potentiality that the memory exists is thought to be in the personal unconscious. The personal unconscious is like a river of life-giving water flowing downstream into the collective unconscious's depths. The collective unconscious is the infinitely deep ocean of our humanity.

In sandplay therapy, which we will discuss more later (Chapter 7), the bottom of the tray is painted blue to represent this digging down to the waters of the unconscious. The entire language of the unconscious (Chapter 5) is considered a symbolic one, filled with images, which is why we use ready-made images, such as miniature figures in sandplay therapy, and encourage art making for life enhancement and treatment. Since the dawn of humanity, we have evidence that we have attempted to understand and express our world through images. It is our common human language. We are creatures of symbols, of stories, and creation. Jung was very interested in the elements that connect us all at the root; he said we emerge from those roots, can get tangled up in them, and yet are also the roots themselves (Jung, 1932). Jung's ideas about our roots are now validated by affective neuroscience, and the popular *The Body Keeps the Score* (van der Kolk, 2014):

> In our fairytale, the natural evil is banished to the "roots", that is, to the earth, in other words, the body.
>
> CW 13, p. 197, § 245

We simply cannot escape our humanity. This is our neverending universal story.

> The universal similarity of human brains leads to the universal possibility of a uniform mental functioning. This functioning is the collective psyche.
>
> CW 7, p. 204, § 235

The idea of the structure of the psyche can assist us in imagining the layers of the conscious and the unconscious mind, as well as a framework for understanding the functions of the psyche, which we will discuss in Chapter 4. By working toward inviting the unconscious to be more conscious, paradoxically, we are at once becoming more ourselves (individuating), less focused on our uniqueness, or egoism, and more holistically human. Confrontation with the Shadow can be terrifying, so people might not want to engage in the therapeutic or a mindful spiritual practice, but as Socrates is credited as saying, the unexamined life is not worth living. Jung recognized that the process might not be for everyone, and warns us to take it seriously, with a downright religious attitude; when someone is in the belly of the whale, uncovering too much too quickly, or if poorly timed, can at best fall on deaf ears, and at worst cause confusion and overwhelm (CW 7). We will talk more about this process in Chapter 8.

Reflections

1. What are some of the "masks" you wear for the "roles you play" in your life? What are some of their characteristics? Feelings that arise in each role? Which roles do you feel most comfortable with? Are there any that don't feel quite aligned with your ego? Self? Are there any that feel stronger or more dominant in your personality? You might consider creating one or more of these "masks".

2. Thinking about anima and animus, make a quick list of characteristics that either you, personally, or a collective aspect of culture (area of the world you are from, live in, work, etc.) might deem as "feminine" and "masculine". After you make the lists, go back and question which of these characteristics "make" these qualities feminine or masculine? Where might these ideas come from? How pervasive or deep are these perceptions? Is there an overlap? Do you notice any contradictions?

3. What do you think makes us human? Does an image come to mind? What is a symbol or an object that might be understood if you showed it to anyone anywhere in the world?

4. What's one of your favorite stories? What culture is it from? How do you know it? Who have you shared it with and in what way? Is there a theme from the story that you can see paralleled in your life?

REFERENCES

American Psychological Association (APA). (2018a). *APA guidelines for psychological practice with boys and men*. www.apa.org/about/policy/boys-men-practice-guidelines.pdf

American Psychological Association (APA). (2018b). *APA guidelines for psychological practice with girls and women*. www.apa.org/about/policy/psychological-practice-girls-women.pdf

Bargh, J. A., & Morsella, E. (2008). The unconscious mind. *Perspectives on Psychological Science*, 3(1), 73–79. https://doi.org/10.1111/j.1745-6916.2008.00064.x

Casement, A. (Ed.). (2018). *Who owns Jung?* Routledge.

Chan Swe, N., Ahmed, S., Eid, M., Poretsky, L., Gianos, E., & Cusano, N. E. (2022). The effects of gender-affirming hormone therapy on cardiovascular and skeletal health: A literature review. *Metabolism Open, 13*, 100173. https://doi.org/10.1016/j. metop. 2022.100173

Choi, S., Hoi-Yun McClintock, C., Lau, E., & Miller, L. (2020). The dynamic universal profiles of spiritual awareness: A latent profile analysis. *Religions, 11*(6), 288. doi:10.3390/rel11060288.

Corbett, L. (2021). *The God-image: From antiquity to Jung.* Chiron Publications.

Eckhardt, J. D. A. (Ed.). (1785). *Secret symbols of the Rosicrucians of the 16th & 17th centuries: First book.* Published by J. D. A. Eckhardt, Book-Printer to H. M. the King of Denmark.

Edinger, E. F. (1972). *Ego and archetype: Individuation and the religious function of the psyche.* Shambhala Publications.

Fuentes, L. A. (2022). Schreber: An approach to soul androgeny. *Journal of Analytical Psychology, 67*(1), 21–32.Jung, C. G. (1932). *The psychology of kundalini yoga: Notes of the Seminar.* Princeton University Press.

Jung, C. G. (1933). *Modern man in search of a soul.* Edinburgh Press.

Jung, C. G. (2023). *The collected works of C. G. Jung: Revised and expanded complete digital edition.* (CW 1–20). G. Adler, W. McGuire, & H. Read (Eds.), R. F. C. Hull (Trans.). Princeton University Press. https://press.princeton.edu/ books/ebook/9780691255194/the-collected-works-of-c-g-jung

Kalsched, D. E. (1996). *The inner world of trauma: Archetypal defenses of the personal spirit.* Routledge.

Landreth, G. (2024). *Play therapy: The art of the relationship* (3rd ed.). Routledge. (Original work published 1991).

Lahav, N., & Neemeh, Z. A. (2022). A relativistic theory of consciousness. *Frontiers in Psychology: Hypothesis and Theory, 12*(704270), 1–25. doi:10.3389/ fpsyg.2021.704270.

Levine, S. B., & Abbruzzese, E. (2023). Current concerns about gender-affirming therapy in adolescents. *Current Sexual Health Reports, 15*, 113–123. https://doi. org/10.1007/s11930-023-00358-x

Maslow, A. (1943). A theory of human motivation. *Psychological Review, 50*, 370–396.

Mbowe, K. (2023, May 28). *The end of men! Soy Boys, Himbos, and Baby Girls unpacked.* [YouTube video]. https://youtu.be/W9G_f4qVyjs

Morsella, E., Godwin, C., Jantz, T., Krieger, S., & Gazzaley, A. (2016). Homing in on consciousness in the nervous system: An action-based synthesis. *Behavioral and Brain Sciences, 39*, E168. doi:10.1017/S0140525X15000643.

Myers, J. E., & Sweeney, T. J. (2007). *Wellness in counseling: An overview* (ACA-PCD-09). American Counseling Association. www.counseling.org/resources/library/ACA%20Digests/ACAPCD-09.pdf#:~:text=Both%20the%20Wheel%20of%20Wellness%20and%20the%20Indivisible,to%20establish%20a%20baseline%20for%20wellness%20counseling%20interventions

Nesbitt-Larking, P. (2022). Constructing narratives of masculinity: Online followers of Jordan B. Peterson. *Psychology of Men & Masculinities, 23*(3), 309–320. https://doi.org/10.1037/men0000394

Newell, Z. (2021). *Flying monkeys, floating stones: Wisdom tales from the Ramayana for modern yogis.* Himalayan Institute Press.

O'Brien, R. (1974). *Don't Dream It, Be It* [Recorded by T. Curry]. The Rocky Horror Picture Show.

Peterson, J. B. (n.d.). *Comment on the APA guidelines for boys and men.* www.jordanbpeterson.com/political-correctness/comment-on-the-apa-guidelines-for-the-treatment-of-boys-and-men/

Pew Research Center. (2009). *Many Americans mix multiple faiths.* www.pewresearch.org/religion/2009/12/09/many-americans-mix-multiple-faiths/#6

Pinna, F., Paribello, P., Somaini, G., Corona, A., Ventriglio, A., Corrias, C., Frau, I., et al. (2022). Mental health in transgender individuals: A systematic review. *International Review of Psychiatry, 34*(3), 292–359. doi:10.1080/09540261.2022.2093629.

Pollard-Wright, H. (2021). A unifying theory of physics and biological information through consciousness. *Communicative & Integrative Biology, 14*(1), 78–110, doi: 10.1080/19420889.2021.1907910.

Rogers, C. (1951). *Client-centered therapy: Its current practice, implications, and theory.* Houghton Mifflin.

Saiz, M. E., & Grez, C. (2022). Inner-outer couple: Anima and animus revisited. New perspectives for a clinical approach in transition. *Journal of Analytical Psychology, 67*(2), 685–700.

Samuels, A., Shorter, B., & Plaut, F. (2013). *A critical dictionary of Jungian analysis.* Routledge.

Schore, A. N. (2003). Guest editorial. *Journal of Analytic Psychology, 48*(2), 3–7.

St. John of the Cross. (1908). *The dark night of the soul.* www.poetryfoundation.org/poems/157984/the-dark-night-of-the-soul. (Original date of publication unknown, approx. 1577–1579).

Takehara, N. K. (2021). Neurobiology of systems memory consolidation. *European Journal of Neuroscience, 54*(8), 6850–6863. https://doi.org/10.1111/ejn.14694

van der Kolk, B. (2014). *The body keeps the score: Mind, brain and body in the transformation of trauma*. Penguin Books.

Visionary Design Group. (2023). *Welcome to Visionary Design Group*. https://visionarydesigngroup.com/

Watts, A. (1970). *Nature, man and woman*. Vintage Books.

Weinrib, E. (2004). *Images of the self: The sandplay therapy process* (2nd ed.). Temenos Press. (Original work published 1983).

Winnicott, D. W. (1971). *Playing and reality*. Basic Books.

4
The Functions of the Psyche

spirit-land = dreamland (the unconscious)
Jung, CW 8, p. 410, § 599

While Jung may be more famous for his outline of the functions of the conscious mind: thought, feeling, intuition, and sensation (see Chapter 2), this
chapter will focus on ideas about the psyche's total functions along with some
contemporary research on the topics. As we mentioned in Chapter 3, "psyche"
refers to the totality of the mind, both the conscious and the unconscious. As
a self-regulating system, psyche is thought to have inherent goals of integrating
unconscious material through the ego-self axis so that we are both well-adjusted
to our environments and true to ourselves. While we will speak more in-depth
about the language of the unconscious in Chapter 5, here will be a broad overview of how the psyche is thought to function, through the additional counseling lens, with a focus on wellness with a spiritual core (CSI, 2023).

One significant area that Jung disagreed with Freud about was what
drives human behavior at a base level. While both Freud and Jung used
the terms "drive", "instinct", and "psychic energy", at times, seemingly
interchangeably, Jung criticized Freud for distilling this down to libido, or
sexual energy, only. Jung found this both confining philosophically, and
inaccurate phenomenologically. Rather, through his work independent of
Freud, Jung proposed five major groups of instinctual factors that he saw
compelling our psyches (CW 8, pp. 159–163, § 236–246): (1) Hunger,
(2) Sexuality, (3) Drive to Activity (including travel, a "love of change",
the "play-instinct", § 240, and restlessness), (4) Reflective Instincts, and
(5) The Creative Instinct (that while he cannot clearly define it, "is
something that deserves special mention", § 162). Jung observed that the
active experience of life, through a healthy fulfillment of the drives, is
how we reach the highest human achievements: our ability to have faith,
experience hope, love, and gain insight (Jung, 1933).

DOI: 10.4324/9781003433736-4

Building upon this idea in today's digital age, where food is processed, definitions of sexuality are in flux, activity is limited, and often meaningless, and we are inundated with corporate-created images, our drive to activity may be both an explanation for "acting out behaviors" as well as an argument for experiential therapies. Before the Industrial Revolution we used our bodies in much more functional ways: carrying things, walking long distances, farming, and creating and washing nearly all of our household items ourselves. Reflecting on, or thinking about, what we need may be considered the basis of how knowledge came into being, as well as the basis of communication, including language, storytelling, and artmaking.

It is undeniable that humans are creative, and that creativity is intertwined with problem solving and mental health, yet HOW exactly is still unknown (McRoberts & Epstein, 2023). However, I have still had to argue this as a creativity researcher both to academic journal editors as well as those who still doubt the science that creative engagement can impact our mental health. Recently, what I am calling the *creative instinct* has been referred to as *the instinct of imagination* by neuroscientists (Alcaro & Carta, 2019); it is essential not only to creativity but also to imagining, making meaning of reflections, as well as relating to ourselves and others. The counseling field, too, has demonstrated that the creative self is a loaded factor of the Indivisible Self, an evidence-based model of wellness based upon the former, and arguably more aesthetically pleasing, Wheel of Wellness; the creative self consists of five components: thinking, emotions, control, sense of humor, and work (Myers & Sweeney, 2004).

Considering that Jung's instinctual factors may be interconnected, I will discuss them here categorized as "the functions of the psyche": the transcendent function, the symbolic function, the religious function, and the reflective function. I'm using my artistic license here. I hope it brings additional cohesion to Jung's distinctive ideas about drives and instincts. I've added in a few surprises, too, that I've discovered along the way.

THE TRANSCENDENT FUNCTION

> The shuttling to and fro of arguments and affects represents the transcendent function of opposites. The confrontation of the two positions generates a tension charged with energy and creates a living, third thing . . . a movement out of the suspension between opposites, a living birth that leads to a new level of being, a new situation. The transcendent function manifests itself as a quality of conjoined opposites.
>
> CW 8, p. 127, § 189–190

As we mentioned in Chapter 3, the psyche is a self-regulating system on a journey called the individuation process. Ideally, the ego's role is to be the seat of our conscious minds, mediating between the Self and the outside world, to identify, hold, and resolve the tension of the opposites. The transcendent function of the psyche refers to that process in and of itself; it is our innate change mechanism. It is a natural inclination to attempt to resolve conflicts with the least amount of damage, physically and relationally. By having access, respect, and understanding of both our conscious and unconscious processes (including our instincts and drives), which I like to call mode-shifting, we can transcend these conflicts, and grow. This concept helps us explain why we might experience psychological distress in the face of duality, how a psychological shift might happen, and what we're attempting to help our clients do when they come in for help to change their own mind.

Humans naturally divide the world into opposites, or more contemporarily, on the binary: right and wrong, good and bad, light and dark, conscious and unconscious, real and fantasy, male and female, young and old, beautiful and ugly. However, none of us are all good or all bad. Many decisions in life do not necessarily have a definitive right or wrong answer. Thinking in this black and white way, though, paradoxically, often leads to distress. As the Buddha taught, it is a truth that we all experience suffering in this life. Thoughts and feelings may become at odds. We may choose to stay silent to get along. We may silently agree to practices or ideas because they are the norm. We all have to grapple with this tension throughout our lives; sometimes it can become overwhelming. We can get stuck.

We might question why bad things happen to innocent children, why we feel so terrible when everything is going so well for us, or how we can love people who've hurt us. How do we both have a strong sense of faith and respect the faith of others? Why is a particular behavior acceptable when coming from one person but not another? How can we understand and empathize with our client's point of view when we don't see them the way they see themselves? What if what we want does not align with what is expected of us by the world around us? Even though our very minds are divided by the conscious and the unconscious, Jung suggests that we find a sense of resolve through a psychological dialogue that cooperates and transcends the binary.

> This function progressively unites the opposites. Psychotherapy makes use of it to heal neurotic dissociations, but this function had already served as the basis of Hermetic philosophy for seventeen centuries. Besides this, it is a natural and spontaneous phenomenon, part of the process of individuation. Psychology has no proof that this process does not unfold itself at the instigation of God's will.
>
> CW 18, p. 690, § 1554

By understanding the transcendent function as a "thing", an actual aspect of the psyche, we can then imagine entrusting this process to resolve conflicts of duality we experience. It can also assist us with commissioning the process and the relationship in activating the transcendent function as we anticipate and observe the change process. In this way, Jungian theory can deepen our understanding for utilizing many cognitive-behavioral techniques, which also encourage this "to and fro of arguments and affects" such as thought challenging. This concept also explains why it may feel better after having an imaginary argument with someone we're mad at. Or why speaking even a bit of truth in a tense situation can relieve the pressure. It also symbolizes the spiritual concept of transcendence, "with an image of instinctive wholeness and freedom" (CW 8, p. 127, § 190).

However, Jung reminds us that knowledge of ego-functioning can be taken for granted, and is often confused with Self-understanding (CW 10). We must remember that the transcendent function is activated, and the real change happens, when we have profound experience with our unconscious.

THE SYMBOLIC FUNCTION

While many Jungians today talk about "the symbolic function", in doing research for this book I could not find a place where he, himself, actually used the phrase "the symbolic function". I only saw one place (a benefit of having the CW as one large ebook!) where he referred to *a symbolic function*. He was discussing the process of detaching ones' energy from

> . . . a real object, its concentration on the symbol and canalization into a **symbolic function** . . . symbol formation, therefore, must obviously be an extremely important biological function . . .
> CW 6, p. 343, § 402 (bolding mine)

Dominique Boukhabza, author of the new book A *Jungian Understanding of the Symbolic Function & Forms* (2023), confirmed it for me: THE symbolic function is not Jung's term, exactly, but it is a JUNGIAN term in that he developed the idea throughout his works, and his legacy continues. Jung also specifically named a **symbol-producing function** (CW 18, p. 223, § 223). Marie von Franz, student of Jung and contributor (after his death) to his only work written for the general public, *Man and His Symbols* (1964), noted:

> C. G. Jung and some of his associates have tried to make clear the role played by the **symbol-creating function** in [our] unconscious psyche

and to point out some fields of application in this newly discovered area of life.

(p. 304 in original; p. 375 in ebook; bolding mine)

Piaget, a pioneering developmental child psychologist, begins to use the phrase *the symbolic function* in one of his early works (1951), referring to the work of French linguist, Gustave Guillaume (1883–1960), and also credits Jung, but because of semantics continues on by referring to the *semiotic function* (2000). This is worth mentioning because he and Jung also distinguish between "symbol" and "sign". Signs relate and refer directly and literally to a signifier and their conscious connection (such as road signs); symbols, on the other hand, are more sacred, expressive, and even figurative (such as a metaphor), and may have latent, or unconscious meanings, personally or collectively, as well as conscious meanings. From a Jungian perspective, as in many organized religions, a symbol may be considered a powerful representation of, and a conduit for connection with the numinous, which also acts as a kind of bridge between us and all that is.

While child psychology was still in its infancy, Piaget suggested that the boundary between the conscious and the unconscious in a child's psyche is even thinner than an adult's, and acknowledged parallels between symbolic play and dreams. Piaget credits Jung at this time, arguing for a case to seek more expansive, less reductionistic meaning of symbols than others in the psychoanalytic school, and inviting a deeper dive into the study of symbols in children's play. While Jung never treated children himself, he did analyze several childhood dreams of adults (Jung, 2008) and inspired the development of sandplay therapy (Kalff, 2020) within his lifetime. Piaget (1951) also acknowledges Jung's innovative conceptualizations of the symbolic function and its importance to the unconscious both personally and collectively, as the language of the Self. So Jung (1973) was validated fairly early on that the unconscious was not just a garbage can.

The symbolic function, as it is broadly understood today, is not only a developmental stage or occurrence, emerging around the second year of life, but an ongoing neuro-cognitive ability to mentally represent objects that are not necessarily in sight; it's involved in the processes of attachment, language, creativity, empathy, and many levels of understanding (APA, 2020; Benedek et al., 2014). It is both a process of discerning "what does this mean?" from any given situation, internally or externally, and the ability to express this meaning. While it is recognized that the symbolic function is essential to the individual and collective development of humanity, there remain controversial discussions, including its ability to be harnessed and measured, whether there are inherent meanings to symbols, and how, exactly, meaning is transferred between people (Iurato, 2016; Quinn et al., 2018; Roesler, 2022; Schmemann, 1973; Veraksa & Veraksa, 2016).

The symbolic function is paradoxically a precursor to language, a language all its own, and a disguise of language. For example, babies often point and gesture to objects they have learned to recognize as pleasurable, both when they want them, and when others say, "Where's. . . the ball? . . . Daddy? . . . your hat?" well before they can talk. "Daddy" may have a general universal meaning but it's also very specific when talking about a particular person whom the baby calls "Daddy". Children might be confused when they realize that other children call their fathers "Daddy" and insist theirs in the REAL Daddy. Even more seemingly banal symbols like "hat" can refer to anything one might wear on the head, but even if someone has several hats, "my hat" may refer to a specific, often favorite one, only known to those most intimate. Jung went so far as to say that

> . . . every psychological expression is a symbol if we assume that it states or signifies something more and other than itself which eludes our present knowledge.
>
> CW 6, p. 655, § 817

While we will discuss symbols more fully in Chapter 5, as an aspect of the language of the unconscious, it should be noted here that both Jung and Piaget agreed on another thing: that an image is a symbol (CW 8; Piaget, 1951). As we have previously discussed, Jung anticipated that we would see an increase of mental health issues as the Industrial Revolution progressed. Not only did people move off of farms and into the city, where their drives for activity were stifled, but with it went aspects of the symbolic life:

> You see, [we are] in need of a symbolic life – badly in need. We only live banal, ordinary, rational, or irrational things – which are naturally also within the scope of rationalism, otherwise you could not call them irrational. But we have no symbolic life. Where do we live symbolically? Nowhere, except where we participate in the ritual of life. But who, among the many, are really participating in the ritual of life? Very few.
>
> CW 18, p. 690, § 625

I wish that Jung was here to see us now. In the digital age, when we are inundated with both banal images and powerful symbols of consumption, and we have multiple social media platforms to create and cultivate our own realities in echo chambers of our own making, how is it that we're worse off than ever before? Some say that we have gone too far in creating our virtual realities . . . to the point of delusion. Perhaps there is a key in that word "participation". Researchers have noted a difference between *passive* and *active* consumption of media effects on mental health and creativity, which is also different among age groups (Lewin et al., 2023; Upshaw et al., 2022). Investigation also needs to continue to discover more precisely how interpersonal interactions form our sense of self, generally our egos, and reality.

A symbolic life today is not always one generated from a well-aligned ego-Self axis. Jung said our *symbol-producing function* may become "twisted and prejudiced" by various factors that stimulate us into repression (CW 18, p. 223, § 512). Being inundated with images, like too much symbolic noise, may overtax our psyche. Many people are unaware of, or unwilling to acknowledge, the power of observing countless images online every day, though there has been discussion for decades about media's representation of bodies, especially, and various psychological impacts. Images carry symbolic messages and are used skillfully and covertly by marketers and content creators. As consumers of digital media, we become the product. Authentic, powerful symbols may arise from the unconscious and overwhelm the unprepared and unexamined ego in response, to get a reaction (see Chapters 3 and 5). Perhaps, too, we need to go a step further, to investigate the "ritual of life" through the religious function.

THE RELIGIOUS FUNCTION

> Since religion is incontestably one of the earliest and most universal expressions of the human mind, it is obvious that any psychology which touches upon the psychological structure of human personality cannot avoid taking note of the fact that religion is not only a sociological and historical phenomenon, but also something of considerable personal concern to a great number of individuals.
>
> CW 11, p. 4, § 1

While today, religious and spiritually integrated practices are considered a multicultural and social justice competency in counseling (ASERVIC, 2023b; Ratts et al., 2016), Jung (CW 11) was one of the first psychologists to acknowledge the individual and collective importance of religious and ritualistic practices. Jung went so far as to say there is an "existence of an authentic religious function in the unconscious" (CW 11, p. 1, § 3) which assists with organizing and making meaning of our lives. The religious function also involves the symbolic function and can assist in activating the transcendent function through "numinous", or spiritually charged, awe-inspiring experience. As a play on the common phrase "spiritual but not religious", the method of pursuing "the symbolic life" (the title of CW 18) on the active path of individuation has been called "religious but not religious" (Smith, 2020). Jungian analysts Edinger (1972) and Corbett (1996) have written extensively about the religious function, which, in light of new research, may be illuminating for counselors more deeply considering cross-cultural implications.

Because of the very philosophy of the psyche in this theoretical orientation, Jungian-oriented counseling may be viewed more as an approach to the numinous than a treatment of psychopathology (von Franz, 1990). Jung reminds us that "psyche", the root word of "psychology", refers not only to the mind, but also the breath, creative lifeforce, or soul, from the Greek "pneuma" (Jung, 1933); similarly, the word "spirituality" comes from "spiritus", Latin for breath, spirit, or soul (ASERVIC, 2023b), which can refer both to an "animating principal" and a "form of entity"; in fact, many cultures' words for the unifying principles of the Self also refer to breathing or wind: *roho* (Swahili), *atman* (Sanscrit), *ruah* (Hebrew), and *ruh* (Arabic) (Main, 2007). In Greek mythology, Psyche was first human and later, through many trials and a descent to the underworld, earned the role of Goddess of the Soul and companion to Eros, the God of Love (Eros: the root of the word "erotic"). This story itself can be seen as a metaphor for the transformation that may occur throughout the individuation process in general, as well as in successful counseling, where one can access and harness creative energy for greater fulfillment in life.

We can also credit Jung and the Jungians for integrating and perpetuating the use of language once only used in religious circles to describe personal disturbances. For instance, the word *demonic*, often carrying connotations of evil and the Christian Devil, shares roots with *daiomai*, which means "to divide", and *daimon*, meaning "spirit" (Diamond, 2014); from a Jungian perspective, if we remember this language, and practice recognizing its symbolic function, we may learn to hold traditional views of "possession", or being "tormented by demons", with the ancient ethical pursuit of *eudaimonia*, which may not be so unlike Jung's idea of *individuation*. Any division in the psyche is considered the root of emotional and psychological disturbance, especially dissociation and psychosis, often correlated with trauma (Kalsched, 1996). The divide may occur in various areas of the psyche, including between personae, a glitch in the ego-Self axis, or between the conscious and the unconscious.

To Jung, observing and publicly acknowledging the religious function and the role of the numinous was of great historical and psychological significance. While Jung feared that psychology would attempt to replace religion, he maintained that he was not attempting to create a religion of his own, as critics have suggested (CW 12; CW 14; Corbett, 1996). However, he did draw parallels to aspects of the religious and the transcendent function that may be activated through psychotherapy. He also humbly noted that there are still many mysteries in life, including what ultimately causes people to grow and heal, which may also be considered divine (CW18). Researchers across scientific disciplines continue to seek answers to these existential questions (Moritz, 2023).

Jung defined religion as the "careful and scrupulous observation of what Rudolf Otto aptly termed the *numinosum* (CW11, p. V, § 6). The Association for Spiritual, Ethical, and Religious Values in Counseling (ASERVIC, 2023a) quotes Corbett's (1990) definition of religion as "an integrated system of belief, lifestyle, ritual activities, and institutions by which individuals give meaning to (or find meaning in their lives by orienting them to what is taken to be sacred, holy, or the highest value" (p. 2). Ancient roots for the word "religion" reference attitudes and practices of respect, consideration, connection, reflection, and revisiting, across time and cultural traditions (CW5; Online Etymology Dictionary, 2023b). Jung observed that it is about having a well-connected "religious attitude", or way of life, and not just a specific formal religion, or religious belief system, that enhances a sense of meaning and satisfaction in life. From a Jungian perspective, "religion is not a reified set of ideas and propositions; religion means attention to the manifestations of the psyche, to its images and affects" (Corbett, 1996, p. 3).

We commonly speak of doing many things "religiously": from attending church on Sunday to brushing our teeth daily. Some rituals may have more overt meaning than others, of course, but they often still serve essential needs, be they physical, social, or emotional. Attachment theory has demonstrated that the religious function also serves practical purposes, namely creating predictable, safe environments we can trust. One of the "building blocks" of attachment is "routines and rituals", as outlined by the evidence-based practice called Attachment Regulation & Competency Framework (ARC; Blaustein & Kinniburgh, 2019). Many parents know this intuitively and attempt to acclimatize their babies to regular feeding, sleeping, and socializing schedules. Many symbols and rituals also accompany those practices, such as bedtime routines with a relaxing bath, a favorite storybook, and tucking in lovies. These practices may also live in the psyche as a symbol for a lifetime, accessed even in adulthood to manage stress. In today's digital age, natural sleep-wake, seasonal, and other patterns dictated by the sun and weather are often treated as nearly obsolete. Parents may work odd hours and children are left to their own devices – literally – which, with their artificial light may interfere with natural cycles, and in turn, mental health (Paksarian et al., 2020). Nevertheless, the religious attitude, or sacred reverence for, and commitment to, the practices and processes that are important to us, is also required. While it is easy to see that attachment is not just about going through the motions of daily routines and rituals, it can be harder to remember in other aspects of life.

Jung was influenced by the work of Rudoff Otto (1923), a theologian and religious scientist, who described the term *numinous*. The root word, *numen*, refers to the powerful feeling or divine presence overseeing a place or experience, by a nodding of the head from *nuere*, "to nod" (Online Etymology Dictionary, 2023a). This nod, an affirming feeling of "yes" can also describe this internalized sense of knowing when something is right or true; we might call this an "Aha! moment", when something finally "sinks in", or we "get it". Three components of a numinous experience include something mysterious or weird (Otto, 1923), a sense of something bigger than oneself, and fascination. This later aspect of fascination may include that sense that a burden has been lifted, new insights are gained, or that one is saved (Lönneker & Maercker, 2021). Numinous experiences may occur at any time or any place. Religious practices may aim to tap into the numinosum to assist with spiritual growth. Another term in the literature akin to *numinous* is *awe*. While the study of awe is still in its infancy, it's suggested that those who experience awe may have a higher capacity to appreciate life's beauty and respond to challenging situations with kindness toward themselves and others (Allen, 2018).

Jung observed, even in his time, that an increased focus on the individual, scientific understanding for religious questions, and progress in the industrial age in turn led to a disinterest and dismissal of past traditions, including important and organizing rituals (Jung, 1933, p. 228). He lamented over the ancient, cross-cultural practice of setting up sacred spaces in the home being moved to churches and then to museums; even in his time he saw the telephone as an interruption to home-based rituals. Many religions warn that a centralization of the ego causes suffering, and that excessive wanting, striving, and desiring disconnects us from "what is" (the tao) or "God". What would he think of us today with our Orwellian "telescreens", especially in the hands of young children? (See Orwell, 2021 for more on this dystopian premonition). With these shifts have come increased stress, emotional disturbance, substance abuse, and feelings of isolation, especially after the COVID-19 pandemic, and especially for our youth, even though we are more digitally connected on a global scale than ever before (Jeffers et al., 2022; Qin et al., 2020; Taylor et al., 2020; Zhao et al., 2023).

In the digital age, too, has come a decrease in formal religious identity, but greater integration of multiple religious beliefs and practices (Pew Research Center, 2009). Most Americans still report believing in God or a higher power, but what that means to each individual may vary considerably; this subjective combination of personal belief and collective theological tradition is what Jungians refer to as *the God-image* (Corbett, 2021). Since the 1990s, American religious demographics have changed dramatically. The number of those identifying as Christian dropped from about 90% to 67%, not because they switched to another religion, but because they don't identify with any one religion; all other religions combined have held steady around 10% (Pew Research Center, 2019, 2022). The research calls this growing population "nones", because when asked about their religious affiliation, they check the box labeled "none". Implications for our society and our counseling practices are immense, and the literature is paradoxical. There is evidence that those who are actively religious tend to be happier (Portnoff et al., 2017; Saad & Hrynowski, 2022), but the levels of reported religious and spiritual trauma are staggering, ranging from nearly half to nearly all study participants, with higher rates found in more marginalized populations (Ellis et al., 2022). This is a spiritual pandemic. Counselors are being called to action (Walsh & Koch, 2023).

With the digital age and the pop-culture phenomenon that is fourth-wave feminism has come an increasing rejection of a historically masculinized God-image, which we haven't seemed to have fully reckoned with. Though we may have attempted to abandon the old gods in favor of new ones, like Media (Fuller et al., 2017–2021; Gaimen, 2001), the sometimes so-called "bad religion" of identity politics (Luminate Media Inc., 2023), or secularism, in its various forms (Berlinerblau, 2021; Schmemann, 1973), a craving for a relationship to the Self and the collective remains. While the idea of the religious function may be unfamiliar to the masses, spirituality is inarguably internationally recognized as a fundamental aspect of our humanity (Puchalski et al., 2014). Even the notoriously outspoken atheist, post-modern critic, and evolutionary biologist, Richard Dawkins, who wrote the New York Times Bestseller, *The God Delusion* (2008), has admitted that there seems to be a common, psychologically rooted, human proclivity toward religion which has yet to be fully identified and explored (Dawkins, 2023; see the 34:39 timestamp for details). In Jungian terms, we call that part of us *the religious function*, and I would like to see that term catch on. Perhaps ironically, Dawkins is also the "father of memes" (Sisyphus 55, 2022), coining the term for how many symbols enter into the collective via the internet. Memes are popular visual representations of common human experiences, or as Jung called them, archetypes. It is still common speech, as it was in Jung's time (CW 9ii), to refer to our psychological problems as our "demons".

After studying 5,000 people from around the world with seven different religious affiliations, researchers have found five cross-cultural dimensions of spiritual capacity (Choi et al., 2020):

1. spiritual reflection and commitment
2. contemplative practice
3. perception of interconnectedness
4. perception of love
5. practice of altruism.

They also identify five levels of spiritual development:

1. non-seeking
2. socially disconnected
3. spiritual emergence
4. virtuous humanist
5. spiritually integrated.

Those who are spiritually integrated, or who have reached *spiritual maturity* (University of the South, 2022), are most protected from mental health issues; those at mid-level, or who are still spiritually emerging, are at the highest risk (Choi et al., 2020). While we do not know exactly what causes this, we speculate that it's because they're in the thick of it. They might be struggling emotionally because they are maturing spiritually (like the saints tormented?), or struggling spiritually because of psychological challenges (a result of modernity or changing relationship with the Divine?). Either way, it's happening. For those who have difficulty bracketing their belief system to work with someone else's, perhaps Jung's psychological explanation of the religious function can be a bridge. And for those who fear betraying their faith, or being accused of being a pantheist, perhaps this science of, shall we say, spiritual common factors can be comforting. Spirituality has always been entwined with our existence. However, while religious and spiritual integrated practices are considered a counseling competency, research on that aspect of our professional identity is lacking (Cashwell &

Young, 2020). We must find a way to make it fit, personally and professionally, in the digital age.

A Jungian idea of having respect and reverence for the religious function of the psyche leaves room for all definitions and practices (CW 18), and parallels common understandings of even the most secular definitions of "spirituality" as a search for connection or meaning (ASERVIC, 2023b; de Brinto Sena et al., 2021). Jung recognized that those who may not overly identify with a particular religion may engage in practices, sometimes unconsciously, in service of attempting to engage the numinous. In CW 11 (§ 7) he names the ancient ritualistic practices of meditation and yoga, specifically, and looks at how popular these two practices have become in mental health today (Bhargav et al., 2023; Kamraju, 2023; Reangsing et al., 2022). We might also consider the possibility that people are seeking out mental health services in droves due in part to the religious function motivating us to fill the "God-shaped hole" in search of meaning, guidance, and ritualized practices on our path to individuation, that for whatever reason people do not feel comfortable seeking within organized religion (Corbett, 1996; Hagedorn & Moorhead, 2010; Johnson, 1991). Maybe parts of us remember the old ways of believing that wisdom may come to us through visions and dreams, or if we trust and still our hearts. It is also important to remember that traumatic incidences of many kinds, including religious and spiritual abuse, domestic violence, child abuse, shaming, isolation, and grief, may impact the religious function, leaving people disillusioned with their traditions, communities, concepts of and relationships with the divine and their sense of Self (Ellis et al., 2022). For this reason, it is important to modify our language when speaking of these concepts to better align with our clients'. In fact, Jung tells us that we can use the word "numinous" when words like "spiritual" or "magical" seem inappropriate (CW 8, p. 267, § 405).

Because Jung believed that it was a religious attitude, or reverence for the numinosity of transformative human experience, that was important for human growth in general, it is also considered an important part of Jungian counselor development to engage in reflective practices on the subject. At a basic level, the idea of *spirit* speaks of both our subjective realities and our innate nature (Main, 2007). While arguably culturally sanctioned, theology has a reputation of bias toward a particular religious study and practice (Collins, 2019). Taking a non-dual, psychological approach to the numinous (see also, mode-shifting) allows us to see and shift between perspectives. As we know from contemporary multicultural, intercultural, and religious and spiritually integrated training models, developing curiosity and cultural humility can be supported through reflection of self and other (Ellis et al., 2022; Kuo, 2020; Pearce et al., 2020).

THE REFLECTIVE FUNCTION

> If we do not fashion for ourselves a picture of the world, we do not see ourselves either, who are the faithful reflections of that world. Only when mirrored in our picture of the world can we see ourselves in the round. Only in our creative acts do we step forth into the light and see ourselves whole and complete.
>
> CW 8, p. 491, § 737

As with the symbolic function, the term *reflective function* has developed out of Jung's work, becoming popular in Jungian circles in the 1990s (Knox, 2004) and hitting the mainstream soon after, especially regarding attachment theory. Jung DID, though, speak much of reflection in general and the *reflective instinct*. The reflective function refers to *mentalization*, the inter- and intra-psychic process of recognizing and imagining emotional states, organizing information, making cohesive meaning of those perceptions, and acting out of value-based judgments. This includes identifying and acting out of feelings, goals, and social norms informed by our awareness of ourselves and others. Through the reflective function we differentiate self and other, see things from various points of view, attempt to resolve conflicts, and engage in the process of discernment (Benbassat, 2020; Fonagy et al., 2016; Knox, 2004). Reflection-IN-action and reflection-OF-action have been considered factors in learning theory for some time now (Schön, 1983). These "spirals of reflection" are how we build, look back upon, and find meaning in learning (Canning & Callan, 2010). However, how exactly these reflective practices are activated and how and to what extent they can be influenced still remain somewhat mysterious.

From a Jungian framework, the reflective function is thought to be an outcome of the transcendent function and interconnected with the symbolic function. When we speak of the "spirit of an age", or the "soul of our practice", we are speaking of the reflective function at work. From a psychological perspective, a Jungian definition of the soul may include our unique capacity to reflect upon the symbolic nature of our existence (Hillman, 1975; CW8). We are able to look back, analyze patterns, and make assessments. I often think about how Jung (CW 12) says we develop as a spiral, radiating out from the center like a mandala; reflection often takes a look across the spiral, and we see ourselves across various points in time, sometimes revisiting old places with new awareness. It may seem we are "right back there again" or that we "have to start over", but it is never exactly the same. Every time we revisit a memory, it is slightly different. Like a labyrinth, too, we may circum-ambulate, or wander around a central idea, until, after reflection, we find our course, and eventually how the pieces fit together into our life (Jung, 1989).

Jung knew that his idea of the reflective instinct may be challenging for those who consider reflection only a cognitive process. He refers to the root of the word reflection as "reflexio" meaning "bending back" (CW 8), referring to how a stimulus becomes for us an experience with meaningful content or, more simply, cohesive thought. I think of how back bending takes flexibility, and can be energizing. This ability to flex speaks of both our attunement with others and personal resilience. "Re-" anything is dif-ficult to define independently because it implies that we are re-fering to or re-vising something. It is through re-flecting, and thereby re-member-ing (re-attaching something dis-membered, lost, or forgotten), re-organ-izing, and re-sponding, that we assimilate information and perhaps even transcend or transform it. We put the pieces together. Reflecting can be like a magic mirror: we can see not only what is, but what was, and what might be. Through observing thought and relationship patterning and our surrounding symbolic language, we develop our wise mind. With greater knowledge of where we have been, how we got there, and back here, we can better imagine ourselves in future scenarios. Our dreams may become clearer, literally and figuratively. Visualizing ourselves in desired situations can assist us in mobilizing movement toward them.

The reflective function is considered a developmental process, like indi-viduation, that, ideally, is activated and nurtured in childhood (Ferreira et al., 2017; Knox, 2004). It is well known that early childhood relation-ships are vital. Mirroring, or reflecting games, are some of the first games experienced by babies and their parents or caregivers. A lack of delight or attuned responsiveness is quickly distressing for babies even in healthy relationships; the longer this dynamic continues, the more damage can be done (Children's Institute, 2017). In the digital age, with so many people's faces in their phones, we lose this literal and precious face-to-face time. We internalize to a large degree the wants, needs, and beliefs of others especially, as well as who we are to them and the messages they send about us. Integrating these stories cohesively into our psyches is key, especially for healthy ego-functioning (Peresso, 2019). Without the ability to think about, and eventually know who we really are, acting from an aligned ego-Self access, we are lost.

If we are not actively engaged in reflection Jung said we will likely be inundated with and bound by unconscious projections by others and ourselves; we are like a boat without a rudder on the sea of the unconscious (CW 8). Having a reflective attitude assists with developing a solid sense of identity, competency, and satisfaction, personally and professionally (Ferreira et al., 2017; Wampold & Imel, 2015). Encouraging reflection, and engaging the reflective function, can be considered at the very heart of both the individuation and the therapeutic process. Through reflecting on past and present experiences, and imagining future ones, through talking and creating, we are invited to observe and be observed, modeling the creation of silent, sacred space to go within, interpret and hear other's interpretations, and transcend areas of inhibition. The reflective function is involved in asking questions about what is working, or not, and why.

Jung observed that a lack of reflectiveness was part of the cause of both psychological disturbance and resistance to treatment (CW 9), areas of ongoing study (Horváth et al., 2023; Johnson et al., 2022). Those whose reflective function is underdeveloped may have difficulty finding meaning in life, be dismissive of symbolic content, experience dependency, lack confidence in themselves or others, or find it difficult to see others' points of view. The reflective function has recently been found to mediate the link between childhood abuse and identity diffusion; identity diffusion refers to a lack of capacity to organize and commit to self-development, including goals, relationships, and even the development of personal values (Penner et al., 2019).

Jung was very forthcoming about his reflective practices and advocated that his students and clients do the same; it is said that he did not ask anything of others that he didn't ask himself (Hannah, 1976). His remarkably candid works include *Memories, Dreams, Reflections* (1989), and the *Red Book* (2009). His active engagement with his reflective function analyzing dreams and experiences inspired drawings, paintings, lectures, books, and changed countless people's lives. Jung continues to be a model for how the counselor's work is never done, because it is a part of who we are, and how we view ourselves and the world. There is always more to explore. In sandplay therapy we often talk about the importance of creating and maintaining a generously attuned sacred space that is both personal and professional. That space begins inside of us, and is a reflection of us.

For counselors, specifically, reflection is also both a primary response skill and a practice of awareness and engagement (Jacobs, 2017; Lambie et al., 2017; Parsons & Zhang, 2014). *Reflective responses* refer to how we mirror back what we perceive and understand. As skills, these include *reflection of feeling, reflection of meaning, paraphrasing,* and *summarizing*. The bulk of our responses as counselors should be reflective, as indicated on the CCS-R, or the Counseling Competencies Scale (Lambie et al., 2017). *Reflective practice* refers to a routine of internal exploration of thoughts, feelings, and behaviors regarding specific events, which may lead to continued self-reflection, increased self-awareness, and self-efficacy, promoting new, more insightful behaviors in the future. Reflective practice is necessary for therapists' professional development, as it encourages critical incident review, personal and professional development, and preparation for future client interactions (Rønnestad & Skovholt, 2003). Though reflective practices are advocated for in the literature in service of personal and professional growth, as well as in preventing and managing impairment in therapists, there is a need for additional research (DeCino et al., 2020). Reflective practices may include a variety of activities such as attending our own counseling, clinical supervision, and engaging in self-care and personal growth, but may also refer to our level of self-awareness and openness to sharing and deriving meaning found within these experiences.

Some in the field have argued that because the reflective function is integrated so deeply into our dispositions, it cannot be taught, nor rebuilt, but nurtured. Creative processes, including play and experiential learning, have been shown to promote reflective practices and increase self-awareness (Bar-On, 2007; Bell et al., 2014; Luke & Kiweewa, 2010; Markos et al., 2008). Self-awareness is thought to be supported by reflective practices; however, there are still challenges, including stigma, surrounding the requirement of them for counselors-in-training (CACREP, 2024; Kalff, 2020; Lees, 2016; Malikiosi-Loizos, 2013).

At the most basic level, it is the reflective function allows us to think. More deeply, it assists us with formulating a story of our lives, where we are both a co-author and a main character. Existentially, it assists us with integration, finding meaning, and a sense of hope. Practically, it is an active, creative process involving the integration of our personal and collective history. In order to exude and inspire creativity, we must embrace the aesthetics of existence and become a living work of art (Foucault, 1984). That requires us to be open to, and eventually fluent in, the language of the unconscious.

Reflections

1. Name one or a few of the important symbols to you in your life. Is there one that has been with you for some time? List all of your associations with that symbol, beginning with free association: just write down anything that comes up . . . no judgment or editing at this point (just associative processes . . . no analysis).
2. When you have given this some time, look up your symbol in a symbol dictionary or on the internet. Search for a fable, fairy tale, or myth with that symbol. Perhaps you remember hearing one as a child. Where are those stories from? What are some other aspects of your symbol that you may have yet to consider? Do any of them seem to fit?
3. What are some of the rituals, beliefs, or traditions that are important to you and/or your community? Describe some of the details involved. Do some research: how far back in history do they go? What connections might they have with another culture?
4. Have you ever had a *numinous* experience? What was it like? How did you feel? How do you explain it? You are invited to share it with someone you trust.

REFERENCES

Alcaro, A., & Carta, S. (2019). The "instinct" of imagination: A neuro-ethological approach to the evolution of the reflective mind and its application to psychotherapy. *Frontiers in Human Neuroscience, 12*, 522. https://doi.org/10.3389/fnhum.2018.00522

Allen, S. (2018). *The science of awe: A white paper prepared for the John Templeton Foundation by the Greater Good Science Center at UC Berkeley.* https://ggsc.berkeley.edu/images/uploads/GGSC-JTF_White_Paper-Awe_FINAL.pdf

American Psychological Association. (2020). *Symbolic function.* https://dictionary.apa.org/symbolic-function

Association for Spiritual, Ethical, and Religious Values in Counseling (ASERVIC). (2023a). ASERVIC white paper. https://aservic.org/aservic-white-paper/

Association for Spiritual, Ethical and Religious Values in Counseling (ASERVIC). (2023b). *Spiritual and religious competencies.* https://aservic.org/spiritual-and-religious-competencies/

Bar-On, T. (2007). A meeting with clay: Individual narratives, self-reflection, and action. *Psychology of Aesthetics, Creativity, and the Arts, 1*(4), 225–236. https://doi.org/10.1037/1931-3896.1.4.225

Bell, H., Limberg, D., Jacobson, L., & Super, J. T. (2014). Enhancing self-awareness through creative experiential-learning play-based activities. *Journal of Creativity in Mental Health, 9*(3), 399–414. https://doi.org/10.1080/15401383.2014.897926

Benbassat, N. (2020). Reflective function: A move to the level of concern. *Theory & Psychology, 30*(5), 657–673. https://doi.org/10.1177/0959354320934182

Benedek, M., Beaty, R., Jauk, E., Koschutnig, K., Fink, A., Silvia, P. J., & Neubauer, A. C. (2014). Creating metaphors: The neural basis of figurative language production. *NeuroImage, 90*, 99–106. http://dx.doi.org/10.1016/j.neuroimage.2013.12.046

Berlinerblau, J. (2021). *Secularism: The basics*. Routledge. https://doi.org/10.4324/9781003140627

Bhargav, H., George, S., & Varambally, S. (2023). Yoga and mental health: What every psychiatrist needs to know. *The British Journal of Psychiatry, 29*(1), 44–55. doi:10.1192/bja.2022.22.

Blaustein, M., & Kinniburgh, K. (2019). *Treating traumatic stress in children and adolescents: How to foster resilience through attachment, self-regulation, and competency*. Guilford Press.

Boukhabza, D. (2023). *A Jungian understanding of symbolic function and forms: The dream series* (1st ed.). Routledge. https://doi.org/10.4324/b23380

Canning, N., & Callan, S. (2010). Heutagogy: Spirals of reflection to empower learners in higher education. *Reflective Practice, 11*(1), 71–82. doi:10.1080/14623940903500069.

Cashwell, C. S., & Young, J. S. (2020). *Integrating spirituality and religion into counseling: A guide to competent practice* (3rd ed.). American Counseling Association.

Children's Institute. (2017). *Still face with dads*. [YouTube video]. https://youtu.be/7Pcr1Rmr1rM

Chi Sigma Iota (CSI). (2023). *Wheel of wellness*. www.csi-net.org/members/group_content_view.asp?group=162835&id=573587

Choi, S., Hoi-Yun McClintock, C., Lau, E., & Miller, L. (2020). The dynamic universal profiles of spiritual awareness: A latent profile analysis. *Religions, 11*(6), 288. doi:10.3390/rel11060288.

Collins, J. J. (2019). *What are biblical values? What the Bible says on key ethical issues*. Yale University Press.

Corbett, L. (1990). *Religion in America*. Prentice Hall.

Corbett, L. (1996). *The religious function of the psyche*. Routledge.

Corbett, L. (2021). *The God-image: From antiquity to Jung*. Chiron Publications.

Council for Accreditation of Counseling and Related Programs (CACREP). (2024). *2024 CACREP standards*. www.cacrep.org/wp-content/uploads/2023/06/2024-Standards-Combined-Version-6.27.23.pdf

Dawkins, R. (2008). *The God delusion*. Mariner Books.

Dawkins, R. (2023). *Richard Dawkins: God, truth, & death*. Triggernometry. [YouTube video]. https://youtu.be/MVq4GLepUwI

de Brinto Sena, M. A., Damiano, R. F., Lucchetti, G., & Peres, M. F. P. (2021). Defining spirituality in healthcare: A systematic review and conceptual framework. *Frontiers in Psychology, 12*. https://doi.org/10.3389/fpsyg.2021.756080

DeCino, D. A., Waalkes, P. L., & Givens, J. (2020). Reflective practice: Counseling students' letters to their younger selves in practicum. *Teaching and Supervision in Counseling, 2*(1), 24–34. https://doi.org/10.7290/tsc020103

Diamond, S. A. (2014). Daimonic. In D. A. Leeming (Eds.), *Encyclopedia of psychology and religion*. Springer. https://doi.org/10.1007/978-1-4614-6086-2_149

Edinger, E. F. (1972). *Ego and archetype: Individuation and the religious function of the psyche*. Shambhala Publications.

Ellis, H. M., Hook, J. N., Zuniga, S., Hodge, A. S., Ford, K. M., Davis, D. E., & Van Tongeren, D. R. (2022). Religious/spiritual abuse and trauma: A systematic review of the empirical literature. *Spirituality in Clinical Practice, 9*(4), 213–231. https://doi.org/10.1037/scp0000301

Ferreira, J. F., Basseches, M., & Vasco, A. B. (2017). Guidelines for reflective practice in psychotherapy: A reflection on the benefits of combining moment-by-moment and phase-by-phase mapping in clinical decision making. *Journal of Psychotherapy Integration, 27*(1), 35–46. https://doi.org/10.1037/int0000047

Fonagy, P., Luyten, P., Moulton-Perkins, A., Lee, Y. W., Warren, F., Howard, S., et al. (2016). Development and validation of a self-report measure of mentalizing: The Reflective Functioning Questionnaire (RFQ). *PLOS ONE, 11*(7). doi:10.1371/journal.pone.0158678.

Foucault, M. (1984). *The Foucault reader*. P. Rainbow (Ed.). Pantheon Books.

Fuller, B., Green, M., Gaimen, N. et al. (Executive Producers). (2017–2021). *American Gods* [TV series]. Starz. www.starz.com/us/en/series/american-gods/31151

Gaimen, N. (2001). *American gods*. William Morrow.

Hagedorn, W. B., & Moorhead, H. J. H. (2010). The God-shaped hole: Addictive disorders and the search for perfection. *Counseling and Values, 55*(1), 63–78. https://doi.org/10.1002/j.2161-007X.2010.tb00022.x

Hannah, B. (1976). *Jung: His life and work: A biographical memoir*. Capricorn Books.

Hillman, J. (1975). *Re-visioning psychology*. Harper and Row.

Horváth, Z., Demetrovics, O., Paksi, B., Unoka, Z., & Demetrovics, Z. (2023). The Reflective Functioning Questionnaire-Revised-7 (RFQ-R-7): A new measurement model assessing hypomentalization. *PLoS One, 18*(2), e0282000. doi:10.1371/journal.pone.0282000.

Iurato, G. (2016). *A psychoanalytic enquiry on symbolic function*. https://hal.science/hal-01361264v1

Jacobs, M. (2017). *Psychodynamic counseling in action*. Sage.

Jeffers, A., Meehan, A. A., Barker, J., Asher, A., Montgomery, M. P., Bautista, G., Ray, C. M., et al. (2022). Impact of social isolation during the COVID-19 pandemic on mental health, substance use, and homelessness: Qualitative interviews with behavioral health providers. *International Journal of Environmental Research and Public Health, 19*(19), 12120. http://dx.doi.org/10.3390/ijerph191912120

Johnson, B. N., Kivity, Y., Rosenstein, L. K., LeBreton, J. M., & Levy, K. N. (2022). The association between mentalizing and psychopathology: A meta-analysis of the reading the mind in the eyes task across psychiatric disorders. *Clinical Psychology: Science and Practice, 29*(4), 423–439. https://doi.org/10.1037/cps0000105.supp

Johnson, R. A. (1991). *Owning your own shadow: Understanding the dark side of the psyche*. HarperOne.

Jung, C. G. (1933). *Modern man in search of a soul*. W. S. Dell & C. F. Baynes (Trans.). Legan Paul, Trench, Trubner & Co.

Jung, C. G. (1964). *Man and his symbols*. (C. G. Jung, Ed., & after his death M. Von Franz, Ed.; D. Hill, Text Ed., M. Kitson. Design Ed., M. Morris, G. Doel, & M. Lloyd, Assistant Eds., M. MacLaren, Research Ed., D. Berwick & N. MacKenzie, Advising Ed.). Ferguson Publishing.

Jung, C. G. (1973). *C. G. Jung Letters: Volume 1: 1906–1950*. G. Adler, A. Jaffe et al. (Eds.), R. F. C. Hull (Trans.). Routledge.

Jung, C. G. (1989). *Memories, dreams, reflections*. A. Jaffe (Ed.), C. Winston & R. Winston (Trans.). Vintage.

Jung, C. G. (2008). *Children's dreams: Notes from the seminar given 1936–1940*. L. Jung & M. Meyer-Grass (Eds.), E. Faizeder & T. Woolfson (Trans.). Princeton University Press.

Jung, C. G. (2009). *The red book: Liber novus*. S. Shamdasani (Ed.), M. Kyburz & J. Peck (Trans.). W. W. Norton & Co.

Jung, C. G. (2023). *The collected works of C. G. Jung: Revised and expanded complete digital edition.* (CW 1–20). G. Adler, W. McGuire, & H. Read (Eds.), R. F. C. Hull (Trans.). Princeton University Press. https://press.princeton.edu/books/ebook/9780691255194/the-collected-works-of-c-g-jung

Kalff, D. M. (2020). *Sandplay: A psychotherapeutic approach to the psyche.* B. L. Matthews (Trans). Analytical Psychology Press, Sandplay Editions. (Original work published 1966).

Kalsched, D. E. (1996). *The inner world of trauma: Archetypal defenses of the personal spirit.* Routledge.

Kamraju, M. (2023). The impact of yoga on mental health. *Indonesian Journal of Community and Special Needs Education, 3*(2), 141–146. www.researchgate.net/profile/M-Kamraju-2/publication/371139056_The_Impact_of_Yoga_on_Mental_Health/links/6475b1446fb1d1682b1bee7a/The-Impact-of-Yoga-on-Mental-Health.pdf

Knox, J. (2004). From archetypes to reflective function. *Journal of Analytical Psychology, 49,* 1–19. https://doi.org/10.1111/j.0021-8774.2004.0437.x

Kuo, B. (2020). Multicultural counseling training and intercultural training: A synthesis. In D. Landis & D. Bhawuk (Eds.), *The Cambridge handbook of intercultural training* (Cambridge Handbooks in Psychology, pp. 407–439). Cambridge University Press. doi:10.1017/9781108854184.016

Lambie, G. W., Mullen, P. R., Swank, J. M., & Blount, A. (2017). The Counseling Competencies Scale (CCS): Validation and refinement. *Measurement and Evaluation in Counseling and Development, 51*(1), 1–15. doi:10.1080/07481756.2017.1358964.

Lees, J. (2016). Microphenomena research, intersubjectivity and client as self-healer. *Psychodynamic Practice: Individuals, Groups and Organizations, 22*(1), 22–37. http://dx.doi.org/10.1080/14753634.2015.1124801

Lewin, K. M., Meshi, D., Schuster, A. M., & Cotten, S. R. (2023). Active and passive social media use are differentially related to depressive symptoms in older adults. *Aging Mental Health, 27*(1), 176–183. doi:10.1080/13607863.2022.2068133.

Lönneker, C., & Maercker, A. (2021). The numinous experience in the context of psychopathology and traumatic stress studies. *Culture & Psychology, 27*(3), 392–416. https://doi.org/10.1177/1354067X20922139

Luke, M., & Kiweewa, J. M. (2010). Personal growth and awareness counseling trainees in an experiential group. *Journal for Specialists in Group Work, 35,* 365–388. http://dx.doi.org/10.1080/01933922.2010.514976

Luminate Media. (2023, February 20). *Konstantin Kisin and the counter-woke revolution.* The Jordan B Peterson Podcast. Episode 333. https://podcasts.apple.

com/us/podcast/333-konstantin-kisin-and-the-counter-woke-revolution/
id1184022695?i=1000600642379

Main, R. (2007). *Revelations of chance: Synchronicity as spiritual experience.* The State University of New York Press.

Malikiosi-Loizos, M. (2013). Personal therapy for future therapists: Reflections on a still debated issue. *The European Journal of Counselling Psychology, 2*(1). doi:10.5964/ejcop.v2i1.4.

Markos, P. A., Coker, J. K., & Jones, W. P. (2008). Play in supervision. *Journal of Creativity in Mental Health, 2*(3), 3–15. doi:10.1300/J456v02n03_02.

McRoberts, R., & Epstein, J. (2023). Creative self-concept, post-traumatic growth, and professional identity resilience in counselors with traumatic experiences: A canonical correlation analysis. *Journal of Creativity in Mental Health,* 1–15. doi:10.1080/15401383.2023.2232730.

Moritz, J. (2023). *Is there a God-shaped hole at the heart of mathematics?* John Templeton Foundation. www.templeton.org/news/is-there-a-god-shaped-hole-at-the-heart-of-mathematics

Myers, J. E., & Sweeney, T. J. (2004). The Indivisible Self: An evidence-based model of wellness. *Journal of Individual Psychology, 60*(3), 234–245.

Online Etymology Dictionary. (2023a). *Numen.* www.etymonline.com/word/numen

Online Etymology Dictionary. (2023b). *Religio-.* www.etymonline.com/word/religio-

Orwell, G. (2021). *Nineteen eighty-four.* Penguin Classics. (Original work published 1949).

Otto, R. (1923). *The idea of the holy: An inquiry into the non-rational factor in the idea of the divine and its relation to the rational.* Oxford University Press. (Original work published 1918).

Paksarian, D., Rudolph, K. E., Stapp, E. K., Dunster, G. P., He, J., Mennitt, D., Hattar, S., Casey, J. A., James, P., & Merikangas, K. R. (2020). Association of outdoor artificial light at night with mental disorders and sleep patterns among US adolescents. *JAMA Psychiatry.* doi:10.1001/jamapsychiatry.2020.1935.

Parsons, R. D., & Zhang, N. (2014). *Counseling theory: Guiding reflective practice.* Sage.

Pearce, M. J., Pargament, K. I., Oxhandler, H. K., Vieten, C., & Wong, S. (2020). Novel online training program improves spiritual competencies in mental health care. *Spirituality in Clinical Practice, 7*(3), 145–161. https://doi.org/10.1037/scp0000208

Penner, F., Gambin, M., & Sharp, C. (2019). Childhood maltreatment and identity diffusion among inpatient adolescents: The role of the reflective function. *Journal of Adolescence, 76,* 65–74. https://doi.org/10.1016/j.adolescence.2019.08.002

Peresso, P. (2019). The analyst and analysand as citizens in the world. *The Journal of Analytical Psychology*, 64(2), 168–188. https://doi.org/10.1111/1468-5922.12477

Pew Research Center. (2009). *Many Americans mix multiple faiths.* www.pewresearch.org/religion/2009/12/09/many-americans-mix-multiple-faiths/#6

Pew Research Center. (2019). *Religion's relationship to happiness, civic engagement and health around the world.* www.pewresearch.org/religion/2019/01/31/religions-relationship-to-happiness-civic-engagement-and-health-around-the-world/

Pew Research Center. (2022). *How US religious composition has changed in recent decades.* www.pewresearch.org/religion/2022/09/13/how-u-s-religious-composition-has-changed-in-recent-decades/

Piaget, J. (1951). *Play, dreams, and imitation in childhood.* Norton.

Portnoff, L., McClintock, C., Lau, E., Choi, S., & Miller, L. (2017). Spirituality cuts in half the relative risk for depression: Findings from the United States, China, and India. *Spirituality in Clinical Practice*, 4(1), 22–31. https://doi.org/10.1037/scp0000127

Puchalski, C. M., Vitillo, R., Hull, S. K., & Reller, N. (2014). Person care: Reaching national and international consensus. *Journal of Palliative Medicine*, 17(6), 642–656. https://doi.org/10.1089/jpm.2014.9427

Qin, F., Song, Y., Nassis, G. P., Zhao, L., Dong, Y., Zhao, C., et al. (2020). Physical activity, screen time, and emotional well-being during the 2019 novel coronavirus outbreak in China. *International Journal of Environmental Research and Public Health*, 17(14), 5170. doi:10.3390/ijerph17145170.

Quinn, S., Donnelly, S., & Kidd, E. (2018). The relationship between symbolic play and language acquisition: A meta-analytic review. *Developmental Review*, 1–15. https://doi.org/10.1016/j.dr.2018.05.005

Ratts, M. J., Singh, A. A., Nassar-McMillan, S., Butler, S. K., & McCullough, J. R. (2016). Multicultural and social justice counseling competencies: Guidelines for the counseling profession. *Journal of Multicultural Counseling and Development*, 44, 28–48. https://doi.org/10.1002/jmcd.12035

Reangsing, C., Lauderman, C., & Schneider, J. K. (2022). Effects of mindfulness meditation intervention on depressive symptoms in emerging adults: A systematic review and meta-analysis. *Journal of Integrative and Complementary Medicine*, 28(1), 6–24. http://doi.org/10.1089/jicm.2021.0036

Roesler, C. (2022). *Development of a reconceptualization of archetype theory: Report to the IAAP.* https://iaap.org/wp-content/uploads/2022/04/Report-Archetype-Theory-Roesler-1.pdf

Rønnestad, M. H., & Skovholt, T. M. (2003). The journey of the counselor and therapist: Research findings and perspectives on professional development. *Journal of Career Development*, 30(1), 5–44. doi:10.1023/A:1025173508081.

Saad, L., & Hrynowski, Z. (2022). *How many Americans believe in God?* Gallup. https://news.gallup.com/poll/268205/americans-believe-god.aspx

Schmemann, A. (1973). *For the life of the world: Sacraments and orthodoxy.* St. Vladimir's Seminary Press.

Schön, D. (1983). *The reflective practitioner: How professionals think in action.* Basic Books.

Sisyphus 55. (2022). *The father of memes: A guide to Richard Dawkins.* [YouTube video]. https://youtu.be/HgdHRZQYPQc

Smith, J. E. (2020). *Religious but not religious: Living a symbolic life.* Chiron Publications.

Taylor, S., Landry, C. A., Paluszek, M. M., Fergus, T. A., McKay, D., & Asmundson, G. J. G. (2020). COVID stress syndrome: Concept, structure, and correlates. *Anxiety and Depression Association of America, 37*, 706–714. https://doi.org/10.1002/da.23071

University of the South. (2022). *Education for Ministry: Reading and reflection guide 2022–2023, Volume B, Living faithfully in a multicultural world.* Church Publishing Incorporated.

Upshaw, J. D., Davis, W. M., & Zabelina, D. L. (2022). iCreate: Social media use, divergent thinking, and real-life creative achievement. *Translational Issues in Psychological Science, 8*(1), 125–136. https://doi.org/10.1037/tps0000306

Veraksa, A., & Veraksa, N. (2016). Symbolic representation in the early years learning: The acquisition of complex notions. *European Early Childhood Education Research Journal, 24*(5), 668–683. https://doi.org/10.1080/1350293X.2015.1035539

von Franz, M.-L. (1990). *Psychotherapy.* Shambhala Publications.

Walsh, D., & Koch, G. (2023, November 15). Helping clients navigate religious trauma. *Counseling Today.* https://ct.counseling.org/2023/11/helping-clients-navigate-religious-trauma/

Wampold, B. E., & Imel, Z. E. (2015). *The great psychotherapy debate: The evidence for what makes psychotherapy work.* Routledge.

Zhao, Y., Paulus, M. P., & Potenza, M. N. (2023). Brain structural co-development is associated with internalizing symptoms two years later in the ABCD cohort. *Journal of Behavioral Addictions, 12*(1), 80–93. https://doi.org/10.1556/2006.2023.00006

5
The Language of the Unconscious

Increased knowledge of the unconscious brings a deeper experience of life and greater consciousness, and therefore confronts us with apparently new situations.
Jung, CW 10, p. 357, § 677

One of the most distinctive factors about humans is that we have a seemingly unique and distinct ability, and inherent need, to symbolize our internal and external reality. We form ideas into images, sounds, words, and movements to make meaning, express ourselves, and communicate with others. Jung focused much of his work around his ideas about the language of the unconscious, and what the unconscious might be saying through its manifested content. His view was that psyche is essentially constructed by and consists of images, and that we need these images as badly as we need our bodies in order to live (CW 8).

Our conscious mind is only in charge of a fraction of our lives, and some may argue it's better that way (Morsella et al., 2016). Even if our egos greatly desire to be in control, we have the unconscious to thank for making it seem effortless: walking, talking, quick thinking, microexpressions, breathing, giving us subtle cues about how we perceive our environment, and respond to it internally with feelings, and externally through behaviors. The "hard problem" of consciousness explains the subjective aspect of our individual lived experiences (Chalmers, 1995). The Jungian counselor highly values the unconscious, language, and problem-solving abilities, often communicated through symbolic material the archetypes hold.

ARCHETYPES

. . . archetypes probably represent typical situations in life.
CW 8, pp. 167–168, § 254

DOI: 10.4324/9781003433736-5

Jung hypothesized that specific aspects and typical patterning of the psyche could be found across time and culture. Without the identification and scientific understanding of these patterns, how could we begin to define what is "normal", "stable", or "healthy" cross-culturally, never mind deviations from the sequence, commonly called "psychopathy"? The question of what an ideal or original form for the patterning the human mind might look like harkens all the way back to Plato in ancient Greece, through the sordid past of evolutionary psychology, to today's neuroscientific study of symbolic interactionism. The word archetype comes from the Greek *arkhetypona*, referring to an original form or pattern from which copies are made, and was one adopted by Jung to talk about these ideas (Online Etymology Dictionary, 2023a). There was some controversy surrounding the discourse of inherited ideas, which Jung clarified as instincts and archetypal images, which he suggested could be found across species, but especially in humans (CW 8). Affective neuroscience took that idea and ran with it, and there is now compelling evidence of this concept (Alcaro et al., 2017).

While it might not be mainstream to talk about symbols and archetypes in the counseling world, it is generally accepted that genetic patterning, social conditions, and our ability to interpret and cope with these intersecting factors accurately all impact our mental health. Long gone is the idea of the tabula rasa, or blank slate; even Jung and Freud agreed upon that long ago. The assumption that we should revisit, parse out, and reorganize memories to make them more tolerable is downright fundamental to trauma treatments, from EMDR to CBT. But the knowledge and the value of the symbolic content embedded in those memories is often ignored there. Jungians focus more on the archetypal elements: the universal, emotionally significant core of imaginable, tangible, symbolic content. However, there remains a lack of research, and contentious debate, even among Jungians, about the definition of archetypes, as well as if, and if so to what degree, genetics and environment play a part in our understanding of them (Goodwyn, 2022; Roesler, 2022, 2024).

Jung's definitions, including "archetypes", did shift throughout his career, and he did not see many of the scientific discoveries we have made about genetic predispositions to mental health. He did talk about a phenomenon which we now know as "intergenerational trauma" (Lucero, 2018; Yehuda & Lehrner, 2018) in several places but he focused on the idea of the life unlived, or repressed from previous generations (CW 6; CW 15; CW17; 1973) versus the more epigenetic exploration being pursued today from the medical model. The brain, particularly our neocortex, is now said to allow us to absorb thousands of previous generations' accumulated and distilled experiences in a single lifetime (Perry, 2004. Two major studies demonstrate some evidence of an innate archetypal symbolic knowledge (Bradshaw & Storm, 2013; Rosen et al., 1991). Others prefer to consider this phenomenon our ancestral knowledge, and how previous generations' wisdom is passed through generations.

Some proposed characteristics of archetypes include:

- They exist a priori, outside of us, or are somehow latent in our psyche which may be biologically, spiritually, and/or relationally/culturally transferred.
- They "are the numinous, structural elements of the psyche" (CW 5, p. 338, § 344). See also Chapter 4 on the structure of the psyche and note the first column of archetypes in Table 5.1 below.
- They "possess a certain autonomy and specific energy which enables them to attract, out of the conscious mind, those contents best suited to themselves" (CW 5, p. 338, § 344).
- They are part of the collective unconscious; they link us to history across time, generations, and cultures.
- They have never been fully consciously known, so they are, will continue to be, arising from the unconscious (CW 8). Hence, the importance of activating the unconscious through the symbolic function and associative process first, delay, and analyze afterward; see also mode-shifting.
- They help to organize our perceptions, ideas, and images into patterns.
- They are represented in the mind as images, characters, or symbols.
- They condense, activate, and direct emotional, psychic, and social phenomena within an individual and interpersonally (Roesler, 2022, 2024).
- They may be helpful in exploring what people idealize, consider a model for socially acceptable behavior or achievement, might set as life goals, and even steps toward growth and healing (Roesler, 2024).
- "Archetypes are complexes of experience that come upon us like fate, and their effects are felt in our most personal life" (CW 9i, p. 30, § 62). Emphasis is added here to note that even archetypes are considered complexes; we may also speak of other complexes having an "archetypal core".

And perhaps most poetically:

- "Psychologically . . . the archetype as an image of instinct is a spiritual goal toward which the whole nature of man strives; it is the sea to which all rivers wend their way, the prize which the hero wrests from the fight with the dragon" (CW 8, p. 276, §415).

Roesler's (2024) recent deconstruction of archetype theory suggests that it may be more prudent for us to clinically apply Jungian hermeneutics as a method of exploration, rather than claiming, or seeking to confirm, a biological, or other definitive answer, about or within them. However, there is compelling evidence of archetypes still emerging from the area of affective-neuroscience (Alcaro et al., 2017). While I do appreciate attempts to come to a definitive definition of archetypes for further scientific study, as a Jungian-oriented counselor, I am more interested in the ongoing exploration of the phenomenon of archetypes. The idea of archetypes inspires us to look at the human experience as a narrative, and not reduce our common history to contemporary ideals of mental health, or worse yet, pathology in need of fixing. Archetypes challenge us to remain humble, curious, open to remembering the wisdom of the past, and to continue looking for the pattern as we work it. If we are evolving, are we not also emotionally evolving? Is our symbolic function not also evolving? This patterning may be intuitive, even instinctual. As Jung said:

> No archetype can be reduced to a simple formula. It is a vessel which we can never empty, and never fill. It has a potential existence only, and when it takes shape in matter it is no longer what it was. It persists throughout the ages and requires interpreting ever anew. The archetypes are imperishable elements of the unconscious, but they change their shape continually.
>
> CW 9i, p. 179, § 301

Archetypes are the parts of a story or image that make it translatable and understood by anyone, anytime, anywhere in the world (Goodwyn, 2022). These include basic aspects of nature, nurturing, life-sustaining or threatening qualities, often with polarizing states, and patterning in general. They also include typical roles or labels put on people from various walks of life (personae) which can also have dual sides, or positive and negative aspects. While archetypal opposites may initially appear divisive, and even perpetuating various -isms, the unifying aspect of the Self reminds us that such separations are an illusion (Brewster, 2020, 2023).

We often see archetypes portrayed as capitalized common words to speak of their universal concepts, such as the Self, the World, Justice, etc. We might say archetypal qualities are the elements that make something "meme-worthy"; "meme" comes from the Greek *mimema* meaning "imitated" (Dawkins, 1976). A meme in the digital age has been copied over and over so much that it is now common knowledge; in Jungian terms, it has become part of the collective. Archetypes simply ARE, while their symbolic form may shift. They are inarguably things that, at least conceptually, exist, are

Table 5.1 Archetypes. (Reprinted with permission. Further reproduction is prohibited without the author's written authorization. All rights reserved. Copyright © 2023 by author, Rachel McRoberts.)

Psyche	Figures / Roles	Situations / States	Settings	Objects	Elemental
Persona	Mother / Father, Queen / King	Birth / Death	Mountain / Valley	Food / Waste	Earth / Air, Fire / Water
Ego	Child / Elder	Chaos / Order	Forest / Glen	Weapon / Tool	Spring / Fall, Summer / Winter
Anima / Animus	Brother / Sister	Rejection / Initiation	Land / Water	Sacred / Profane	Hot / Cold
Self	Creator / Destroyer	Hunger / Satisfaction	Home / Strange Land	Clothes / Adornments	Day / Night
Shadow	Hero / Villain	Lost / Found	Safe / Danger	Medicine / Poison	Hard / Soft
Light / Dark					
Personal Unconscious	Trickster / Nurturer	Sick / Healed	Work / Leisure	Bridge / Great Divide	Thought / Emotion
Collective Unconscious	Wounded Healer / Servant Leader	Conflict / Resolution	Heaven / the Pit	Bed / Car	Top / Bottom

experienced, and we attempt to know and understand them by representing them symbolically.

> The archetypes too . . . are as much found as invented: they are discovered inasmuch as one did not know of their unconscious autonomous existence, and invented inasmuch as their presence was inferred from analogous representational structures.
>
> CW 8, p. 584, § 871

Though Jung warned us that it "is no use at all to learn a list of archetypes by heart" (CW 9i, p. 30, § 62), some great resources are out there to get us started. Over the past 80 years, the Archive for Research in Archetypal Symbolism (ARAS, 2023) has cataloged and cross-indexed over 18,000 images from around the world, with over 46,000 searchable keywords, making it one of the most comprehensive resources. There is also a quick reference list of several hundred archetypes (Jeffery, 2018), and archetype cards (Myss, 2003); clients and I both love the cards because, while they are all figures, they represent people of a range of skin tones and also have a brief light/shadow aspect of each. Table 5.1 contains several for those who want to contemplate a few archetypes.

You might notice that archetypes relate to play themes observed in counseling and elsewhere (Landreth, 2024; Ray, 2004). They are also involved in the Hero's Journey, or monomyth, discovered and developed by Joseph Campbell (2008) and adopted by famous Hollywood story consultant Christopher Vogler (2020); beyond a narrative template, the Hero's Journey is an archetype all its own. These themes and the meeting of archetypal characters along the Hero's Journey make up the outline of ancient and contemporary epic stories. I highly recommend both the Campbell and Vogler texts for depth and reference.

All of the archetypes speak symbolically, or what some consider to be our common human language. Like archetypes, symbols resist concrete definitions, and may shift or hold multiple meanings across the personal and collective. Nonetheless, they remain significant, containing images and wisdom stories of the ages. We are called to dive in and attempt to begin understanding while suspending judgment (Turner, 2005).

SYMBOLS

> As a plan produces its flower, so the psyche creates its symbols.
>
> CW 18, p. 223, § 512

We live immediately only in a world of images.

CW 8, p. 423, § 624

The word "symbol" is derived from the Greek *symbolon*: *sym* meaning "together" and *ballein* meaning "to throw" (Stevens, 1998). A *symbolon* originally was a physical object used to ritualize an agreement, or signify a relationship. The object, such as a bone, would be broken and the halves given to two people, to be brought together at another time as a kind of identity verification (like, bona fide). This conjunction, or bringing together what has been thrown apart, implies a bridging, or connecting gaps in the psyche. The importance of symbols has been known since ancient times, and is now studied with the symbolic function as vital to our process of developing a self-identity and our ability to relate to those in the world.

As discussed in Chapter 4, the symbolic function of the psyche is a vital developmental and ongoing process. While signs stand in for something concretely specific, living symbols are "pregnant with meaning" (CW 6, p. 654 § 816–817). Symbols bridge the unconscious and the conscious psyche and help us relate to others, the world, and purposefulness in our lives. A "poverty of associations" (CW 3, p. 27, § 22) can lead to a variety of unpleasant experiences and may be at the root of many disturbances in the psyche. Symbols bring richness and nuance to our existence while carrying archetypal themes. While there may be symbolic patterning in the collective, symbols also often have a very personal nuance. For a more detailed example of this, you might want to read my article on the white rabbit, which is available online (McRoberts, 2023).

Many things may have a symbolic charge, attitude, meaning, association, or value, often through the emotions evoked (Franks, 2003; Stevens, 1998), but only occasionally have an overt "intellectual or aesthetic interest" (CW 6, p. 656, § 819). Jung thought that the way the unconscious chooses to manifest the symbol is "the best possible description or formulation of a relatively unknown face, which is nonetheless known to exist or is postulated as existing" (CW 6, p. 653, §814). This is why we should allow lots of space for curious, creative exploration, and be well versed in the language of the unconscious. Symbolic content may emerge at any time and if we are attuned, much can be learned. Jung identified that most "associations are thinly veiled expressions of complexes" (CW 3, p. 148, § 208) and that being lost in or numb to them in a poverty of associations could be a factor in disturbances of attention and understanding. This poverty of associations often looks like not wanting to take a deeper look at things at all, avoiding identifying, discussing, or naming things, finding life meaningless or overly anxiety

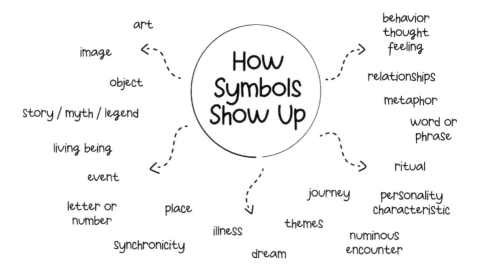

Figure 5.1 Symbols. (Reprinted with permission. Further reproduction is prohibited without the author's written authorization. All rights reserved. Copyright © 2023 by author, Rachel McRoberts.)

provoking, having an intolerance for or aversion to people or situations, or, in other words, being stuck in analytic mode (see mode-shifting theory).

This is a very broad definition of symbol (see Figure 5.1). In this way, almost anything might be symbolic: from an apple to a birth to a panic attack . . . so it all might mean something else, yet unconsciously, and vary from person to person? Yes! We must be very cautious in interpreting symbols, especially as counselors. One symbol dictionary is never enough and will never fully describe the impact of a symbol manifesting for someone. (However, I do recommend collecting them!). Symbols, like archetypes, from our perspective carry a numinous quality, and may have an archetypal core which may give them greater meaning. While all language is symbolic, and may reference concrete objects in the world meant for ease of communication (i.e., water, body, cat, etc.) it is often taken for granted that even words hold a great deal of room for nuance that may be misunderstood. Living symbols, when they well up, may resonate with emotion, and be shared and understood, when well attuned; like a plucked harp, if you are sitting close enough, you not only hear it, you literally feel it. Let's not be too quick to judge.

Symbols emerge through associative processes, so we really want to stay with them and encourage exploration before beginning the analysis (see mode-shifting). That requires us to be open, curious, and actively engaged. It also requires us to make sure we are doing our own work, especially knowing our own associations with symbolic content, and practicing cultural humility (Loue, 2015). A working example is avoiding labeling things for others, especially our clients. To label something and call it "this" or "that" is a manifestation of power, more so if we are sitting in a position of authority caring for a child, or anyone asking for our help. It may be as innocent and seemingly obvious as giving a common name for an object like a "cup", gendering a doll, or calling a monster "bad", but it is nonetheless assuming and may throw our client off. We don't know what we don't know. Our own personal and cultural frames of reference likely bind our biases for or against symbolic content. While our biases may be understandable generalizations, and may assist us in relating to the world, including communicating verbally, sharing space, and empathizing, they also need to be challenged and expanded upon. Remember, true symbols do not have one definitive meaning, so our interpretations should always be held lightly. As we say in counseling, we want to take a non-judgmental stance; from a Jungian perspective, that looks like having a symbolic attitude. In order to truly listen to the complex meaning of symbols, we need to be knowledgeable and receptive to how the unconscious speaks.

HOW THE UNCONSCIOUS SPEAKS

> Whenever contents of the collective unconscious become activated, they have a disturbing effect on the conscious mind, and contusion ensues. If the activation is due to the collapse of the individual's hopes and expectations, there is a danger that the collective unconscious may take the place of reality. This state would be pathological. If, on the other hand, the activation is the result of psychological processes in the unconscious of the people, the individual may feel threatened or at any rate disoriented, but the resultant state is not pathological, at least so far as the individual is concerned.
>
> CW 8, p. 407, § 595

The language of the unconscious is composed of archetypes and symbols. The process of that unconscious material becoming conscious is what we will refer to here as HOW the unconscious speaks. Jung (CW 12) noted that this is a developmental process that might circumambulate, moving or spiraling around a central symbol, image or theme; it may seem to grow from a known center, like a spiderweb, or we may feel pulled toward it, like circling a drain. In the mental health field, I have honestly more often heard the term "spiraling" used to describe decompensation. This speaks to the general disinformation about and undervalue of the unconscious, a lack of theoretical understanding about the purpose of mental health disturbance, as well as our collective fear of "spiraling out of control". Here, in further describing how the unconscious speaks, we will address a few topics of particular relevance:

- Dreams
- Synchronicity
- Complexes and Defenses
- The Hero's Journey in Stages

Dreams

> It is only in modern times that the dream, this fleeting and insignificant-looking product of the psyche, has met with such profound contempt. Formerly it was esteemed as a harbinger of fate, a portent and comforter, a messenger of the gods. Now we see it as the emissary of the unconscious, whose task it is to reveal the secrets that are hidden from the conscious mind, and this it does with astounding completeness.
>
> CW 7, p. 354, §433

In a recent interview, when asked what dreaming is for, Deirdre Barret responded by turning the question around, asking what conscious thought was for, and pointing out the seeming absurdity of that question (World Science Festival, 2022). The fact remains that dreams, their function, and interpretation, while meaningful and important, still are shrouded in mystery. Dream interpretation is an ancient practice and probably most famously introduced by Freud in his *Interpretation of Dreams* (1955). While Jung agreed with Freud that dreams may sometimes be a veiled narrative about compensations, he also inherently valued and was open to the possibility that they may provide hints about solutions. Jung was also adamant that the dreamer knows themselves best, and while analysis might be helpful, it was to be a collaborative process.

While contemporary neuroscientists may not see the value in attempting to code and accurately interpret dreams objectively, it remains agreed upon that dreams can be very meaningful for the dreamers and are vital for everyone, regardless of if they remember their dreams or not. REM sleep, or the rapid eye movement stage of sleep, when dreams most often occur, is now commonly understood as necessary to assist in thought and emotional regulation. Research also suggests that dreams reflect our waking lives and play a role in interpreting and encoding thoughts and memories, including learning and emotional growth, first suggested by Jung (Hoss, 2018). There is also ongoing investigation into social- and threat-simulation theories of dreaming, suggesting that because dreaming is such an ancient part of our brains, it likely serves an evolutionary and adaptive function to anticipate and rehearse possible or imminent waking life scenarios. Nightmares continue to be under-reported and unrecognized by mental health providers, which could lead to increased risk factors, but when treated, may save lives (Cromer et al., 2022).

Today, dreams remain a cross-cultural and cross-disciplinary topic, spanning the study of neuroscience, religion, art, and ourselves. The International Association for the Study of Dreams (2023) is a rabbit hole of all things dreaming, with several journals, an annual conference, books, links, including to the Sleep and Dream Database, and more. I was delighted to see Jung's name mentioned several times, crediting his foundational contributions to the field.

Dreams may be the mind's comments or criticisms regarding the day's events, a past or future event, or a pattern in our lives. Dreams may indicate that the unconscious is for, against, or neutral about the dreamer's current state (Jung, 1974). There are several ways of deconstructing and analyzing dreams, now backed by empirical data (Roesler, 2020). Jung identified five types of dreams and a basic dream structure involving four stages, which we will discuss more in Chapter 7 on Creative Techniques. For now, let us address a naturally occurring phenomenon that can seem like a waking dream.

Synchronicity

> Synchronicity . . . means the simultaneous occurrence of a certain psychic state with one or more external events which appear as meaningful parallels to the momentary subjective state – and, in certain cases, vice versa.
>
> CW 8, p. 565, § 850

While you may have heard the term "synchronicity" in movies, songs, or in reference to astrological events, Jung invented the term over the course of 50 years to describe a phenomenon that he and many others have experienced which is still not a fully understood or explainable psychological happening (Etter, 2020). "Synchronicity" is one of the most widely recognized Jungian words (Sacco, 2019), contrived from the Latin *synchronus*, or "simultaneous", combining the Greek roots, *syn-*, meaning "together", or "joined with", and *khronos* meaning "time", referring to events occurring at the same time (Hocoy, 2012; Online Etymology Dictionary, 2023c).

Jung imagined an archetypal patterning where psyche and matter become one with an "ascasal connecting principal" (CW 8, p. 538). Jung went on to develop the concept of synchronicity in collaboration with quantum physics pioneer, and 1945 Nobel Prize winner, Wolfgang Pauli, sometimes referred to as the "Pauli-Jung Conjecture" (Atmanspacher & Fuchs, 2014). Jung added to the classic physics triad of space, time, and causality a fourth principle he called *synchronicity*, developing "a *quaternio* which makes possible a whole judgment" (CW 8, p. 647, § 961).

> . . . it seems to me necessary to introduce, alongside time, space and causality, a category which not only enables us to understand synchronistic phenomena as a special class of natural events, but also takes the contingent partly as a universal factor existing from all eternity, and partly as the sum of countless individual acts of creation occurring in time.
>
> CW 8, p. 654, § 968

Jung stated that synchronicity is a ". . . meaningful coincidence of two or more events, where something other than the probability of chance is involved" (CW 8, p. 655, § 969), and "consists of two factors", each "as puzzling as the other" (CW 8, p. 573, § 858):

1. "An unconscious image comes into consciousness either directly (i.e., literally) or indirectly (symbolized or suggested) in the form of a dream, idea, or premonition . . ."
2. "An objective situation coincides with this content . . ."

Synchronicity has recently been defined in the research literature as meaningful connections made between internalized and externalized phenomena, which may occur or be reflected upon simultaneously (Roxburgh et al., 2016; Sacco, 2019). Some synchronistic events (SE) may occur within a certain limited timeframe, while others may only be realized in hindsight. For example, one woman reported that after her grandmother's death, she asked for a sign that she was alright; at that moment, a little bird flew up to the window, and the woman then saw the bird periodically and it brought her great comfort.

Synchronistic events refer to happenings which are too significant to be "just a coincidence". They may align with a numinous feeling, like déjà vu. They may appear as recurrences or alliances in dreams, symbols that appear in waking life, in conversation, or other events. They are often associated with being "sent a message" from the divine, the Self, the "other side", or the unconscious, on our path to individuation. They may be seen as a "sign" that we are "on the right track" or a warning that danger is ahead. The phenomenon may seem like someone is somehow psychic, or at least very connected to another person or event. Jung suggested that associations and amplifications of archetypal material may also be considered an aspect of synchronicity (CW 18). Synchronicity, whether called such or not, may also be a factor in the study of experiences of the paranormal, hypnosis, and those separated from loved ones at birth, sometimes called parapsychology or psi (Main, 2007).

Synchronistic events are prevalent in the general population (see the definition of archetypes above). Reinforcing Jung's initial declaration that this is an archetypal experience, it has been suggested that this may be because we are meaning-making creatures, preferring order over chaos, and seeking out ways to make it all make sense. While some have found correlations between reports of synchronicity and psychotic symptoms, experiencing intense emotions, or going through major transitions in life (Beitman, 2011), others suggest that it is the connection with the unconscious that may be more significant (Pasciuti, 2011; Roxburgh et al., 2016). In one study, nearly half of the surveyed mental health clinicians reported experiencing synchronicity in the therapy office, and more than half thought it could be helpful to the therapeutic process; not surprisingly, counselors and psychotherapists were found to be more likely than psychologists to think that synchronicity may be experienced because of unconscious material needing to be expressed, and all dispelled "fate" or "divine intervention" as the explanation (Roxburgh et al., 2016, p. 50). Curiously, a spiritual connection has been cited elsewhere as the main explanation of SE (Allison, 2019; Main, 2007).

The REM Model (Russo-Netzer & Icekson, 2022) outlines a three-step process involved in synchronistic experiences: (R) receptiveness, or openness to the thoughts and feelings about the external cues, (E) the exceptional encounter, often sudden and echoing an internal state with "perfect timing", often when "a sign" seemed needed, and (M) meaning is detected. People tend to look both internally to explain external events as well as externally to find explanations for internal experiences, and may self-select details to create meaning (Colman, 2011). It has been suggested that those high in traits of openness, training in unconscious material, as well as belief and/or previous experience with SE and other psi phenomena, may influence the experience (Cardeña, 2018; Sacco, 2019).

> Synchronistic phenomena are found to occur – experimentally – with some degree of regularity and frequency in the intuitive, "magical" procedures, where they are subjectively convincing but are extremely difficult to verify objectively and cannot be statistically evaluated (at least at present).
>
> CW 8, pp. 645–646, § 958

The prediction and benefit of SE continue to be explored. Jung suggested that the Fibonacci sequence of numbers (each the sum of the proceeding two), commonly found in nature, could play a role in SE dynamics (Jung, 1976). This theory has recently been tested, finding it statistically significant that the Fibonacci Harmonic Model can predict the frequency of SEs in the Jungian analyst population (Sacco, 2019); more than half of the analysts rated these experiences 10/10 meaningful, with feelings of "surprise" and "trust" being the most prominent. Though research on the therapeutic benefits of SE is limited, most UK surveyed providers report that SE may assist with overcoming resistance and impasses, and increase personal insight and growth (Roxburgh et al., 2016).

Notably, the religious or secular worldview does not seem to impact the frequency of the experience of synchronistic events, nor the comforting emotions, increased sense of purpose, gratitude, meaning, or cohesiveness, but does vary on the explanation of them, namely, divine intervention versus a yet unknown aspect of the order of things. Either way, it reinforces a pervasive idea that we are connected, that "everything happens for a reason", or the common counseling goal of creating a coherent narrative integrating the internal and external, or in other words, finding meaning. SE has the potential to bring a sense of existential comfort, if not direct evidence, by demonstrating the interconnectedness in the way of things. Inspired by both the mind/matter connection as well as philosophies from East and West, Jung used the term *unus mundus* or "one world" (CW 10, p. 409, § 778), to describe this concept of an ordered universe. Jung has inspired several quantum physicists in their search for answers to the hard problem of consciousness, namely how it is that we have subjective experiences in an objective world (Bohm & Peat, 1987; Gullatz & Gildersleeve, 2018).

Synchronicity has been defined as a "spiritual path" in our secular, digital age (Allison, 2019). Jung said that the word spirit is "synonymous with 'mind'", with connotations of

> . . . courage, liveliness, or wit, or it may mean a ghost; it can also represent an unconscious complex that causes spiritualistic phenomena like table-turning, automatic writings, rappings, etc. In a metaphorical sense it may refer to the dominant attitude in a particular social group – the spirit that prevailed there . . . in a material sense as spirits of wine, spirits of ammonia, and spirituous liquors in general.
>
> CW 8, pp. 412–413, § 602

While "evidence-based research" tends to value quantitative (statistics) over qualitative (the study of the lived experience, or subjective reality, of participants), both psychodynamically oriented psychotherapists and counselors tend to be drawn to our clients' reports as well as the therapeutic relationship itself. With those factors comes the idea of trusting our intuitive knowledge: ours and others. While some get hung up on the idea of acausality being unscientific (Main, 2007), I argue that Jung's idea of archetypal patterning as an organizing principle in the psyche takes into account human creation, and our meaning-making ability, which fits into our counseling values of empowerment and Servant Leadership (Greenleaf, 1970). Jung writes freedom into the ontology of his study of phenomenology, conceptualization of consciousness, as well as his psychotherapy, making the idea of archetypes even more probable (Gullatz & Gildersleeve, 2018) and perhaps more palatable for those with a lower tolerance for ambiguity.

We frequently talk about intangibles in counseling like "intuition", "hunches", and assumptions like assuming to know about someone's internal processes, "reflecting empathy", or knowing "when the time is right", to make a "gut decision" (Russo-Netzer & Icekson, 2022; Shapiro & Marks-Tarlow, 2021). Jung argued that even the most harsh tangibles of objective reality can only be known through the subjective experience of the mind (CW 8). While we may not have all the answers yet, even basic knowledge of mirror neurons suggests that there may be more to thought transference, intersubjective fields, or energy exchanges within the therapeutic relationship, referred to in the literature as "local intuition" and perhaps most popularly as "interpersonal neurobiology"(Shapiro & Marks-Tarlow, 2021). The word intuition comes from the Latin *intueri*, suggesting both taking a look inside and having a high regard for the process (Latdict, 2023).

Though the idea of synchronicity, and the quantum mechanics involved, might be considered "woo-woo", "fringe science", or parapsychology (psi), it is nonetheless worthy of further discussion and inquiry. Just because a cause of the experience cannot be proven does not make these experiences less "real". Are "paranormal" truly "para"-normal if it is perfectly normal, based on the high numbers of people experiencing them? It may be of note that while the Greek *para* refers to "alongside, beyond; altered; contrary; irregular, abnormal", the Latin refers to preparing to defend, or "that which protects from", like parachute or parasol (Online Etymology Dictionary, 2023b). To add clout to the argument, the American Psychological Association is still publishing on psi, advertising a meta-analysis with significant findings and promoting the call for more rigorous study of these phenomena (Cardeña, 2018). While psi may be challenging to explain and study, the fact remains that many people report these experiences and find them significant. It is still unknown what causes them, or many other mind/body, subjective/objective, I/thou experiences. While counselors and other mental health providers are trained to read people and be aware of typical patterns (. . . archetypes?) we still do not claim to be able to predict the future for a particular client, nor even give advice. We simply cannot know the outcome of anyone's life, nor the "best" path. There is still so much that is a mystery, and that deserves our humble respect.

> Synchronicity designates the parallelism of time and meaning between psychic and psychophysical events, which scientific knowledge so far has been unable to reduce to a common principle. The term explains nothing, it simply formulates the occurrence of meaningful coincidences which, in themselves, are chance happenings, but are so improbable that we must assume them to be based on some kind of principle, or on some property of the empirical world . . . Synchronicity is a modern differentiation of the obsolete concept of correspondence, sympathy, and harmony. It is based not on philosophical assumptions but on empirical experience and experimentation.
>
> CW 8, p. 669, § 995

Complexes & Defenses

> Neurosis is always a substitute for legitimate suffering.
>
> CW 11, p. 105, § 129

Jung was interested in conceptualizing the internal structure of the psyche and how splitting, formation of complexes, and emotional and behavioral disturbances arise from the unconscious through symbolic representation and action (Jung, 1958). While the word "complex" has found its way into the pop-psychology lexicon, it is not as commonly used clinically. Nonetheless, it is conceptually relevant when discussing how and why symptoms emerge after a stressful experience.

If the psyche is a self-regulating system, why would we develop mental health issues? From a Jungian perspective, there must be a good reason. Because we hold the psyche and the unconscious in high regard, the very things we might call "symptoms" or "diagnosis" in the general mental health field are valued as serious attempts with an inherent meaning all their own. The disturbance is trying to tell us that the unconscious may have the answer and is trying to get our attention. However, the word "complex" itself is not pathologizing like "symptom". A complex, more broadly, is a cluster of ideas or images we have about a certain thing, with an archetypal core and emotional tone; when complexes are activated, or constellated, this is where we experience or witness a disturbance of some kind (Samuels et al., 2013). Jung considered complexes our "weak spots" (CW 6). They speak of our deepest loves as well as our deepest fears, and our emotional tones in between.

> . . . complexes are focal or nodal points of psychic life which we would not wish to do without; indeed, they should not be missing, for otherwise psychic activity would come to a fatal standstill.
>
> CW 6, p. 720, § 925

A complex is thought to be created and activated as a set of psychological schemas comprising the experience and memory of events, with subsequent thoughts, sensations, emotions, symbols, and their perceived meanings. It behaves autonomously and temporarily overtakes the conscious personality. A complex may be activated by a *stimulus word* (CW 11), like in Jung's Word Association Test, now more commonly known as a *trigger* (Siegel, 2007; van der Kolk, 2014), or a quick reminder to the parasympathetic nervous system that danger may be at hand. It was also Jung's contention that complexes play a crucial role in the structure and content of our way of knowing, remembering, patterning, and dream material (CW3; Jung, 2008) now recognized as a significant cultural consideration (Yakushko et al., 2016). There is a good deal of wisdom and history in a complex. Complexes are attempts to satisfy urges of the drives and allow us to generalize information enough to function (see Chapter 4), linking biological, cognitive, and emotional neuropathways (Escamilla et al., 2018). While they aid in our understanding of the world, complexes may also emotionally disturb, and develop into what has historically been called a *neurosis* (CW 3).

> A neurosis, as I have said, consists of two things: infantile unwillingness and a willingness to adapt.
>
> CW 10, p. 169, § 359

While ego-defenses are considered self-healing, protecting psychic material from becoming overwhelming, in cases where there is marked trauma, these complexes can become rigid, or stuck, because of their dual nature. The tension of the opposites needs to be mitigated. This defense against toxic flooding by numbing feelings aligns with even early attachment theory

(Winnicott, 1971), which has come to be known in Jungian circles as *psyche's archetypal self-care system* (Kalsched, 1996). This system is considered archetypal because it may emerge before an ego has developed, it seems to act out of control of the ego, and is found among people as an aspect of experiencing trauma around the world.

A complex can be considered our thoughts and feelings that come up around something with an archetypal core, a widespread pattern known as something that is likely a word or phrase found in many languages worldwide. For example, we know from learning and attachment theory that our earliest experiences about people and situations shape our thoughts and behavior. So it is not surprising that many complexes, or perceptions about the world, form around everyday personal experiences, like our relationship with our parents or caregivers, which ultimately forms our psychic understanding of what a Mother is, or even a Woman. We may or may not have conscious memories of our mother, but the idea of a mother is one experienced around the world. There are many different kinds of mothers. Mothers may look, feel, sound, and act very differently and be experienced in many different ways. While the thought and feeling of "mother" may be different for two people, even if they are from vastly different places, psychically or physically, there is a common idea of the phenomenon being talked about. There is an ongoing discussion in the collective right now attempting to define what a woman is (I'll not reference it here, but it's easily found on the internet). While we may be reductionistic and say that "a woman is an adult human female", the idea of a Woman is archetypal and, for many, goes beyond a simple medical definition, like Mother (also see anima in Chapter 3). While there are some common, positive, healthy associations with, say, Mother – love, home, hugs, etc. – there might be more negative associations such as abandonment, coldness, or harm, depending on individual experience.

In general, psychological defenses are vital in order to both get our needs met and be socialized creatures. Jung recognized that a certain amount of withdrawal from the external world was periodically necessary and healing, especially in times of distress, and for introverts, but only up to a point; a significant disconnect between us and the world, the conscious and unconscious mind, especially if there is a misalignment with the Self, causes suffering (CW 11). Different defense mechanisms may arise through different personae as we move through the world in our various roles. Contemporary Jungians may refer to the *archetypal defense system* when speaking of the nature and wisdom of trauma responses (Kalsched, 1996, 2013).

Several (but certainly not all) defense mechanisms are categorized in the Defense Style Questionnaire (DSQ; Andrews et al., 1993). The DSQ is used as a diagnostic tool by some in the psychodynamic world, categorizing the defenses as (1) Immature, (2) Neurotic, (3) Mature. I have taught this model several times and have to add some caveats in addition to my Jungian perspective. While we may not often hear the term "neurotic" used in most counseling circles today, it was, and still is, foundational in psychodynamic theory. It also helps explain the phenomenon of feeling, being diagnosed with, and treated for anxiety and depression together (though that practice is controversial and out of the scope of this chapter, the following studies provide more information on the phenomenon: Kaiser et al., 2021; Moncrieff et al., 2022; Mossman et al., 2021). The categorical terms "mature" and "immature" are somewhat misleading; they imply that a developmental process has occurred when that might not be true. For example, most will agree that the inappropriate use of humor is certainly not mature, as the DSQ categorizes it. Experiencing anxiety through anticipation is not necessarily more mature than somatic symptoms. Perhaps we might shift our thinking toward how conscious, integrated, adaptive, or functional a defense mechanism is. Below are several of the defense mechanisms outlined in the DSQ in three categories with notes from Jung's CW and my own musings:

1.

- *Anticipation* – We think ourselves very clever to be able to imagine and anticipate future events based on our knowledge of historical patterns of behavior, especially as counselors. This ego-centric defense mechanism is thinly guised worry at best, and fortune-telling at its worst. "As a matter of fact, most fantasies consist of anticipations. They are for the most part preparatory acts, or even psychic exercises for dealing with certain future realities" (CW 8, p. 531 § 808).
- *Humor* – Speaking of worry, Jung observed that there is a "very common displacement, and that is the disguising of a complex by the super-imposition of a contrasting mood. We frequently meet this phenomenon in people who have to banish some chronic worry. Among these people we often find the best wits, the finest humorists, whose jokes however are spiced with a grain of bitterness. Others hide their pain under a forced, convulsive cheerfulness, which because of its noisiness and artificiality ("lack of affect") makes everybody uncomfortable. (CW 3, p. 72, § 13). (Note that "displacement", though, is considered immature by the DSQ).

- *Suppression* – It is interesting to note that Jung distinguished between *suppression* and *repression* (repression is not mentioned in the DSQ but is very significant for Jungians). Suppression is more conscious, and an act of the will through ego-functioning (CW 8). "Suppression may cause worry, conflict and suffering, but it never causes a neurosis" (CW 11, p. 75, § 129). "Repression is a process that begins in early childhood under the moral influence of the environment and continues through life" (CW 7, p. 177, § 202). "Repression . . . should be clearly distinguished from suppression. Whenever you want to switch your attention from something in order to concentrate it on something else, you have to suppress the previously existing contents of consciousness, because, if you cannot disregard them, you will not be able to change your object of interest. Normally you can go back to the suppressed contents any time you like; they are always recoverable. But if they resist recovery, it may be a case of repression" (CW 17, p. 109, § 199). What is repressed is said to be cast into Shadow. (See also dissociation).
- *Sublimation* – While sublimation is typically considered the transformation of an unacceptable urge into productivity, Jung did not think this was very impressive, especially if it was unconscious. "This transfer of sexual libido from the sexual sphere to subsidiary functions is still taking place . . . Wherever this operation occurs without detriment to the adaptation of the individual we call it 'sublimation', and 'repression' when the attempt fails" (CW 4, p. 182, § 286); ". . . in other words, . . . apply it non-sexually, in the practice of an art, perhaps, or in some other good or useful activity. According to this view, it is possible for the patient, from free choice or inclination, to achieve the sublimation of his instinctual forces" (CW 7, p. 78, § 71). "When there is no need and no inexorable necessity, the 'sublimation' is merely a self-deception, a new and somewhat more subtle form of repression" (CW 8, p. 473, § 704).

2.

- *Pseudo-altruism* – Jung calls this defense *abnormal altruism.*

The main danger is direct and indirect egotism, i.e., unconsciousness of the ultimate equality of our fellow men. Indirect egotism manifests itself chiefly in an abnormal altruism, which is even capable of forcing something that seems right or good to us upon our neighbor under the disguise of Christian love, humanity and mutual help. Egotism always has the character of greed, which shows itself chiefly in three ways: the power-drive, lust, and moral laziness. These three moral evils are supplemented by a fourth which is the most powerful of all – stupidity.

CW 18, p. 612, § 1398

That's pretty harsh, but it also reinforces his firm belief that we need to do our own work before and while helping others. Jung (CW 16) first proposed the idea which has been come to be known in the mental health literature as the Wounded Healer, a dynamic that impacts the parallel process in counseling (Burton, 2021; St. Arnaud, 2017). In the ancient Greek myth, Chiron, the wise centaur (namesake of the constellation Sagittarius), was a great teacher and healer but suffered from chronic wounds. The now familiar phrase "physician heal thyself" is an ancient and multicultural one, also quoted in the Bible, and referenced by Rumi, the great Sufi poet. It speaks to us specifically as counselors because we not only tend to have a history of trauma, but put ourselves in emotional harm's way by sitting in the pain with others (McRoberts & Epstein, 2023). We can aim to work to heal these wounds and become Servant Leaders (Greenleaf, 1970).

- *Idealization* – The act of imagining the iconic version of someone or something, or holding it to an ideal, suggests a disconnect from what is, and a rejection of the Shadow. "Idealization is a hidden apotropaism; one idealizes whenever there is a secret fear to be exorcized. What is feared is the unconscious and its magical influence" (CW 9i, p. 106, § 192).

- *Reaction formation* – While Jung did not use this term specifically, he did write extensively on the tension of the opposites, polarities, and the role of the unconscious in attempting to compensate for the unlived or inauthentic life. For example:

> . . . instinctive forces influence the activity of consciousness. Whether that influence is for better or worse depends on the actual contents of the unconscious. If it contains too many things that normally ought to be conscious, then its function becomes twisted and prejudiced; motives appear that are not based on true instincts, but owe their activity to the fact that they have been consigned to the unconscious by repression or neglect. They overlay, as it were, the normal unconscious psyche and distort its natural symbol-producing function.
>
> CW 18, p. 223, § 512

3.

- *Devaluation & Denial* – In CW 7 Jung addresses the widespread devaluation and denial of the unconscious and the religious function in favor of rationalism to the great detriment of the individual and collective psyche. Denial can be at the base of many defense mechanisms, as it rejects some phenomenon to the point of refusing to acknowledge its very existence despite significant disturbance.

To push something into Shadow is to devalue it. "This mechanism of deprecation and denial naturally has to be reckoned with if one wants to adopt an objective attitude" (CW 7, p. 277, § 323).

- *Dissociation* – "Civilized life today demands concentrated, directed conscious functioning, and this entails the risk of a considerable dissociation from the unconscious. The further we are able to remove ourselves from the unconscious through directed functioning, the more readily a powerful counter-position can build up in the unconscious, and when this breaks out it may have disagreeable consequences" (CW 8, p. 100, § 139). "Repression causes what is called a *systematic amnesia*, where only specific memories or groups of ideas are withdrawn from recollection. In such cases a certain attitude or tendency can be detected on the part of the conscious mind, a deliberate intention to avoid even the bare possibility of recollection, for the very good reason that it would be painful or disagreeable (CW 17, p. 109, § 199).
- *Projection* – Jung discusses projections extensively throughout most of the CW.

> If you imagine someone who is brave enough to withdraw all his projections, then you get an individual who is conscious of a pretty thick shadow. Such a man has saddled himself with new problems and conflicts. He has become a serious problem to himself, as he is now unable to say that they do this or that, they are wrong, and they must be fought against . . . Such a man knows that whatever is wrong in the world is in himself, and if he only learns to deal with his own shadow he has done something real for the world. He has succeeded in shouldering at least an infinitesimal part of the gigantic, unsolved social problems of our day.
>
> CW 11, p. 83, § 140

Not so fast, though. Empathy is also arguably a projection (CW 7). It is an emotionally toned imagining of what another person is feeling. Empathy can be dangerous if our perceptions are skewed by our unresolved experiences, but can be a salve if it comes from a place of wisdom.

- *Somatization* – Jung discusses several cases, including patients suffering with a psychosomatic fever, psoriasis, and a distended colon: "Such experiences make it exceedingly difficult to believe that the psyche is nothing, or that an imaginary fact is unreal" (CW 11, p. 12, § 16). While somatization, from hysteria to contemporary conversion disorder, has a controversial reputation, we have a great deal of research, and a popular option that the body does, indeed, keep the score of individual and collective trauma (Maguire-Jack et al., 2019; van der Kolk, 2014).

- *Splitting* – ". . . splitting is an analytical depotentiation for the purpose of preventing too powerful impressions" (CW 4, § 106, p. 69). Splitting can occur within the psyche (such as with dissociation) or as a projection onto others (a common phenomenon in borderline personalities, or even those with black-and-white thinking, where people or situations are deemed all-good or all-bad).

Though not listed on the DSQ, Jung frequently suggests that one of the most dangerous defenses is that of exclusive *rationalism* (CW 7, CW 8), otherwise known as *concrete thinking*, *over-intellectualization*, or being stuck in *analytic mode*. Being stuck in analytic mode cuts us off from our unconscious, the richness of the associative processes, including our feelings, instincts, and wisdom of the collective. It is isolating and uprooting. Without an emotional tone or larger interpersonal context, facts in and of themselves can distort reality. The greater the hold on overt rationalism, especially in times of turmoil, the greater the potential is to form negative attitudes; the more we are dissociated from our psychic content, the more likely it is to frighten us when confronted with it, and the more likely we are to project it onto others (CW 13). Many people are actually rewarded for utilizing this defense: being rational, calm, controlled, and logical is valued in many contemporary societies. Counselors, medical doctors, and other helpers are trained to respond in this way in the face of clinical emergencies; it is also a trauma response, as we see in children who appear precocious after critical incidents. In this way, over-intellectualization can be considered a gateway, or core defense, as well as one that can easily be hidden in plain sight.

As Jungian-oriented counselors, we are to be wary of our own over-intellectualization. We are to remain aware that everyone has defense mechanisms, and respect that, but question, both in ourselves and our clients, are they more helping or hindering? How might they be related to our current level of suffering? A major task in this work is to act as a translator between the experiential-associative system and rational-analytic system (Kahneman, 2011; Shapiro & Marks-Tarlow, 2021), otherwise known as mode-shifting (see Chapter 2). We do this by actively placing ourselves in situations where that projection may take place and be worked through in the context of our relationships, including within the context of the therapeutic relationship.

Therefore, we all need to value and be aware of the language of the unconscious. Resistance may not be resistance at all but a preference for not moving forward in a relationship, or letting go of defenses (CW 3). It might also mean that our situation "rests on false assumptions" (CW 16, p. 116, § 237), such as a misaligned theoretical orientation or a misattuned therapeutic relationship. It can be frightening to even think of letting go of our defenses, to take off the mask. We could be risking everything: our livelihood, our relationships, our sense of self. That risk is very real. In order to truly let go, we need to have something better in mind, and it has to be worth it. It is important to remember that for our own work as well as our clients' as Jungian counselors. While we may earn our credentials and begin each therapeutic relationship with the end in mind, our work is never done. We must actively engage in the symbolic life on the path to individuation. To remain open, curious, and responsive to the numinous, we must also be vigilant in listening to the Self and uncovering our own Shadow material. Our profession involves our personhood. Our ethical duty is to see that our professional persona is well aligned with the Self; this requires ongoing reflective practices both individually and collectively. In order to be able to really hear what the unconscious has to say, we need to practice listening deeply. It is calling us to embark on adventures.

The Hero's Journey in Stages

As mentioned in Chapter 2, we often forget that our first nature is to seek harmony, oriented around a spiritual core, as we are becoming ourselves. We are each to be the hero of our own story on the path to individuation, which involves conflict, collaboration, integration, and growth. While counselors may be familiar with therapeutic goal setting, the unconscious has its own goals and means of getting there, too, which we, as Jungians, respect, seek to understand, and collaborate with. We have come to know that fighting what is with our egos can bring additional suffering; the Self holds deeper wisdom and peace. As a client once said to me: "Psyche don't care!".

Jung (CW 16) first introduced his four stage change model in 1929, which has been further explored by other Jungians, including analysts and art and sandplay therapists (Allan, 1988; Swan-Foster, 2018; Turner, 2005): *confession, elucidation, education,* and *transformation.* Not all Jungians conceptualize the therapeutic process in this way. However, I introduce it here to illustrate and help concretize what can sometimes seem like a long, rambling, and elusive process, both in life and in the counseling office. It is important to remember, though, that this cycle is not necessarily linear, often repeats throughout our lives, and that symbols, even those presented here, do not have definitive meanings and may not apply to everyone. Jung was also clear that this process was not to be undertaken to become "normal" or try to fix our Self. It is an adventure!

The imagining of the stages was initially influenced by *alchemy*, and the alchemical process, which can be considered the basis of both modern chemistry and psychology. This term is a stumbling block for some, though, as it conjures images of medieval, occult pseudo-science, and is sometimes taken too literally. For Jung, the alchemical process was a metaphor for both the individuation process as well as the therapeutic relationship, and reminds us today to hold the witnessing of experience with mystery: counseling is both science and art, and many hold it in in the realm of the spiritual. Alchemists may be best known for their attempts to turn *prima materia* into gold, or creating the elixir of life; remember the first book in the Harry Potter series (Rowling, 1999)? When seen symbolically, this is what we attempt to do when we decide to enter counseling: we take the raw material (*prima materia*, the elements) of our experience (known and unknown) and attempt to transform it into something that can bring about a sense of renewal that we can take forward into our lives (transmutation of the elements).

In counseling and other nurturing relationships, we think of doing this in the *vas*, or carefully chosen vessel, which acts as a kind of *holding environment* (as the attachment folks call it), a sacred space known in ancient Greek as *temenos* (CW 18; Turner, 2005; Winnicott, 1971). Here, the material may be contained, explored, and observed by the "good-enough" counselor (mimicking the good-enough mother from developmental theory). It speaks of performing experiments, a building block for learning. Ideally, this allows for a safe, dreamy, associative process of inviting up unconscious material to play with. Our role as counselors is to create a sense of "reverie" for our clients. Reverie has been described as the caregiver's role of interpreting a baby's needs so that the baby then begins to know and trust both their internal cues, and the factors that get their needs met, including relationship dynamics, that bring comfort and understanding (Knox, 2004). We must increase our tolerance for and ability to hold the "tension of the opposites" as we are presented with feelings, thoughts, and actions that may be seemingly at odds, creating unwanted chemical reactions.

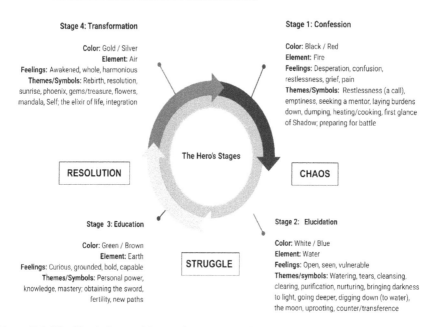

Figure 5.2 The Hero's Stages. (Copyright © R. McRoberts, 2023. Reprinted with permission. All rights reserved.)

Ultimately, though, like raising a child, we aim for the client to feel "good enough" and be aware of and maintain their own inner vas.

However, outside of the therapeutic relationship, the path to individuation has also come to be known as the Hero's Journey (Campbell, 2008; Vogler, 2020). It has been discovered to be the flexible foundation of all great myths, legends, stories, and now, movies. It is also a framework for taking the empowering perspective that we are the main character in our own life, not a bit part in someone else's story. In the diagram below (see Figure 5.2), I have illustrated Jung's four stages, along with how I see Johnathan Allan's (1988) more simplified version for children: Chaos, Struggle, and Resolution integrated in.

Confession

The act of confession can be seen in many ancient traditions, and is one of the most evident links between spiritual and psychotherapeutic practices. An act of confession may be seen as an archetypal pattern of responding to a call from the Self, embarking on a new adventure, taking on a difficult task, embracing change, asking for help, holding ourselves accountable, or becoming initiated into a new order. This confession is often needed before a ritualistic cleansing, or catharsis. An individual who feels compelled to confess something is attempting to be relieved of their burdens by laying them down in the presence of another. They have become too heavy to carry. The confessor may be overwhelmed, confused, tormented, restless, scared, grief stricken, directionless, tired, or simply bored. They may have been suffering in silence for some time and are at the point of reaching out, sometimes in desperation, in search of freedom. While we know that early intervention for traumatic incidents is ideal, it is not always the case; after a traumatic incident, or other life-changing event, it may take time for psyche to digest and make some meaning of it by allowing Shadow material to become activated.

When someone feels compelled to reach out to a Counselor, a Mentor, or Teacher (capitalized here because they are all archetypes), in an initial act of confession, we might think of Shadow material having become activated, or as we say in common American speech, "things got heated". Those first interactions may be heavily defended, very analytical, where people try to be on their best behavior and simply ask for professional opinions or specific techniques. More often, though, we see a lot of "dumping". This is often very literal with children, as they dump over baskets of toys, often into the sand. It may be more metaphorical with adults, involving several waves of various emotions. For this reason, counselors may choose not to give formal assessments in the earliest sessions, or even at all. Even though we know that people may feel relief just from reaching out, so a delayed assessment may not capture the pre-treatment data, from a Jungian perspective that is beside the point. The process involves focusing on the client's point of view, tapping into the unconscious. It may be counter-productive, then, to attempt to collect seemingly objective, quantifiable data from someone we have not built a trusting relationship with; that is incongruent with Jungian theory and counselor values.

Aspects of the Shadow may not only be repressed feelings and thoughts, but also bright aspects of the Self that have been denied in service of ego preservation. For example, this may be "telling on" something or someone we love, by speaking the truth, or giving our perspective, when the message (overtly or covertly) has been not to; to do so would be a betrayal of the current status quo of the ego or other system. It is risky, like opening up a Pandora's box, conducting a new experiment, or traveling to an unknown land. One change may lead to another, but the outcome is unknown.

Confession can bring up feelings of fear, being out of control, and wanting confirmation that we aren't "crazy" or "bad". We may not want to go deeper at first; we may just want to "tell on" ourselves and experience "symptoms", hoping act of confession will be enough. I have seen this derail some counselors utilizing CBT, when a client engages in confession right away, or again and again early on; they may call this the "crisis of the week" (insensitively, but officially known as COWS), try to get clients to save part of their story for later, or want to jump ahead to psychoeducation or other "fix it" measures. It is hard to know which way to go, what is rational or irrational, before the situation is more fully explored, consciously and unconsciously. That takes time and hard work. Unfortunately, this is the stage when a mental health diagnosis is often given, which may be premature given it is often a time of crisis and over-exposure. From a Jungian perspective, we attempt to get to know, understand, and integrate our Shadow, beyond the surface-level trauma narrative.

As the psychic alchemical process continues in the therapeutic relationship, the situation surrounding the confession continues to "cook" and may become charred or "blackened". Yes, it may burn, but this blackening is not "bad". We might think of it as a ritualistic fire, a phoenix burning before it's reborn from the ashes, or cooking techniques like spice blends adding depth of flavor and heat. We may resist going deeper into the next phase for some time, especially if a large change is anticipated. It can be hard to admit, let alone let go of, perceptions, behaviors, and relationships that have seemed to work for so long but have somehow grown intolerable. Leaving home for the first time is scary, even in the best of conditions. Shame may be infused; the idea that we are to blame for our suffering seductively suggests that we may be able to do something about it. While it may be a stumbling block, this can be a place to begin. It is often helpful to gather the support of others around us during this time and gather supplies, as one might do when planning a great journey or event. It is not uncommon for people to be either scared off, never to return again, or miraculously feel better directly after confession. Jung is said to have thought that this phase encapsulates Freud's method entirely. However, it is important to remember that confessions may happen periodically throughout our lives, and the therapeutic process, as layers of understanding develop, new opportunities present themselves, and routines and rituals emerge through the cycle.

Elucidation

During the elucidation stage, the situation becomes clearer, like moonlight shining on water in the darkness. Though the darkness might be frightening, we begin to feel a bit braver and go exploring, sometimes to places that we can only go alone. Mysteries begin to reveal themselves. Being present and reflective makes the psyche feel safer, and invited to open and align more fully. Stones dropped in the water may cause ripples radiating from the center. For example, a client might allude to situations they are not ready to discuss; a counselor may drop a feeling word that resonates with a client. Tears may be shed, sometimes without knowing the full reason why. Children may play in the water, want to wash themselves or toys. We can imagine this as a type of ritualistic cleansing. However, intrusive thoughts and feelings may not be washed away; they may only be more revealed.

Elucidate comes from the word to "draw out", and Jung notes that Adler's model of the mind starts here, on the threshold of education. It is the stage where engaging in activities and interventions may eventually lead to greater insight, but Jung cautions us that the journey still belongs to the hero and it is not over. Drawing inferences too quickly may lead to a superficial understanding of things. This is true for the Hero on their own, the client, or the counselor. After the confession, clients may be able to see the pieces more clearly and start putting them together in new ways. I often use the metaphor of clearing out the closets, skeletons and all; after things have been spread out all over the floor we can begin to decide what things are, what might be garbage that needs to be thrown out, what can be given away, and what the client wants to keep. Counselors and others on the path may feel the urge to jump in and do the work for the Hero: organizing, labeling, and giving too many directions. Jung warns that this is tempting for many, but ultimately short-sighted, and disempowering.

It is a phase where the heart of the matter ideally becomes revealed in its own time. Digging up the roots of a plant to see how it's growing is not recommended. However, the counselor's questions and directive interventions at this point often are doing just that: leaving the client truly over-exposed and vulnerable. Trying to "find out" or "figure out" where the Hero has come from or what they are doing so that we can be more helpful is often the opposite; it can be shocking, uprooting, and disorienting to be told about oneself. The Hero must struggle to grow, and deserves to be tended to, but Jung says "no amount of confession and no amount of explaining can make the crooked plant grow straight, but that it must be trained upon the trellis of the norm by the gardener's art" (CW 16, p. 68, § 153). When I read this, in the context of Jung's question of attempts of authority over the Self, whether that be, say, the ego of the Hero, the norms of society, the method employed, or the counselor themselves, I wonder who the gardener is. Like most symbols, I think it may be complex and hold multiple meanings. People may get stuck in the confession phase and fail to grow; this may happen for many reasons: because they are not in the right environment or are not being tended properly, either by negligence, ignorance, or will. The nature of the process must be known, and details are important to reveal, but all in good time.

Education

The stage of education is sometimes overlooked completely by some Jungians, or is not formally accounted for. However, for those already working within an Adlerian, CBT, or trauma-informed model of counselor, or from our own educational experiences, we tend to value it. Education can be empowering. Knowledge can ground us. While a Jungian perspective highly values the unconscious, it also acknowledges that we live, move, and interact with the world around us, and need egos familiar with this knowledge. Psychoeducation can be helpful in understanding both the "why" and "how" of our experiences. It can help give words to sensations never before described, normalize experiences, and provide procedures for practicing new skills which can be empowering. Education can be grounding, validating, normalizing, and empowering. Psychoeducation topics may include:

- identifying thoughts, feelings, and behaviors (which fits well into a TF/CBT model)
- providing greater knowledge of the counseling process: the therapeutic powers of play, dynamics of healthy relationships, how art may be helpful, why we value the unconscious, etc.
- treatment planning
- dream journaling/analysis
- active imagination
- archetypal and symbolic content in stories, myths, fairy tales, current events
- coping skills (grounding/relaxation techniques, thought stopping, mindfulness)
- assertive communication skills

- psychopharmacology – encouraging clients to speak with their providers
- research on topics that arise.

In addition, clients may show interest in educating us about their interests. Like the old adage goes, if you want to really learn something, teach it. By allowing space for clients to be the expert during sessions, they may reinforce their desire to engage in that process. Our response of interest and curiosity may also assist in this reinforcement. Education can serve as a foundation for unconscious material to take root in the conscious mind. Any gardener knows that different plants require different soil conditions, preparing and tending the beds accordingly for optimal growth.

It is important to note, though, that Jung did not agree with Adler's method of focusing too much on education in psychotherapy, nor the medicalized model that was developing and contributing to a generalized favoring of the conscious over the unconscious in society; Jung did, though appreciate developments that were happening in the areas of self-education, and saw his method as being an approach to wellness (CW 16). Jung made significant contributions to the self-help movement, the history of women becoming analysts (Kirsch, 2000), and I'd argue, by proxy, counselors. This Jungian tradition of treating the well, though, and questioning of the medical model, which has been continued to this day, I think has been a double edged sword: it could be argued that it has both led an aura of exclusivity around Jungian analysis and pushed the Jungian value of the scientific into Shadow. Remember, Jung considered himself more a scientist than a philosopher, valuing the systematic study of phenomenology. The reduction of his work to largely the treatment of potential analysts-in-training and self-help gurus, in addition to the resistance of the Jungian movement on a whole to embrace quality research methods has, unfortunately, resulted in a general devaluing of his work in the American mental health field. As readers will note across this book I see Jungian concepts being researched without giving him credit, perhaps because of the stigma that to mention his name is somehow unprofessional or unscientific.

Like a lot of self-help, while it can seem, and be, empowering, there's also a lot of junk out there, and people doing psycho-spiritual work without formal training calling themselves Jungians. Jung suggested that self-improvement should take precedence over compulsion, but in the digital age, with endless access to information, self-improvement has *become* a compulsion. "Being taught" isn't the same as "learning". Real education is not just about consuming data collected from anywhere; it's a process that takes discernment, discipline, critical thinking, practical application, and mentorship. It's about following the path, being led by the Self, exploring possibilities that are interesting to us, learning from experience and wise teachers. Education, ideally, leads to integration and transformation.

Transformation

The last stage is transformation. The quest has been completed. We've been met with many challenges, learned valuable lessons, and have encountered, found, and been reunited with our Self. Here, unconscious material is consciously assimilated. We no longer need to be either/or; we can be both/and. We accept that we all have light and dark sides. We acknowledge that we have a body, mind, and spirit and through the work toward developing harmony, may feel more integrated. We might imagine a newborn phoenix rising from the ashes. We might feel like we've come up for air, can breathe again, feel lighter, relieved, and free of old habits and burdens. There's a great sense of peace. We might attempt to spread our wings and fly again, returning home only to leave the nest again. This is not always the end of the story, nor the end of counseling. As we say in the field of addictions, we never really "arrive". Our conscious awareness of unconscious material is an ongoing process that requires maintenance. To paraphrase Jung, we can never be cured of our human experience, including our suffering; the only real "cure" is change, along the path of individuation (CW 16).

Jung suggests that we all go through this process, and as those who treat others, are ethically bound to be mindful of that (CW 16). As counselors, we experience and interpret another's happening subjectively which requires us to continue to do our own work. Just because we may know about the process, and take the responsibility, even, to respond to others on their journey appropriately and with empathy, does not excuse us from going on our own journeys. In fact, Jungians embrace the fact that if we are open to the experience, the therapeutic process is truly a dialectic – both the client and the counselor are transformed. We are called to continue to seek and be refreshed in our awareness, so as not to forget, and continue living the symbolic life. As Jungian counselors we are faced now with a challenge: to continue to become the people we are meant to become, as we walk with others doing the same.

Reflections

1. Choose an active, accessible symbol from your life. It may be one that has been with you since childhood. What is it? When do you access it? How? What about it might change or stay the same? Have you had any dreams about it? You might choose to draw, paint, or look up pictures of it. You might also imagine what it might say to you. Does it have a message it wants you to hear?

2. Have you ever experienced a synchronicity? How about someone you know? If so, you might consider writing down everything you remember about it. Give time and attention to the feeling tone and perceived meaning of the event. What were the paralleling events (inner and outer)? What images or other symbolic material was involved?

3. Taking a look at the list of defense mechanisms above which might be one of yours? Where do you think you learned how to do it? How has it served you well? How might it be getting in your way?

4. Do you think you've been on a Hero's Journey? If so, I encourage you to map it out a bit. Who were the characters in your story? What were the challenges, lessons learned, and resolution?

REFERENCES

Alcaro, A., Carta, S., & Panksepp, J. (2017). The affective core of the Self: A neuro-archetypical perspective on the foundations of human (and animal) subjectivity. *Frontiers in Psychology*, 8(1424), 1–13. https://doi.org/10.3389/fpsyg.2017.01424

Allan, J. (1988). *Inscapes of the child's world: Jungian counseling in schools and clinics.* Spring Publications.

Allison, J. E. (2019). *Revelations of spirit: Synchronicity as a spiritual path in a secular age.* [Doctoral dissertation]. ProQuest: 13815167. https://media.proquest.com/media/hms/ORIG/2/HpkiH?_s=xMEDYK4uMiHwod4V5btruXZIkuY%3D

Andrews, G., Singh, M., & Bond, M. (1993). The Defense Style Questionnaire. *Journal of Nervous and Mental Diseases, 181*(4), 246–256. doi:10.1097/00005053-199304000-00006.

Archive for Research on Archetypal Symbolism (ARAS). (2023). About. https://aras.org/about

Atmanspacher, H., & Fuchs, C. A. (Eds.). (2014). *The Pauli–Jung conjecture and its impact today*. Imprint Academic.

Beitman, B. D. (2011). Coincidence studies. *Psychiatric Annals, 41*, 561–571. doi:10.3928/00485713-20111104-03.

Bohm, D., & Peat, F. D. (1987). *Science, order and creativity*. Bantam Books.

Bradshaw, S. & Storm, L. (2013) Archetypes, symbols and the apprehension of meaning. *International Journal of Jungian Studies, 5*(2), 154–176. doi:10.1080/1 9409052.2012.685662

Brewster, F. (2020). The racial complex: A Jungian perspective on culture and race. Routledge.

Brewster, F. (2023). *Race and the unconscious*. Routledge.

Burton, N. (2021, February 20). The myth of Chiron, the wounded healer. *Psychology Today*. www.psychologytoday.com/us/blog/hide-and-seek/202102/the-myth-chiron-the-wounded-healer

Campbell, J. (2008). *The hero with a thousand faces* (3rd ed.). New World Library. (Original work published 1949).

Cardeña, E. (2018). The experimental evidence for parapsychological phenomena: A review. *American Psychologist, 73*(5), 663–677. https://doi.org/10.1037/ amp0000236

Chalmers, D. J. (1995). Facing up to the problem of consciousness. *Journal of Consciousness Studies, 2*(3), 200–219. https://consc.net/papers/facing.html

Colman, W. (2011). Synchronicity and the meaning-making psyche. *The Journal of Analytical Psychology, 56*(4), 471–491. https://doi.org/10.1111/j.1468-5922. 2011.01924.x

Cromer, L. D., Stimson, J. R., Rischard, M. E., & Buck, T. R. (2022). Nightmare prevalence in an outpatient pediatric psychiatry population: A brief report. *Dreaming, 32*(4), 353–355. https://doi.org/10.1037/drm0000225

Dawkins, R. (1976). *The selfish gene*. Oxford University Press.

Escamilla, M., Sandoval, H., Calhoun, V., & Ramirez, M. (2018). Brain activation patterns in response to complex triggers in the Word Association Test: Results from a new study in the United States. *The Journal of Analytical Psychology, 63*(4), 484–509. https://doi.org/10.1111/1468-5922.12430

Etter, H. F. (2020). Synchronicity and "being endowed with meaning". *Psychological Perspectives, 63*, 106–115. doi:10.1080/00332925.2020.1739469.

Franks, D. D. (2003). Mutual interests, different lenses: Current neuroscience and symbolic interaction. *Symbolic Interaction, 26*(4), 613–630. https://doi. org/10.1525/si.2003.26.4.613

Freud, S. (1955). *The interpretation of dreams*. Basic Books.

Goodwyn, E. (2022). Archetypes and clinical application: How the genome responds to experience. *Journal of Analytical Psychology, 67*(3), 838–859. doi:10.1111/1468-5922.12821.

Greenleaf, R. (1970). *The servant as leader*. www.greenleaf.org/products-page/the-servant-as-leader/

Gullatz, S., & Gildersleeve, M. (2018). Freedom and the psychoanalytic ontology of quantum physics. *The Journal of Analytical Psychology, 63*(1), 85–105. https://doi.org/10.1111/1468-5922.12381

Hocoy, D. (2012). Sixty years later: The enduring allure of synchronicity. *Journal of Humanistic Psychology, 52*(4), 467–478. https://doi.org/ 10.1177/0022167812436427

Hoss, R. J. (2018). *Learning in dreams: Psychological growth*. The International Association for the Study of Dreams: Brain Awareness Week. www.asdreams.org/baw-learningindreams/

International Association for the Study of Dreams. (2023). Home page. www.asdreams.org/

Jeffery, S. (2018). *The ultimate list of archetypes*. https://scottjeffrey.com/archetypes-list/#Jungian_Archetypes_List

Jung, C. G. (1958). *Psyche and symbol*. V. S. de Laszlo (Ed.). Doubleday & Company.

Jung, C. G. (1973). *C.G. Jung Letters: Volume 1, 1906–1950*. G. Adler, A. Jaffe et al. (Eds.), R. F. C. Hull (Trans.). Routledge.

Jung, C. G. (1974). *Dreams*. R. F. C. Hul. (Trans.). Princeton University Press.

Jung, C. G. (1976). *Letters of C. G. Jung, Volume 2*. Routledge and Kegan Paul.

Jung, C. G. (2008). *Children's dreams: Notes from the seminar given in 1936–1940*. L. Jung & M. Meyer-Gress (Eds.). Princeton University Press.

Jung, C. G. (2023). *The collected works of C. G. Jung: Revised and expanded complete digital edition*. (CW 1–20). G. Adler, W. McGuire, & H. Read (Eds.), R. F. C. Hull (Trans.). Princeton University Press. https://press.princeton.edu/books/ebook/9780691255194/the-collected-works-of-c-g-jung

Kahneman, D. (2011). *Thinking, fast and slow*. Farrar, Straus and Giroux.

Kaiser, T., Herzog, P., Voderholzer, U., & Brakemeier, E. (2021). Unraveling the comorbidity of depression and anxiety in a large inpatient sample: Network analysis to examine bridge symptoms. *Depression and Anxiety, 38*, 307–317. https://doi.org/10.1002/da.23136

Kalsched, D. (1996). *The inner world of trauma: Archetypal defenses of the personal spirit*. Routledge.

Kalsched, D. (2013). *Trauma and the soul: A psycho-spiritual approach to human development and its interruption.* Routledge.

Kirsch, T. S. (2000). *The Jungians: A comparative and historical perspective.* Routledge.

Knox, J. (2004). From archetypes to reflective function. *Journal of Analytical Psychology, 49,* 1–19. https://doi.org/10.1111/j.0021-8774.2004.0437.x

Landreth, G. (2024). *Play therapy: The art of the relationship.* Routledge. (Original work published 1991).

Latdict. (2023). *Latin definition for: intueor, intueri, intuitus.* Latin Dictionary and Grammar Resources. https://latin-dictionary.net/definition/24587/intueor-intueri-intuitus

Loue, S. (2015) Ethical issues in sandplay research. In Loue S. (eds.) *Ethical issues in sandplay therapy practice and research.* Springer. https://doi.org/10.1007/978-3-319-14118-3_5

Lucero, I. (2018). Written in the body? Healing the epigenetic molecular wounds of complex trauma through empathy and kindness. *Journal of Child and Adolescent Trauma, 11,* 443–455. doi:10.1007/s40653-018-0205-0.

Maguire-Jack, K., Lanier, P., & Lombardi, B. (2019). Investigating racial differences in clusters of adverse childhood experiences. *American Journal of Orthopsychiatry, 90*(1), 106–114. https://doi.org/10.1037/ort0000405

Main, R. (2007). *Revelations of chance: Synchronicity as spiritual experience.* The State University of New York Press.

McRoberts, R. (2023). The white rabbit: Sacred & subversive. The Archive for Research in Archetypal Symbolism. *ARAS Connections: Image and Archetype, 2,* 1–32. https://aras.org/newsletters/aras-connections-image-and-archetype-2023-issue-2

McRoberts, R., & Epstein, J. (2023). Creative self-concept, post-traumatic growth, and professional identity resilience in counselors with traumatic experiences: A canonical correlation analysis. *Journal of Creativity in Mental Health.* doi:10.1080/15401383.2023.2232730

Moncrieff, J., Cooper, R. E., Stockmann, T., et al. (2022). The serotonin theory of depression: A systematic umbrella review of the evidence. *Molecular Psychiatry.* https://doi.org/10.1038/s41380-022-01661-0

Morsella, E., Godwin, C., Jantz, T., Krieger, S., & Gazzaley, A. (2016). Homing in on consciousness in the nervous system: An action-based synthesis. *Behavioral and Brain Sciences, 39,* E168. doi:10.1017/S0140525X15000643.

Mossman, S. A., Mills, J. A., Walkup, J. T., & Strawn, J. R. (2021). The impact of failed antidepressant trials on outcomes in children and adolescents with anxiety and depression: A systematic review and meta-analysis. *Journal of Child and Adolescent Psychopharmacology, 31*(4), 259–267. https://doi.org/10.1089/cap.2020.0195

Myss, C. (2003). *Archetype cards.* Hay House.

Online Etymology Dictionary. (2023a). *Archetype.* www.etymonline.com/word/archetype#etymonline_v_16958

Online Etymology Dictionary. (2023b). *Para-.* www.etymonline.com/word/para-?ref=etymonline_crossreference#etymonline_v_7162

Online Etymology Dictionary. (2023c). *Synchronous.* www.etymonline.com/word/synchronous?ref=etymonline_crossreference

Pasciuti, F. (2011). Measurement of synchronicity in a clinical context. *Psychiatric Annals, 41*(12), 590–597. doi:10.3928/00485713-20111104-07.

Perry, B. D. (2004) *Understanding traumatized and maltreated children: The core concepts.* Video Training Series 1. The Child Trauma Academy. www.childtrauma.org

Ray, D. (2004). Supervision of basic and advanced skills in play therapy. *Journal of Professional Counseling Practice, Theory, and Research, 32*(2), 28–41.

Roesler, C. (2020). *Structural dream analysis: Manual and case illustration.* https://iaap.org/wp-content/uploads/2020/01/Manual-Structural-dream-analysis-engl-2.pdf

Roesler, C. (2022). *Development of a reconceptualization of archetype theory: Report to the IAAP.* https://iaap.org/wp-content/uploads/2022/04/Report-Archetype-Theory-Roesler-1.pdf

Roesler, C. (2024). *Deconstructing archetype theory: A critical analysis of Jungian ideas.* Routledge.

Rosen, D. H., Smith, S. M., Huston, H. L., & Gonzalez, G. (1991). Empirical study of associations between symbols and their meanings: Evidence of collective unconscious (archetypal) memory. *The Journal of Analytical Psychology, 36*(2), 211–228. https://doi.org/10.1111/j.1465-5922.1991.00211.x

Rowling, J. K. (1999). *Harry Potter and the sorcerer's stone.* Scholastic.

Roxburgh, E. C., Ridgway, S., & Roe, C. A. (2016). Synchronicity in the therapeutic setting: A survey of practitioners. *Counselling & Psychotherapy Research, 16*(1), 44–53. https://doi.org/10.1002/capr.12057

Russo-Netzer, P., & Icekson, T. (2022). Engaging with life: Synchronicity experiences as a pathway to meaning and personal growth. *Current Psychology: A Journal for Diverse Perspectives on Diverse Psychological Issues, 41*(2), 597–610. https://doi.org/10.1007/s12144-019-00595-1

Sacco, R. G. (2019). The predictability of synchronicity experience: Results from a survey of Jungian analysts. *International Journal of Psychological Studies, 11*(3), 46–62. doi:10.5539/ijps.v11n3p46

Samuels, A., Shorter, B., & Plaut, F. (2013). *A critical dictionary of Jungian analysis.* Routledge.

Shapiro, Y., & Marks-Tarlow, T. (2021). Varieties of clinical intuition: Explicit, implicit, and nonlocal neurodynamics. *Psychoanalytic Dialogues, 31*(3), 262–281. https://doi.org/10.1080/10481885.2021.1902744

Siegel, D. (2007). *The mindful brain.* Norton.

St. Arnaud, K. O. (2017). Encountering the wounded healer: Parallel process and supervision. *Canadian Journal of Counseling and Psychotherapy, 51*(2), 131–144. https://cjc-rcc.ucalgary.ca/article/view/61147

Stevens, A. (1998). *Ariadne's clue: A guide to the symbols of humankind.* Princeton University Press.

Swan-Foster, N. (2018). *Jungian art therapy: A guide to dreams, images, and analytical psychology.* Routledge.

Turner, B. A. (2005). *The handbook of sandplay therapy.* Temenos Press.

van der Kolk, B. (2014). *The body keeps the score: Mind, brain and body in the transformation of trauma.* Penguin Books.

Vogler, C. (2020). *The writer's journey: Mythic structure for writers.* Michael Wiese Productions. (Original work published 1998).

Winnicott, D. W. (1971). *Playing and reality.* Basic Books.

World Science Festival. (2022, November 17). *The dreaming mind: Waking the mysteries of sleep.* Big Ideas Series, John Templeton Foundation. https://youtu.be/wvvovktKKa4

Yakushko, O., Miles, P., Rajan, I., Bujko, B., & Thomas, D. (2016). Cultural unconscious in research: Integrating multicultural and depth paradigms in qualitative research. *The Journal of Analytical Psychology, 61*(5), 656–675. http://dx.doi.org/10.1111/1468-5922.12257

Yehuda, R., & Lehrner, A. (2018). Intergenerational transmission of trauma effects: Putative role of epigenetic mechanisms. *World Psychiatry, 17*(3), 243–257. doi:10.1002/wps.20568.

6
Space & Time Together

The Role of the Counselor

The process is "a dialectical relationship . . . It is an encounter, a discussion between two psychic wholes, in which knowledge is used only as a tool. The goal is transformation – not one that is predetermined, but rather an indeterminable change.
Jung, CW 11, p. 554, § 904

As we discussed briefly in Chapters 2 and 5, the therapeutic process begins with the relationship and the safe container which we may refer to as the vas.

> The bottle is an artificial human product and thus signifies the intellectual purposefulness and artificiality of the procedure, whose obvious aim is to isolate the spirit from the surrounding medium. As the vas Hermeticum of alchemy, it was "hermetically" sealed (i.e., sealed with the sign of Hermes); it had to be made of glass, and had also to be as round as possible, since it was meant to represent the cosmos in which the earth was created. Transparent glass is something like solidified water or air, both of which are synonyms for spirit. The alchemical retort is therefore equivalent to the anima mundi, which according to an old alchemical conception surrounds the cosmos. Caesarius of Heisterbach (thirteenth century) mentions a vision in which the soul appeared as a spherical glass vessel. Likewise the "spiritual" or "ethereal" (aethereus) Philosophers' Stone is a precious vitrum (sometimes described as malleabile) which was often equated with the gold glass (aurum vitreum) of the heavenly Jerusalem (Rev. 21: 21)
>
> CW 13 pp. 197–198, § 245

We might say that the vas, the "bottle", or the holding space of the therapeutic relationship/process is, indeed, "artificial" in that, while as real as any other relationship, it is a unique and professional one, with transparency, "hermetically sealed" with purposeful, protective, ethical boundaries. Counselors are to provide adequate space ("as round as possible") for

DOI: 10.4324/9781003433736-6

the client to listen to their Self, and not impose our own will, no matter how well-intentioned.

> Through imitation, one's own values become reactivated. If the way to imitation is cut off, they are nipped in the bud. The result is helpless anxiety. If the imitation is a demand made by the analyst, i.e., if it is a demand for the sake of adaptation, this again leads to a destruction of the patient's values, because imitation is an automatic process that follows its own laws, and lasts as long and goes as far as is necessary. It has quite definite limits which the analyst can never know. Through imitation the patient learns individuation, because it reactivates his own values.
>
> CW 18, p. 453, § 1100

This describes the importance of unconditional positive regard (from a humanistic perspective) or mirroring (interpersonal neurobiology) for our client. We are to reflect on what we see in our clients without an agenda so they might engage their own reflective function (Penner et al., 2019). At the same time, we know that people turn to counselors for "answers"; even though we might attest that we don't give advice, that we're not a model for living, clients will listen to us as an authority because they have chosen to trust in us, and perhaps the authority of our State-issued credentials. That is power to be used wisely. This is to occur even, and especially, when our client is "being resistant", playing around, or seemingly being phony (remember what Jung said about the personae). At this point, counselors may confront their clients, thinking they are wasting time, or otherwise not ready to do the work. The Jungian-oriented counselor may be more hip to the ego's defenses here, and not push our agenda that a client should behave a certain way in counseling. It's their time. The unconscious cannot be rushed. This also reflects the American Counseling Association's (ACA, 2014) expectation that we not impose our values and beliefs onto our clients. This is their journey, their process; we are merely hired guides and co-travelers for a time.

Briefly, though, we're soon to run into another parallel between Jungian and person-centered counseling theory: counselors, especially those in training, often have difficulty believing in their core that their clients can solve their own problems, and trusting that they, the counselors, are "doing enough" by "just" assisting in creating the vas, or sacred, safe space and providing nurturing support and engaging in empathic confrontation. They, like others in the world, feel a pressure to DO MORE and BE MORE, but are encouraged to do so with their egos: by attempting to control the performance of their lives, by achieving, by pleasing others.

On the most basic level, inspired by counselor professional ethics and Jungian play therapist JP Lilly (2015) I see the primary responsibilities of the Jungian-oriented counselor to be:

1. a witness
2. a container (the *vas*; what sandplay therapists call *the safe and protected space*; and what other psychodynamic folks call *setting* or *holding the frame*)
3. a collaborator and co-interpreter.

The foundation of the therapeutic relationship begins ideally begins in a relaxed state, known in Jungian terms as *reverie* (Bravesmith, 2008; CW 16), and the safe, protected space (Kalff, 2020) of the therapeutic relationship, more widely known as *temenos* (CW 18; Turner, 2005). The word temenos goes back to the ancient Greek, sharing a root with the word *temple*, denoting a sacred space set apart from common land, a place of sanctuary for refuge, reverence, and quiet contemplation (Online Etymology Dictionary, 2023). The therapeutic relationship is ideally accepting of awareness and containment, first in the therapist's mind and then in the client's, much like an attentive caregiver's awareness and meeting of an infant's needs.

To truly collaborate with our clients, they need to be able to consent to the relationship and be informed about what that means. That involves knowing a bit about who we are, an idea about what to expect, and that they have the freedom to participate in or refuse activities with us. Both client-centered and Jungian approaches recognize that this is a process that can take time. Clients need to feel safe in order to allow defenses to drop so they can be seen. The ability for us to safely hold professional boundaries and contain psychic discharge in the relationship starts from the beginning, with informed consent.

INFORMED CONSENT & SAFETY

Informed consent should be both a formal document (see below) as well as an ongoing process. One of my favorite definitions for informed consent is from the Tennessee Department of Mental Health and Substance Abuse Services (2013, p. 363) which states that it should be:

voluntarily given in writing after sufficient explanation and disclosure of the subject matter involved to enable the person whose consent is sought to make a knowing and willful decision without an element of force, fraud, deceit, duress, or other form of constraint or coercion.

In most states, "informed consent" is a legal definition, and in more than half the states, minors, usually teenagers, legally may give their own informed consent or refuse voluntary mental health treatment (World Population Review, 2023). I wrote an article for the *Play Therapy Magazine* (McRoberts, 2018) about how I think it is important to obtain not only the LEGAL informed consent document, but the ETHICAL assent, or the child's agreement to engage in counseling. That requires us to respect the child client as a person, and make sure that we explain the counseling process at a developmental level they can understand, offer choices in the playroom, and see that we keep the relationship sacred (APT, 2022).

Informed consent begins with the counselor disclosing who they are, their credentials, what services they provide, how they determine the course of treatment, and what that might look like, including risks and benefits. It should be made clear verbally and in writing that the client has the right to refuse any treatment, activity, or intervention at any time. This includes children! We need to make sure that people regardless of age know who we are, that they are free to say or do whatever they like in our office (within certain limits), and that we will respect their privacy (within certain limits). For a young child that may sound like:

"Hi. My name is ___. I'm a [counselor and a play therapist]. That means that kids come to me and can talk about whatever they want and play with the toys in my office here almost any way they want to. I keep whatever the kids say to me private. But the kids can tell whomever they want what they say and do in the playroom. Sometimes I'll let you know if I think it's a good idea to tell your [mom/dad/caregiver] something, or if they want to have a meeting. We can talk about what you want me to say or not say. The only time I HAVE to tell is if I think someone has gotten hurt or could get hurt. Do you have any questions?". If they don't, then I ask them to sign their name, or make a mark if they can't write yet, right next to their parent or guardian's name; most kids love this part!

Sometimes a child may be brought to counseling against their will. I've had clients say they were "forced" or even "tricked" into coming to my office for the first time; one client said they thought they were just being taken somewhere to get something to eat! I don't think this is ok and I let them know that. I apologize, and often will ask, after I tell them who I am, why their parents or other grown-up in their life might have brought them to see me. Most of the time they have some idea. Then I explain my informed consent form. I let them know that we can spend our time together almost however they want. Then I ask them if they want to stay. Most kids say "yes".

Informed consent defines the boundaries and purpose of the counseling relationship, which in turn helps to create a sense of safety, for both the counselor and the client. This sense of safety is the foundation for building the therapeutic alliance.

THE THERAPEUTIC ALLIANCE

The therapeutic alliance, sometimes called the "working alliance" or "therapeutic relationship", is everything and begins from the first moment of interaction. It cannot exist without informed consent, safety, and buy-in from our clients. There is some discussion in the field if there is a distinction between the two; if we can parse out what is essentially Us and what it is that we do in the context of the relationship (O'Connor & Ray, 2023). Nonetheless, we need to buy what we're selling. And don't be selling junk! The youngest of clients, and especially those who've experienced trauma, can smell a fake a mile away. Counseling is a relationship. It's professional, but it better be a REAL relationship. Without alignment, the relationship is not working.

Clients may spend a good deal of time looking for the right counselor. These days, that happens quite often online. They may ask their friends on social media, do a broad internet search, or go onto various platforms seeking their idea of the ideal counselor. What they find online about their potential counselor and those initial meetings can have a real impact. It has been recognized for some time that people may be more likely to trust someone who looks like them, shares their culture or values, or that they assume will be more likely to relate to them (Meyer & Zane, 2013). For these reasons we need to be mindful about our online presence, and our level of comfortable alignment with the personal and professional. Who are we reaching out to and why? Are we showing up on platforms where they can find us?

Clients are also becoming savvy consumers. Some agencies even call their clients "consumers" though I don't prefer the term. Nonetheless, our method is part of our "brand", along with who we are. Clients may have never been to counseling before and don't know what to expect. Or, they may have tried various methods before and want more of that, or another. However they find us, we know that we have to believe in our method ourselves, not only because Jung suggests it, but because the clients need to feel safe and secure enough to buy into the process. In other words, we need to buy what we're selling. This installation of hope, that we believe that the method works, and therefore believe in ourselves, not only builds up the therapeutic alliance but is one of the best predictors of positive outcomes in therapy (Wampold & Imel, 2015).

We have an obligation to let clients in on what they're signing up for. That means describing what a therapeutic relationship looks like. We cannot assume that the client will know or feel comfortable just figuring it out. It's not empowering to keep someone guessing. Allan (1988) identifies a framework for a Jungian way of being in therapeutic relationship which includes:

- believing that talking about situations, thoughts, and feelings is helpful
- active observation of thoughts, behaviors, and affect
- the use of active listening
- the selective and minimal use of questioning and limit setting
- the use of the therapist's sense of self, communicating thoughts, feelings, and perceptions timed appropriately, in service of the client.

This framework is clear, straightforward, and could easily be added to intake paperwork to describe what a client might expect in counseling (along with policies and procedures, including HIPAA guidelines). The inclusion of developing routines and rituals together, especially around beginnings and endings, is recommended, to engage the religious function. When well attuned, this tends to happen naturally. We might notice how a client tends to prefer to start and stop sessions. It can be as simple as taking a quiet moment and a deep breath; lighting or blowing out a carefully placed candle; an inside joke; finishing a cup of tea; or a pinky-promise to be a safe person and see you next week.

In-Person & Online

The space that we create to invite our clients and potential clients into matters. Today, the first time a client reaches out to a new counselor is online. We should consider elements found on the site and choose them intentionally, remembering that visual communication is symbolic. You may ask yourself why you chose each element as well as what other cultures or individuals might think or feel about them. What is both true and comfortable to you and your style, while being considerate of others? A word we might imagine is "hospitable". Some considerations are as follows:

- Do you prefer warm, cool, or neutral colors? There is no "right" color, but some can be over (vibrant/clashing) or under (deep/muddy) stimulating. Consider your population as well as your own tastes. Pops of color, such as throw pillows or even the toys/miniatures on the shelves might be enough in an otherwise neutral palette.

- Does the space feel more cozy or airy? Lived-in or clear? Wide open spaces can sometimes feel too vacuous; overcrowded spaces can prompt anxiety. A well-planned break up of space, with activity nooks (art, sand, books, snacks), is ideal for in-person. Having some items in baskets, behind curtains or cupboard doors can also aid in organization and overstimulation. Avoid sitting behind a desk or with your back to your client or the door. Lighting should be soft, so overheads and bright fluorescents should be avoided.

- Seating and our body posture should also be considered. In-person, clients of various body types should feel free to sit comfortably. A bit of variety is ideal: beanbags are popular with children and teens, loveseats and slipper chairs can accommodate larger bodies or multiple people. Does your seat provide you with both adequate support and freedom of movement? Online, consider how far you are sitting from the computer. Does it mirror how close you would sit to someone in-person? Observe others' conversational distance and accommodate based on preferences you feel and notice. Where are you in the frame of the camera? Aim to be near the center to avoid looking up or down at the client.

- What materials do you have for your clients to use? These materials should be selected carefully based on your training, conditions of the environment, preferences, and client's needs. They may range from art supplies to sandtrays and a collection of miniatures (see Chapter 7 for further discussion). Are materials out for clients to use freely or are they tucked away for when you think the client may be ready for them? These decisions may be made based on the age range of your clients, additional preparation needed for messy projects, or your integration of other therapist-led interventions.

Presence & Value

> Values are chiefly created by the quality of one's subjective reactions. This is not to deny the existence of "objective" values altogether; only, their validity depends upon the consensus of opinion.
>
> CW 5, p. 150, § 126

A Jungian perspective to counseling focuses on the presence and value of the counselor, the client, and, perhaps most uniquely, the unconscious processes and symbolic material. The counselor must be able to hold the space and be receptive both to the client and the symbolic material. It deserves a greater mention that the ongoing maintenance of overall wellness and ego-Self alignment is important for the counselor as well as the client.

Counseling itself is not value free. ACA (2014) lists the following core professional values as the foundation of our ethical practice:

1. enhancing human development throughout the life span
2. honoring diversity and embracing a multicultural approach in support of worth, dignity, potential
3. uniqueness of people within their social and cultural contexts
4. promoting social justice
5. safeguarding the integrity of the counselor–client relationship
6. practicing in a competent and ethical manner.

The Jungian approach also shares these values. It's been suggested many Jungians would not even want another book attempting to pin down a Jungian method because it is so individually tailored to personality, preferences, and needs (Kottman, 2014). These values extend from the counselor to the client, how the client experiences the counselor (Meyer & Zane, 2013), and the symbolic material from the unconscious; the values of our ancestors from generations ago may also emerge.

Before we begin to practice counseling from a Jungian perspective we need to know who we are and intentionally craft a description of our practice. Writing this out not only can assist us in becoming clearer ourselves, but is ethical, and can also serve as vital pieces of our documentation and define the boundaries of our therapeutic frame. Professional dispositions are often elusive, reflecting personality traits, values, and skills, but are emerging as assessments in CACREP programs (Christensen et al., 2018). The ACA Code of Ethics (2014) encourages us to explore our own cultural identities and values and utilize methods that are well aligned and grounded in theory. Our Multicultural & Social Justice Competencies in Counseling (MCSCC; Ratts et al., 2016) go further in describing what these are and how to remain culturally alert. Hanging out in Jungian circles, as well as engaging in reflective and creative practices, can inspire us to continue to dig deeper and remain curious. For example, I continue to struggle with the word "Caucasian". I don't identify with it as a white woman, and find myself educating people about it at least once a semester. Here's some history: German doctor Johann Blumenbach developed the first official human taxonomy in the late 1700s, which was first introduced to us in English in 1807 through a translation by Dr. William Lawrence (Painter, 2003). Blumenbach examined the skulls and skin of people from around the world, categorizing and ranking them by his own aesthetics and interpretation of theology, with "Caucasians" at the top. It was Blumenbach's assessment that because the Christian myth claims in the book of Genesis that Noah's Arc landed in the Mountains of Ararat, known today as the Caucasus Mountains, where Mount Ararat, in Eastern Turkey, is located, that white people were the first humans. While the story remains, the science widely accepted today suggests otherwise. Nonetheless, the people of the Caucasus are a diverse indigenous population, including dozens of distinct ethnicities and languages in the region between Eastern Europe and Asia; the area, about as big as California, includes parts of Armenia, Azerbaijan, Georgia, Iran, Turkey, and Russia (Hays, 2016; Internet Encyclopedia of Ukraine, 2023; Transcaucasian Trail, 2019). While many white people in America might identify as Caucasian, or state so in medicalized settings to sound more formal, further consideration of the social justice implications for counselors continuing to perpetuate the standardization of this taxonomy is warranted, as is being done in the medical community (Shamambo & Henry, 2022). Calls for more culture-centered (Phillips, 2021) and antiracist (Shand-Lubbers, 2023) counseling are being heard from the field. The continued use of the word "Caucasian" as a synonym for "white" because it is considered more "official" or "medicalized" is concerning for me as a counselor, scientist, advocate, and a human.

I find myself asking, and ask others as well, who's making the boxes and how free are people to not check them, especially if they don't know their own history? How are we, individually, and as counselors, going to hold ourselves accountable to truly work from an anti-racist model when we can't even accurately describe who WE are? The 'white savior complex' dominating mental health is an ongoing national problem (Kim, 2022). How are we working to systematically work towards greater self-knowledge when we still can't even say "white" or openly explore what "white culture" is (National Museum of African History and Culture, 2024; Potapchuck, 2012)? We are only beginning to understand this phenomenon as a part of counselors' professional identity development (Shand-Lubbers, 2023); there is a lot of wounding all around that needs to be brought to light, explored, and shared. Jung knew we had a lot to learn, and that we are never to stop learning. As we say in recovery, "We never arrive". If we're wanting to help others, we must first help ourselves.

> The analyst must go on learning endlessly, and never forget that each new case brings new problems to light and thus gives rise to unconscious assumptions that have never before been constellated. We could say, without too much exaggeration, that a good half of every treatment that probes at all deeply consists in the doctor's examining himself, for only what he can put right in himself can he hope to put right in the patient. It is no loss, either, if he feels that the patient is hitting him, or even scoring off him: it is his own hurt that gives the measure of his power to heal. This, and nothing else, is the meaning of the Greek myth of the **wounded physician**.
>
> CW 16, p. 116, § 239 (bolding mine)

While we may be Wounded Healers, we aim to be Servant Leaders. A concept seemingly as old as time, reflected in great religious leaders around the world, the term "servant leader" was coined by Robert Greenleaf (1970) a businessman inspired by the novel *The Journey to the East* (Hesse & Rosner, 1956), whose mission is now taught through the Robert K. Greenleaf Center for Servant Leadership (2021), and is a value found in the counseling profession. Greenleaf admitted that this idea came to him from his unconscious, and remains rooted there, as intuition. Servant Leaders intuitively have a sense of knowing the way and point to it. The way is not the ego alone. A Servant Leader recognizes that their sense of wholeness, or alignment of their ego-Self axis, and creative expression are fulfilled through humble service. Like Jung, and the counseling profession, this concept embodies the value of a spiritual core, common among all peoples, and a desire to help without coercion. We must be aware of the power dynamics involved in the counseling relationship and keep ourselves in check. Our position is one of privilege, especially when serving the most vulnerable; we are accepting and empathize. We must hold that position humbly as we serve our clients, and use that position as power when advocating for them within systems that may aim to exploit. This is why knowing ourselves and using appropriate personal disclosures, such as in our professional identity statements and other paperwork, are encouraged, so that clients can truly make an informed decision as to if they want to work with us.

There are nine professional dispositional behaviors assessed in counselor training which are especially important to the Jungian-oriented counselor: Conscientiousness, Coping and Self-Care, Openness, Cooperativeness, Moral Reasoning, Interpersonal Skills, Cultural Sensitivity, Self-Awareness, and Emotional Stability (Garner et al., 2016, 2020). We must realize that being a minority theory in the field can be a disadvantage and requires extra attention to our ethical considerations, reflective practices, and advocacy efforts. Being aware of the similarities and differences between the history and practice from a Jungian perspective is important. We are responsible for doing our own work to care for our mental health, creativity, and spiritual life so we can give to our clients (see also the Wheel of Wellness). We may have, or need, daily, weekly, monthly, and annual practices. We may choose to continue in Jungian analysis, attend worship services, study sacred texts, join dance troupes, and spend long hours in our art studios. Edith Kramer, the great art therapist, suggested to me when I was in training to make sure to balance client and art-making time. I know that may be a financial sacrifice or reflection of our privilege to be able to do, especially for a counselor earlier in their career. Openness has been correlated with valuing and engaging in creative, playful exploration (Holland, 1997; Karwowski & Kaufman, 2017; Kelly, 2006). It is important to work on being open to possibilities and comfortable with not knowing when encountering the unconscious. Openness also invites collaboration with our clients, which is foundational to our counselor identity.

One of the reasons it is important to identify a theory of practice is because they all begin with a set of assumptions. For Jungian counseling, we might identify these assumptions as:

1. The structure and function of the psyche is self-regulating and largely governed by the personal and collective unconscious.
2. The language of the unconscious is symbolic and valuable.
3. Both associative and analytic functions are needed to access and interpret symbolic material in order to make sense of it and find meaning.
4. Mental health is an ongoing process of becoming ourselves. It involves understanding and listening to ourselves, more than trying to actively change our behavior through our will alone.
5. The client's experience and interpretation is more important than the counselor's assessment.

Jungian-oriented counseling may assist with meaning making and healing through:

1. the therapeutic relationship itself (represented by the vas, or container)
2. supporting and uncovering unconscious material
3. inviting associative and analytic processing
4. psychoeducation.

Time Together

The concept of time is one of great relevance in the therapeutic relationship. We often speak of beginning with the end in mind, or anticipating how long treatment may last; clients often ask this question, and it is recommended to address this to a degree at intake, and have a statement in the paperwork. Both client-centered and Jungian theory acknowledge that while benefits may be felt quickly, the relationship may last longer. While we don't want to "foster dependency" in the therapeutic relationship, we are a resource and can be an important part of someone's wellness plan. Because we are coming to the table from a wellness perspective, we may not be so quick to independently judge when we think someone is done with counseling. This is a collaborative relationship. A part of most Jungian analytic training programs is to remain in analysis throughout. Similarly, our client may be a mental health professional, or someone with a long history of mental health concerns, who wants to attend weekly or monthly counseling as "maintenance".

I have met counselors who are uncomfortable with seeing people irregularly for a variety of reasons: from wanting their schedules to be more predictable, to not wanting to hold "too many" people's stories. It can be a real gift to clients, though, when the relationship can be revisited if needed. I have one client whom I saw as a young child who returned as a teenager and then a young adult; I knew her story, she felt safe with me, and expressed gratitude for being able to pick up where she left off. Many clients have said that they have avoided treatment because they didn't want to have to "start over" with a new therapist. The therapeutic relationship is a real relationship. How long "should" that last? Ideally, the client holds the keys. Frequently, it's negotiated between the client and the counselor. Too often, though, time together is dictated by financial limitations, managed care, and the courts. These are conversations worth having early on, and as situations arise. Each session counts.

Counselors must develop the ability to feel and hold to a typical "clinical hour" which is usually 45–50 minutes. Starting and ending well are important rituals to establish. It's common to initially ask how someone is, but a warm "welcome back" can be less directive. Counselors can also broach discussions about how a client might like to begin and plan for future sessions. There are various opinions about having clocks and timers in the counseling office. Some say that an obvious clock, especially a ticking one, can draw the client's attention to it and away from the "real work" of the counseling session. Losing track of time, or *temporal distortion*, though, is a frequent phenomenon, especially in the mental health world, which can be exacerbated by not being able to easily check (Blom et al., 2021; Holman et al., 2023). This is commonly exploited in shopping centers and casinos. Because I want clients to feel at ease, stay safely grounded in the here and now, and anticipate when it is almost time to go, I have more often chosen to have a large ticking clock in my office. I have felt waves of both anxiety and ease in sessions where there is no clock, but only when the time frame was flexible; that is an uncommon structure for counseling sessions, though, which is why I tend to prefer a clock.

Broaching is also a topic related to time. Broaching refers to anticipating, being open to, and sensitively bringing up salient aspects of culture that may be relevant to the therapeutic relationship (Day-Vines et al., 2007). The timing of these discussions is important. While some may bring up "demographic" information once, usually upon intake this may be considered an avoidant broaching style; instead, we are encouraged to infuse broaching throughout our therapeutic relationship. We may take it for granted that counselors are comfortable with having difficult discussions, and emphatically confronting our clients, but broaching intersecting topics of race, ethnicity, religious and spiritual issues, and sexuality are notoriously difficult, even when we consider ourselves culturally aware, humble, and competent (Erby & White, 2020).

SETTING & HOLDING THE FRAME: PSYCHIC ENERGY & BOUNDARIES

> I cannot regard the transference merely as a projection of infantile-erotic fantasies. No doubt that is what it is from one standpoint, but I also see in it, as I said in an earlier letter, **a process of empathy and adaptation.**
>
> CW 4, p. 394, § 662 (bolding is mine)

By the time many counselors-in-training make it to me as their clinical supervisor, they have gained the impression that somehow transference and countertransference are "bad" things in therapy. I'm not exactly sure where this comes from since counseling is built on a foundation of empathy and the importance of the therapeutic relationship. How can we feel with someone if we don't have feelings toward them? How can we expect a real relationship to form, albeit a professional one, if we don't expect, encourage, or allow our clients to have feelings about us? I suspect this comes from Shadow material from other historical counseling values. Perhaps it is leftover from the early over-analytic psychodynamic days, where therapists were only supposed to be objective observers. Perhaps, too, it is a shallow interpretation of the person-centered value of "unconditional positive regard", suggesting that we are to only delight in our clients. As I see it, and read in Jung, the only way to truly be able to hold someone in positive regard is to be able to also see and accept those things in ourselves that have been pushed into Shadow; only then may they eventually come to light. By only acknowledging the "positive", I argue we are taking a dualistic, judgmental stance, and are likely being inauthentic.

Let's start with some definitions. On the most basic level, from the standard psychodynamic perspective, transference is how our clients may feel about us at any given time. Countertransference is how we feel about our client. Co-transference, though, is a sense of being with, and comes out of the developmental Jungian movement (Bradway & McCoard, 1997); it is similar to concordant countertransference (Cabaniss et al., 2016). All types of transference hold aspects of how the people involved experience attachment, trust, and boundaries. This often includes expectations, power dynamics, and communication within the relationship. However, it is our responsibility as counselors to *set and hold the frame*, or the boundaries of the therapeutic relationship, and contain the psychic energy therein. This involves being transparent about our professional identity, ethical guidelines, limits of time and confidentiality, scope of practice. It also requires us to elegantly navigate the waters that bubble up within the relationship.

Transference

Transference is classically divided into *positive transference* and *negative transference* (Cabaniss et al., 2016). While this reflects the dual nature of transference, it can be unhelpful to divide them in such a polarizing way, especially if coming from outside a Jungian orientation, and contradictory to the DSQ, often taught alongside it in psychodynamic circles. Let's deconstruct these dualistic ideas a bit:

"Positive" transference, including *idealization, eroticism,* and *parentification* of the counselor might absolutely get in the way of a client's therapeutic progress if it gets *amplified* (or, as we say in the field of addictions, "co-signed"), or goes unrecognized by the counselor, and continues to be unconscious in either psyche. If mishandled by the counselor, "positive transference" is anything but, and can quickly turn "negative". A client may not make progress in therapy because they look to us for all the answers and neglect looking deep within; counseling may turn into the dreaded "advice giving" unless the counselor can temper that need and work toward empowerment. Clients may become distracted by their erotic feelings for their counselor if we fail to see how those feelings might be displaced, libidinal, or vital creative energy; we are obligated to hold the frame of the therapeutic relationship, including our boundaries, to protect us both and help the client reclaim their lives.

"Negative" transference can be overt or covert, and look like anger or hostility coming at us, clients expressing that they're feeling judged, over-exposed, humiliated, abandoned, victimized, or disrespected by us or in the context of the therapeutic relationship. I think that as Jungian counselors, we are to suspend our judgment and avoid labeling this as "negative" too quickly in the first place. We also have the responsibility for creating an atmosphere of transparency and safety, which includes owning what's ours, especially when we violate the terms of our arrangement (see also "informed consent").

Therefore, it is my perspective that transference is necessary, purposeful, and transformative. It encompasses all the feelings a client may have toward us within the context of the therapeutic relationship, both conscious and unconscious. These feelings are necessary for the material to be worked through within the relationship. Without a feeling tone, there is no relationship.

Jung says that dealing directly with transference often happens during the elucidation phase, after the initial confession, as unconscious material is emerging and may be confusing to the client (CW 16). Counselors generally aim for an egalitarian and collaborative relationship with our clients. However, we must also be aware that many clients have experienced vulnerability and disempowerment in their relationships with authority figures. It is common for clients to look to us for answers and project feelings about their loved ones onto us. While we need to come to accept this, we are also ethically called to remind the client of the boundaries of our relationship as outlined in the ACA Code (2014) and manage our countertransference, which is bound to happen.

Countertransference

Countertransference, or the therapist's feelings toward their client, is traditionally understood as objective, subjective, and client-induced, but from a Jungian perspective we add one other: co-transference. Our feelings toward our clients are involved in every aspect of the counseling relationship. They are necessary in order to feel, and are worthy of identification and exploration as an active part of ongoing reflective practices.

1. *Objective Countertransference* is the kind of reaction "anyone" might have. This is often considered an appropriate emotional response to a client's behavior but may need to be tempered according to professional standards. For example, if a client is consistently late, the counselor may naturally feel somewhat irritated; however, to manage this well, the counselor should identify the feeling, perhaps process it in supervision, discuss the lateness with the client, and remind them of the policy regarding starting the session on time.

2. *Counselor-Induced Countertransference* (also frequently called *Subjective, Therapist/Counselor Induced*, or *Negative*) – We might also call this being "triggered" by our clients. This is when we might see our client through a distorted, negative, or harsh way because our past experiences and biases may be in the way. This is our "subjective" view which is an aspect of our relationship with the archetype of the Wounded Healer on our journey to become Servant Leaders.

3. *Client-Induced Countertransference* (sometimes just called "induced" countertransference in the literature) – This experience can be quite unnerving and confusing for counselors and may even have a numinous quality. Counselors may feel strangely toward their client, in a way that initially does not make overt logical sense. We might find ourselves intensely or subtly angry, rejecting, preoccupied, or otherwise "counter" to our conscious processing of the situation. Because the therapeutic relationship may be used to recreate and play out previous relationships in the client's life, this process may therefore be "client-induced", where the unconscious dynamics and needs are evoked in the unconscious of the counselor. If we suspect this may be occurring, we might ask ourselves:

Who in the client's life may have felt this way about them? When? What might the client have needed instead?

4. *Co-Transference* – Co-transference is a distinctive, non-pathologizing approach of observing, valuing, joining with, and being open to the transformative power of the therapeutic relationship. Jung identified rapport as a "relationship of mutual confidence, on which the therapeutic success ultimately depends" (CW 16, p. 116, § 239). This Jungian view of expanded, deepened rapport, or therapeutic alliance, was coined by sandplay therapist Kay Bradway (Bradway & McCoard, 1997). Co-transference can also be related to healthy attunement, and *co-regulation*, terms used in attachment therapy to describe the necessity of the caregiver to be a safe, understanding, well-regulated container for the dysregulated child/client to process trauma with and through (Blaustein & Kinniburgh, 2019). Through this process, the *tension of the opposites*, or *conjunctio*, is witnessed and respected. When knowledge and felt experience are shared and tolerated, the ruptures and repairs, or breaks in connection, of the past and present, can be more easily and deeply explored; this process is considered a fundamental healing experiential in and of itself (Circle of Security International, 2023; Wilkinson, 2005). Elizabeth Urban (1996), a child Jungian analyst, expanded on Winnicott's (1971) idea of the internalized "good-enough" mother, or a sense of me- and we-ness that is aimed to be symbolically recreated in the therapeutic relationship, assisting with the re-establishing of the ability to tolerate psychic material. This process is supported by neuro-scientific research in mirror neurons, or the building of self-regulation through co-regulation with a safe caregiver first, and the client having the freedom to look away when distress or intensity becomes too much for the system to self-regulate (Wilkinson, 2006). This *reverie* (CW 16) in the therapeutic relationship is not so much interpretation. Still, it is both safe and accepting awareness and containment, first in the therapist's mind, then in the client's, much as a loving and attentive caregiver's awareness and meeting of an infant's needs (Willemsen, 2014). This non-verbal, sometimes unconscious processing and communication within dyads has been validated by the neuroscientific study of mirror neurons, and may be vital to the development of empathy, socialization, and self-esteem (Leader, 2015; McRoberts, 2018). This co-transference may be experienced by increased frequency of finishing each other's sentences (Samuels, 1985), a shared sense of knowing, or an overall peace or ease in the relationship.

Navigating these abstract, subjective moving parts requires what we call "countertransference management" to have clear, deep working relationships (Metcalf, 2003; Nissen-Lie et al., 2017). Countertransference must be carefully observed and crafted, as it is considered transformative; the counselors must not only possess knowledge of psyche, symbol, and clinical practice, but also demonstrate the ability to connect with their own inner dialogues, through personal and professional reflective practice, in service of themselves and their clients (Steinhardt, 2012). For example, Jung (CW 17) stressed the importance of adults working with children to avoid an authoritarianism and projection through their own individuation process; sometimes we need a mirror in order to really see ourselves in situations like this. While we know of the benefits, there are also barriers to counselors being open to reflective practices with their supervisors.

THE PARALLEL PROCESS & USE OF SUPERVISION

I inquire, I do not assert; I do not here determine anything with final assurance; I conjecture, try, compare, attempt, ask . . .

CW 16, p. 164

Open reflective practices with supervisors can make us feel vulnerable, but are a vital part of the parallel process. We expect our clients to be open and honest, and so we must, in turn, do the same, with a trusted supervisor or colleague. Holding onto our feelings about our clients is unhealthy for us, our clients, and the therapeutic relationship in the short term, and can have serious, long-term consequences for our physical and emotional health, as well as our careers. By entering into a supervisory process as an act of self-advocacy, we also provide the opportunity to amplify our voices, and in turn, our clients'. These reflective practices may assist us in developing and maintaining our professional dispositions, cultural responsiveness, and advocacy competencies (Garner et al., 2016; Lewis et al., 2018; Ratts et al., 2016).

The term *parallel process* was introduced by Searles (1955), building upon psychoanalytic concepts of counter/co/transference to specifically include the reflective process of bringing issues between the client and therapist to supervision. The concept developed into considering the mutuality beyond the power dynamics involved and now includes the emotionality, influence, and transformational potentiality between any of the three collaborative professional relationships: client, counselor, and supervisor. All three have both conscious and unconscious processes, and relate to each other in both ways. As we work together, we all may develop or revisit our inter- and intra-psychic material. To use Jung's (CW 12) spiral metaphor, we grow out of and around a central structure, but may also find ourselves looking across the spiral, noticing patterns and associations. In this way, expect that we are all circumambulating the ideas and emotions that emerge in the process.

With respect to unconscious processes and symbology, the Jungian-oriented counselor's ability to share a sacred space parallels the neurobiological evidence of the importance and healing benefits of *resonance*, or shared circuitry, through mindfulness practices (Balfour, 2013; Keysers, 2011; Siegel, 2007). Research also suggests that it is important for the treatment provider to be as aware as possible of one's own internal processes and possible associations in order to engage empathetically (Petchkovsky et al., 2013), paralleling the Jungian concept of reciprocal individuation (von Franz, 1980).

While up to 60% of communication occurs non-verbally (Burgoon, 1985), young children especially may lack the verbal and cognitive capacity for modalities that do not utilize play (Kestly, 2014; Landreth, 2024; Stewart et al., 2016). Those who have experienced a trauma may especially benefit from largely non-verbal creative therapies that tap directly into memory and somatic responses with lower levels of perceived threat (Perryman et al., 2019). Activating mirror neurons through a safe, empathetic relationship may account for up to 30% of therapy outcomes through enhancing neuroplasticity (Lambert & Barley, 2001); additionally, clients may be supported in finding their neuroplastic "sweet spot" through non-directive play therapies that co-create "wordless narratives of self-awareness and transformation" supporting "attention, awareness, and consciousness" (Stewart et al., 2016, pp. 5–6).

How countertransference is managed in clinical supervision has limited research. Though countertransference has been identified as key to meaning making and client care outcomes (Francis, 1995; Gil & Rubin, 2005; Metcalf, 2003), there is surprisingly little research on therapist countertransference management in general, or, in a similar vein of reflective practice, therapists' personal psychotherapy (Gold et al., 2015; Malikiosi-Loizos, 2013; Pastner et al., 2014; Viado, 2015). Low responses rates of countertransference management may be due to lack of knowledge or importance of the issue (Fall et al., 2007). Research on empathy training in counseling also remains limited (Ziff et al., 2017), but the creative arts have been used to assist in skill development (Elliott et al., 2011; Potash & Chen, 2014). Creative processes, including play (Bar-On, 2007; Lennie, 2007; Luke

& Kiweewa, 2010; Markos et al., 2007) and experiential learning (Bell et al., 2014), have promoted reflective practice and increased self-awareness. Self-awareness is an essential factor of effective countertransference management in the therapeutic relationship (Metcalf, 2003; Robbins & Jolkovski, 1987; Van Wagoner et al., 1991). However, across models of supervision, research suggests that therapists may have difficulty revealing insecurities about personal issues and skills both to themselves and supervisors due to fears about showing vulnerability (Eryılmaz & Mutlu, 2017). The use of a wide range of expressive arts and play therapy techniques in counseling and supervision is increasingly popular with all ages and has been shown to positively influence the parallel process (Yoo, 2011).

The therapist's self-concept and exploration of countertransference issues can be sensitively explored through the parallel process within experiential supervision, positively influencing the supervisory relationship, outcomes of supervisees' professional development as well as client care outcomes (Stillo, 2018; Yoo, 2011). Sandtrays have been utilized in play therapy supervision, often integrated with other models, to support the supervisory relationship, build group cohesion, and creatively explore personal and professional development through the visualization of experience, goals, and growth (Anekstein et al., 2014; Markos et al., 2008; McCurdy & Owen, 2008; Mullen et al., 2007; Paone et al., 2015). Use of the sandtray, specifically, can help identify unconscious bias, creating feelings of safety and unity, as well as increasing awareness and self-reflection (Doyle & Magor-Blatch, 2017; Loue, 2015; Paone et al., 2015).

Research on post-traumatic growth indicates that therapists' countertransference management when working with clients who have experienced trauma, as many play therapists do, is of particular significance due to the initial strong emotional reactions that emerge within the therapeutic relationship (Bartoskova, 2015). Research suggests that therapists employing positive coping in their own lives positively affects treatment outcomes (Nissen-Lie et al., 2017).

Emphasis on creatively and curiously seeking out personally meaningful ways of processing the traumatic material has been noted as significant to therapists' personal and professional identity (Bartoskova, 2015). Therapist's countertransference associated with vicarious trauma is also correlated with compassion fatigue (Figley, 2002; McCann & Pearlman, 1990; Pearlman & MacIan, 1995), a factor leading to burnout, and a direct threat to one's professional identity, professional self-efficacy, and client care out-comes (Brooks, 2015; Lammers et al., 2013). Perspective taking, or the capacity to see another's point of view, has been found to be stimulated through imagination and creativity (Glăveanu et al., 2018). The very environment that the therapist creates, known in sandplay as the "free and protected space" (Kalff, 2020; Steinhardt, 2012), is thought to communi-cate both the conscious and unconscious beliefs of the therapist, through metacommunication, including levels of resilience, acceptance, tolerance, and present control.

Too often, counselors-in-training encounter "lousy" supervision. Yes, that's the official term in the literature (Bernard & Goodyear, 2014). While we might think that whoever's our boss is inevitably our clinical supervisor, this may not be enough, especially for the Jungian-oriented counselor and play therapist. I have always had to seek out additional supervisors with more specific training, knowledge, and goodness-of-fit with my areas of interest and clinical focus. While this may be frustrating and a bur-densome expense, I cannot imagine being where I am now without that support. While counselors-in-training may receive supervision from any independently licensed therapist in many instances to meet State require-ments (LCSW, LMFT, etc.), a licensed counselor is preferred; those vary by state and may include: Licensed Professional Counselor (LPC), Licensed Mental Health Counselor (LMHC), Licensed Professional Counselor – Mental Health Service Provider (LPC-MHSP), Licensed Clinical Coun-selor (LCC). Also, if one is pursuing credentialing from the Association for Play Therapy, or the Sandplay Therapists of America, the supervi-sion or consultation must be from someone holding appropriate creden-tials from those organizations. Knowing who we are, what we do, what we need, and going out to find mentorship is vital for a healthy personal and professional identity.

Despite our knowledge of the importance of creativity, supervision, and eth-ics, there is a remarkable gap in the recent literature, especially in the field of play therapy (Yee et al., 2019). While supervision is a requirement for state licensure as a counselor, not everyone training in play therapy will seek out the additional requirement of play therapy specific supervision. However, this specific aspect of training is essential to address ongoing professional identity concerns, including theoretically conceptualizing and documenting symbolic manifestations of unconscious material.

DOCUMENTATION

I have stressed the need for more extensive individualization of the method of treatment and for an irrationalization of its aims – especially the latter, which would ensure the greatest possible freedom from prejudice. In dealing with psychological developments, the doctor should, as a matter of principle, let nature rule and himself do his utmost to avoid influencing the patient in the direction of his own philosophical, social, and political bent.

CW 16, p. 26, § 42

We communicate with our clients through the first questions we ask them, often on our forms. While collecting biopsychosocial information is considered best practice, we must also hold ourselves accountable to any assumptions we make or prejudices we might have based on the information we receive (APT, 2022). Jungian orientation should be integrated throughout our documentation. This includes our Informed Consent document, any assessments we might use, both informal and formal, in our collaborative goal setting, or treatment planning, and in our notes.

Informed Consent

As stated above, informed consent begins with clients knowing who we are and what they might expect when they agree to enter into a professional relationship with us. Professional identity statements should be a part of our Informed Consent document. The Professional Identity Statement should include the ethical guidelines of the state and organizations to which the counselor belongs. We may adopt the guidelines for crafting a one minute professional identity statement (Burns, 2017) according to our specific needs:

1. Speak directly to potential clients: Language should be professionally presented, yet warm and relatable. Remembering that the people reading your statement are likely under a great deal of stress and may not have a long attention span, nor understand clinical jargon.
2. Identifying information: This includes our legal and preferred names, title, and credentials, as well as where we practice.
3. Professional philosophy, values, and practices.
4. Scope of practice and qualification.
5. Client demographics.

Assessments

Assessments include both formal and informal assessments. I often remind counselors-in-training of this when they say they do not use assessments at their site. What they often mean is that they do not use formal assessments, otherwise known as *measures* or *instruments*, *inventories*, or *psychological tests*. Many of these instruments are now free or integrated into EMRs (electronic medical records). From a Jungian perspective, formal assessments may be required, helpful, or, quite honestly, unhelpful.

While Jung is credited in the development and trend of using various formal assessments, we must also consider that they may be weaponized against clients and employees. Some agencies require that counselors use formal assessments to aid in diagnosing and justifying treatment. However, if we take the perspective that clients are free to attend counseling despite a mental health diagnosis, they may be unnecessary. While the outcomes of an assessment, including a diagnosis or other type of score, may be helpful, they may also be a kind of self-fulfilling prophecy, where clients and counselors alike may hold too tightly to a definition or expectations of what a client "should" be doing. Diagnosis can be subjective. In my practice, I've met many clients with multiple diagnoses from multiple providers because their situation was assessed differently. I've also worked with clients who have felt pigeonholed at work by various assessments given by their employers, and even experienced legal issues because the court accessed their formal assessments. Speaking out against this type of weaponization has been going on for some time (Caplan, 2012; Lewis, 2021).

The fact is, there is not a single formal assessment that captures the totality of a person. We're just too complex. Formal assessments are generally given as a standard part of intake, such as to screen for current suicidal ideation, and informed by the counselor's initial informal assessment. That is, we often need an inkling that someone might be experiencing anxiety to think to give an anxiety assessment. Like the idea of evidence-based practice in general, a full clinical assessment is, ideally, made up of multiple factors such as what information is presented by the client, other sources, as well as what the counselor observes, perceives, their area of specialization, as well as the integration of any formal assessments, and their interpretations. I am quite hesitant to be definitive in my assessment because I, as a person, am fallible. Formal assessments are also often self-reported, which has received a great deal of criticism about their "objective" validity; they can change depending on various factors impacting a client's day, and even if the measure has been found to be statistically significantly valid and reliable, mental disorders as a "thing" are still questionable (Jablensky, 2016). Some counselors choose to give measures periodically to track progress. Most Jungians I know, though, honestly, don't tend to utilize formal assessments very often, except on intake or if they are conducting research. Of particular relevance to Jungian-oriented counseling, though, is the suggestion that it is best practice that all assessments, formal or informal, especially regarding religious and spiritual integration, be reflective, person-centered, and periodically revisited (Cashwell & Young, 2020).

Informal assessments are active and ongoing, though, in any therapeutic relationship. What we notice about all aspects of case conceptualization as well as each session is included:

- how our client looks, acts, sounds, etc.
- their report of how they've been feeling, thinking, acting
- their dreams, current life events, and meaning making
- what they choose to talk about, play, create, or avoid
- what others have said, or reported about how they've been
- our impressions of their progress.

Collaborative Goal Setting

Many clients have reported to me that they never set goals with the therapist before, that they didn't know what they were, and even when I have developed a treatment plan with them, that they have forgotten their goals. In this way I think of goals like consent: ideally it is ongoing and revisited often. Clear, collaborative goals are not only ethical best practice, but may help develop a working alliance that empowers clients, prevents dependency, helps navigate the treatment process, and improves outcomes (ACA, 2014; Gerhart 2016; Geurtzen et al., 2020).

Collaborative goal setting begins with our first interactions with the potential client. By sharing who we are, what we do, and how we might be helpful, we set the frame for the counseling process by making our boundaries clear. When we are able to create this safe container, or vas, then the client may be more free to enter more fully into the process. Then we listen to what the client is looking for.

While a treatment plan may not be a Jungian counselor's first priority, they are often necessary when working in an agency setting, or to even begin writing progress notes in many electronic medical records (EMR). More importantly, it is part of our ethical practice guidelines to work collaboratively with our clients on treatment plans that offer:

> . . . reasonable promise of success and are consistent with the abilities, temperament, developmental level, and circumstances of clients. Counselors and clients regularly review and revise counseling plans to assess their continued viability and effectiveness, respecting clients' freedom of choice.
>
> (ACA, 2014, A. 1. C. Counseling Plans, p. 4)

We are to create the treatment plan with our clients, regardless of age. THIS MEANS CHILDREN, TOO. Some counselors are hesitant to do this because children are often brought to counseling against their will, or are the scapegoat for a dysfunctional family. I think this is ample justification for why we are called to collaboratively create the plan with the children. Returning to the ACA Code of Ethics, our professional values extend to the foundational principles of ethical behavior which I also think aligns directly with Jungian principals:

- honoring autonomy, the right of an individual to control the direction of their own life
- avoiding harm (non-maleficence)
- working for the good of the individual and collective (beneficence)
- treating people fairly, with respect and dignity (justice)
- being truthful and forthcoming about our professional practices (veracity)
- keeping our promises and fulfilling our responsibilities (fidelity).

The plan is not about making sure the client is "compliant" with treatment (according to parents, teachers, institutions, or our own counselor agendas), or even making progress (thought that is important); it's to hold us as counselors accountable and show our clients, regardless of their age, that we are there for them as Servant Leaders. We must look at the world through our client's eyes and join with them in order to truly see their perspective and help them find their way to their goal.

Yes, people come to counseling because they are suffering and want to change. But as Jung said, "neurosis is always a substitute for legitimate suffering" (CW 11, p. 75, § 129). The counseling process can be terrifying, can hurt more before it gets better, and change is risky. The unconscious has produced defenses against real stressors in the world. It takes bravery, scaffolding, and trust in a well-trained guide to navigate the unconscious. We might think we know what is best for the client, or what the evidence says is more likely to get them from here to there, but we hold to our values that it's THEIR CHOICE, THEIR JOURNEY, every step of the way.

The plan should clearly reflect what the client wants (goals), long and short term, what they're willing to do, one step at a time (objectives), building upon what is already working, from a wellness perspective (non-pathologizing), and what we will do to help them get there (interventions). Let's discuss each a bit more below.

I encourage my students to start with the clients' own words about what they want to get out of counseling. If a child or teen says they don't even want to be there, we might find a goal in the client's report of why they were "made to come here" or what their parents said about why they want them to come to counseling. Adult clients may be equally confused about what is "wrong" with them but they are reaching out for help. Some counselors may be required at their site to use "more clinical" language, or jargon, in their treatment plans and show the use of "evidence-based practices". SMART goals, first developed for the field of management (Doran, 1981) are also commonly required, especially when working with managed care for insurance billing (Beacon Health Options, 2021), which stands for *specific, measurable, achievable, realistic,* and *time bound.* (Though this connection between the field of management and how some counselors embrace the term "behavioral management" for what we do is not my favorite.) It is also considered best practice to build on the client's strengths, what is already working, and at least one wellness-based goal (Gibson et al., 2021; Myers et al., 1996). Strengths or areas of desired growth may be linked to one or more aspects of the Wheel of Wellness (Myers et al., 1996). Wellness counseling may be distilled into five domains: mind, body, spirit, emotion, and connection (Ohrt et al., 2019). Remember: wellness is a way of life. And don't forget that spiritual core. Adding in a spiritual assessment, deeply listening, and actively engaging in discussion about the spiritual aspects of both the distress and possible solutions have been found to significantly reduce both spiritual and emotional disturbance (Jolley, 2023).

My "cheat sheet" for building collaborative goals:

1. Goal – In the client's words. What do they say they want? What do they want more or less of in their life?
2. Objective – What will the CLIENT do?
3. Intervention – Literally, how will the COUNSELOR "intervene"?

1. Goal – (**Big picture**) Listen to the client. What do they really want? What brought them to counseling? The goal should be *directly related* to their reported problem. Use their own words when possible and avoid jargon. Because these are more subjective, or client reported, we might not be able to see these things but can trust the client to say when they may be there. This is often expressed as a want or a need, or more or less of something.

   > For example: "I want to feel like myself again". "I need to be a better mom to my kids". "I want to feel less anxious". "I need to get over this trauma". "I want to enjoy life more".

2. Objective – (**CLIENT** will . . .) What is ONE NEXT STEP the client is able and willing to take? What is really "do-able"? This should be something observable or measurable, built upon their strengths, and ideally what they're already doing, taking their overall wellness into account (see the Wheel of Wellness). They might start with words such as:

   • increase/decrease
   • continue
   • attend
   • engage in
   • develop
   • verbalize
   • practice
   • consider
   • implement.

   For example: Client will . . . **increase frequency** of and honesty in communication with their support system; **decrease engagement** with xyz; **continue to** keep a dream journal next to the bed and utilize it at least once a week; **explore** roles, values, and symbols that appear salient; **attend** meeting/group/individual counseling session x times per week/month; **engage in** creative/relaxing/physical activity x times weekly/monthly; **develop routines/rituals** around bedtime, meals, work schedule, spiritual practices, meditation, etc.; identify holidays and anniversaries that are of particular importance and plan to keep the day . . .

3. Intervention – (**COUNSELOR** will . . .) How will the COUNSELOR intervene to support this step? Reflection is a primary counseling skill

and should be the focus. These should start with words that reflect our values and theoretical orientation such as:

- reflect (feeling, content, meaning)
- assist
- co-develop/strategize
- collaborate with
- support
- inquire
- follow up
- provide
- review
- introduce
- explore.

For example: Counselor will . . . **maintain** therapeutic boundaries to assist increasing feelings of safety in the relationship; **support** client through active listening and collaborative problem solving; **inquire** about the week's dreams; **provide** art and play materials for symbolic expression with delayed interpretation; **remind** client of strengths; **introduce** psychoeducation about mindfulness practices; **review** goals and progress by x date.

4. Termination Plan: Begin with the end in mind. While we will discuss this topic more fully in Chapter 8, let's put a placeholder for consideration here. When will the plan be reviewed to see if goals have been met? What happens when they meet their goal? What if you're an intern, the semester ends, and you leave; what is the transition plan? What if they leave before their goals are met; can they come back? Are there a predetermined number of sessions? What referrals might you provide?

Those looking for additional evidence-based treatment planning tips may be interested in the Jongsma (2021, 2023) series for adolescents and adults; more about play therapy specific documentation can be found in Homeyer and Bennett's (2023) latest work.

Notes

Jungian-oriented counseling involves awareness that the counselor is also having a subjective experience and we are not the ultimate authority in clients' analytic process (CW 16); they are. Therefore, it is my position that we have a responsibility to self-critique what others might consider simply "objective". For example affective content in a session is commonly considered objective; however, I do not assume to know what a client is feeling, even if I see a particular behavior or expression. I consider it my interpretation that someone might be feeling sad if I see them crying; in this case, the crying may be considered objective, but I would need confirmation from my client that they indeed felt sad.

Common progress note formats include the SOAP (subjective, objective, assessment, progress) and more the condensed DAP (data, assessment, plan), which removes the pesky subjective/objective dilemma. Minimal documentation requirements vary from state and agency, but generally should contain the client's name, date and length of the session, a brief description of the session, others involved in the session, a diagnosis (if applicable), the date of next session, and a signature; a mini risk assessment is now also becoming standard practice to more frequently screen for homicidal and suicidal ideation. While psychodynamically oriented providers are notorious for describing sessions at length, counselors and play therapists generally avoid this. We aim to be as brief as possible in addressing the content, themes, materials, interventions, progress, and ongoing planning (Homeyer & Bennett, 2023; Ray, 2011). We may also choose to use more Jungian specific language such as archetypes seemingly "awakened" or engaged, as well as a "soft hypothesis" in the assessment section, and if applicable, the type(s) of play observed, such as isolative, associative, or competitive (Lilly & Gaskill, 2023). Because clients have a legal right to see their medical records, including progress notes, counselors are advised to be as concise and clear as possible, and to avoid sharing information that might cause harm (OpenNotes, 2023). Supervisors may develop a note based on agency requirements that contain checkboxes of frequently used topics and interventions with optional open text boxes when further details are needed. However, special consideration should be given to the experiential nature of Jungian-oriented art- and play-based interventions. While the process is more relevant to the product we must address how to care for creations manifested during session.

Photographing & Storing the Work

Written permission must be obtained before recording the counseling process in any way, including photographing a client's physical remains of the work, be that art, play, journaling, or the like. STA provides a "sandplay therapy note form" in their sandplay research guidelines (STA, 2024), but it does not meet many of the standard requirements for a progress note. There is some debate if these supplemental documents are considered part of the medical record, or are "psychotherapy notes" to be kept separate. Where and how are they kept, though? For ethical and legal reasons, the decision to record the expressive remnants of the session should not be taken lightly. It has been my professional experience that the untrained eye is likely to inaccurately read into symbolic work; for this reason I tend to protect client images even from my own records, especially if the case is likely to go to court. Unless it's been a training requirement, I generally just describe the physical elements of the work in the progress note and don't photograph or keep client artwork.

Clients may delight in taking their artwork home, and in the digital age, even the youngest clients have requested to take a cellphone photo. I was taught by several members of STA that sandplay therapists disallow their clients from photographing their trays, but the therapist does, and keeps them for a final review upon termination. Former guidelines (from STA, 2012, now removed from their website) mostly addressed the importance of taking photos from multiple angles and indicating the position of the client and the therapist, not how or where to store the photos. While I understand the sentiment of "not allowing" clients to take photos of their work so that the image might be digested by the client's psyche, it's always made me uncomfortable, so it's not a "rule" in my playroom. The aesthetics of existence attest that the creative work belongs to the maker; it's their image. My clients know that all sandtrays are disassembled, and all play materials are put away after the session, because those belong to "the playroom", but usually, more honestly, "me". Some clients choose to disassemble the tray; again, I think that's their choice, but I know many others don't. Either way, the sandtray image will eventually be no more. If it's that important to them to have a photo, so be it. I would never tell a client not to write down what they remember about a session, not to take a picture of the appointment card I gave them, or the like.

The same goes for their artwork. Sometimes clients have a plan to give the piece to someone but want to keep a photo. That's their choice. Large, wet paintings may be temporarily stored on drying racks or on top of a bookshelf in the office, if those are available, which should be double locked, like all client records. Those are generally returned to a client the next week. I am generally against displaying client artwork in the office because it is so private and so not mine to exploit. I know "exploit" is a harsh word, but what else might be call decorating one's office with a vulnerable person's sacred images? There are times, though, when a client asks us to hang something up, or when a client wants to share their work as an act of advocacy; in these rare cases, if we're going to entertain that idea, we should have a policy on hand, benefits and risks should be explicitly discussed with the client, and a release of information should be obtained. We should never solicit client artwork to use for self-promotion. I'm generally uncomfortable doing so even for educational purposes. As a professor teaching clinicals, we generally require all images and recordings to be destroyed after being reviewed with the supervisor. I think we have an ethical obligation to take a hard, honest, and ongoing look at why and how frequently client images are taken and used for our own professional gain, be that teaching, research, or publication, especially as Jungian-oriented counselors, play therapists, and sandplay therapists.

REMEMBERING OUR ROLE

There's a popular quote on the internet attributed to Jung that says something like: the World will ask you who you are and if you don't know, it will tell you. He didn't *quite* say that in *Memories, Dreams, Reflections* (1989, p. 382), but he says:

> The meaning of my existence is that life has addressed a question to me. Or, conversely, I myself am a question which is addressed to the world, and I must communicate my answer, for otherwise I am dependent upon the world's answer.

This is relevant for all people, but let's consider it specifically in the counseling and play therapy profession. Clients, parents, agencies, insurance companies, schools, the justice system: everyone will have some idea of what they think a counselor is, what our role is, especially if they're looking for something from us, such as asking, or demanding, help. It is our role to know who we are, what we stand for, what we do, and conversely, what we won't do. I know some people disagree with me, but our theoretical orientation is the foundation on which we stand when examining ethical and legal codes, personal and professional boundaries. Theory comes from the Greek root, *theoria*, meaning "to look at", "behold", or "creatively contemplate" (The Dictionary of Spiritual Terms, n.d.). Our primary duty is to support and protect the dignity and privacy of ourselves and our clients.

If I am to not impose my values nor an agenda onto my clients, I think that means I need to be transparent about what those agendas are, including how I offer and hold space for people to come in and heal. This means disclosing my Jungian theoretical orientation, and my professional identity as a counselor and play therapist. It's my ethical duty to explain that in terms my client can understand, so that they might make an informed decision about if they want to work with me, and to hold the frame of our relationship. How about you? What do you think?

Reflections

1. What are some of your thoughts and feelings about relationships, including therapeutic relationships, occurring in person vs online? What are some possible similarities, differences, and challenges? Why might someone prefer one over the other?
2. Tell a story about your supervision history. You might choose symbols to represent you and your supervisor or supervisee. Does the story mirror another from your life? What were their messages about counter/co/transference? How did you grow or change? What did you learn? Did you get what you needed? Who do you turn to now for guidance?
3. Practice developing a life goal with objectives and interventions. How might you support yourself or ask for help with the interventions?
4. What are your top three core values right now? Are they different personally or professionally? You might do an internet search for a list of values to assist you.

REFERENCES

Allan, J. (1988). *Inscapes of the child's world: Jungian counseling in schools and clinics.* Spring Publications.

American Counseling Association (ACA). (2014). *ACA code of ethics.* www.counseling.org/resources/aca-code-of-ethics.pdf

Anekstein, A. M., Hoskins, W. J., Astramovich, R. L., Garner, D., & Terry, J. (2014). "Sandtray supervision": Integrating supervision models and sandtray therapy. *Journal of Creativity in Mental Health, 9,* 122–134. doi:10.1080/15401383.2014.876885

Association for Play Therapy (APT). (2022). *Play therapy best practices: Clinical, professional & ethical issues.* https://cdn.ymaws.com/www.a4pt.org/resource/resmgr/publications/best_practices.pdf

Balfour, R. N. (2013). Sandplay therapy: From alchemy to neuroscience. *Journal of Sandplay Therapy, 22*(1), 101–116. www.sandplay.org/journal/abstracts/volume-22-number-1/balfour-rosa-napoliello-sandplay-therapy-from-alchemy-to-neuroscience/

Bar-On, T. (2007). A meeting with clay: Individual narratives, self-reflection, and action. *Psychology of Aesthetics, Creativity, and the Arts, 1*(4), 225–236. https://doi.org/10.1037/1931-3896.1.4.225

Bartoskova, L. (2015). Research into post-traumatic growth in therapists: A critical literature review. *Counselling Psychology Review, 30*(3), 57–68.

Beacon Health Options. (2021). *SMART goal planning for behavioral health.* https://s21151.pcdn.co/wp-content/uploads/SMART-Goal-Planning-for-Behavioral-Health-Slides.pdf

Bell, H., Limberg, D., Jacobson, L., & Super, J. T. (2014). Enhancing self-awareness through creative experiential-learning play-based activities. *Journal of Creativity in Mental Health, 9*(3), 399–414. https://doi.org/10.1080/15401383.2014.897926

Bernard, J. M., & Goodyear, R. K. (2014). *Fundamentals of clinical supervision* (5th ed.). Pearson Allyn & Bacon.

Blaustein, M., & Kinniburgh, K. (2019). *Treating traumatic stress in children and adolescents: How to foster resilience through attachment, self regulation, and competency.* Guilford Press.

Blom, J. D., Nanuashvili, N., & Waters, F. (2021). *Time distortions: A systematic review of cases characteristic of Alice in Wonderland Syndrome. Frontiers in Psychiatry, 12,* 668633. https://doi.org/10.3389/fpsyt.2021.668633

Bradway, K., & McCoard, B. (1997). *Sandplay: Silent workshop of the psyche.* Routledge.

Bravesmith, A. (2008). Supervision and imagination. *The Journal of Analytical Psychology, 53*(1), 101–117. http://dx.doi.org/10.1111/j.1468-5922.2007.00704.x

Brooks, T. P. (2015). *How therapy affects the counselor: Development through play therapy practice and supervision.* [Doctoral dissertation]. https://trace.tennessee.edu/utk_graddiss/3561

Burgoon, J. K. (1985). Nonverbal signals. In M. L. Knapp & C. R. Miller (Eds.), *Handbook of inter-personal communication* (pp. 344–390). Sage.

Burns, S. T. (2017). Crafting a one-minute professional identity statement. *Journal of Counselor Leadership and Advocacy, 4*(1), 66–76. doi:10.1080/2326716X.2017.1284623.

Cabaniss, D. L., Cherry, S., Douglas, C. J., & Schwartz, A. R. (2016). *Psychodynamic psychotherapy: A clinical manual* (2nd ed.). Wiley.

Caplan, P. J. (2012, November 11). *APA does not care about weaponized diagnosis*. Psychology Today. www.psychologytoday.com/us/blog/science-isnt-golden/201211/apa-does-not-care-about-weaponized-diagnosis

Cashwell, C. S., & Young, J. S. (2020). *Integrating spirituality and religion into counseling: A guide to competent practice* (3rd ed.). American Counseling Association.

Christensen, J., Dickerman, C., & Dorn-Medeiros, C. (2018). Building a consensus of the professional dispositions of counseling students. *Journal of Counseling Preparation and Supervision, 11*(1). https://digitalcommons.sacredheart.edu/jcps/vol11/iss1/2

Circle of Security International. (2023). *Rupture and repair*. www.circleofsecurityinternational.com/tag/rupture-and-repair/

Day-Vines, N. L., Wood, S., Grothaus, T., Craigen, L., Holman, A., Dotson-Blake, K., & Douglass, M. J. (2007). Broaching the subjects of race, ethnicity, and culture during the counseling process. *Journal of Counseling and Development, 84*(4), 401–409. doi:10.1002/j.1556-6678.2007.tb00608.x.

The Dictionary of Spiritual Terms. (n.d.). *Definition of "theoria"*. www.dictionaryof-spiritualterms.com/public/Glossaries/terms.aspx?ID=358

Doran, G. T. (1981). There's a SMART way to write management goals and objectives. *Management Review, 70*(11), 35–36.

Doyle, K., & Magor-Blatch, L.E. (2017). Even adults need to play: Sandplay therapy with adult survivor of childhood abuse. *International Journal of Play Therapy, 26*(1), 12–22. http://dx.doi.org/10.1037/pla0000042

Elliott, R., Bohart, A. C., Watson, J. C., & Greenberg, L. S. (2011). Empathy. *Psychotherapy, 48*, 43–49. doi:10.1037/a0022187

Erby, A. N., & White, M. E. (2020). Broaching partially-shared identities: Critically interrogating power and intragroup dynamics in counseling practice with trans people of color. International Journal of Transgender Health, 23(1–2), 122–132. https://doi.org/10.1080/26895269.2020.1838389

Eryılmaz, A., & Mutlu, T. (2017). Developing the four-stage supervision model for counselor trainees. *Educational Sciences: Theory & Practice, 17*, 597–629. http://dx.doi.org/10.12738/estp.2017.2.2253

Fall, M., Drew, D., Chute, A., & Moore, A. (2007). The voices of registered play therapists as supervisors. *International Journal of Play Therapy, 16*, 133–146. http://dx.doi.org/10.1037/1555-6824.16.2.133

Figley, C. R. (2002). Compassion fatigue: Psychotherapists' chronic lack of self care. *Journal of Clinical Psychology, 58*(11), 1433–1441.

Francis, C. (1995). The therapeutic issues of transference and countertransference in the play therapy world. In B. Mark & J. Incorvaia (Eds.), *Handbook of infant, child, and adolescent psychotherapy: A guide to diagnosis and treatment* (6th ed., pp. 305–341). Aronson.

Garner, C., Freeman, B. J., & Lee, L. E. (2016). Assessment of student dispositions: The development and psychometric properties of the professional disposition competence assessment (PDCA). *Vistas, 52*, 1–14. www.counseling.org/knowledge-center/vistas/by-subject2/vistas-assessment/docs/default-source/vistas/article_5235f227f16116603abcacff0000bee5e7

Garner, C., Freeman, B., Stewart, R., & Coll, K. (2020). Assessment of dispositions in program admissions: The Professional Disposition Competence Assessment – Revised Admission (PDCA-RA). *The Professional Counselor, 10*(3). https://tpc-journal.nbcc.org/tag/dispositions/#:~:text=The%20nine%20dispositions%20assessed%20in,%2DAwareness%2C%20and%20Emotional%20Stability

Gerhart, D. R. (2016). *Theory and treatment planning in counseling and psychotherapy.* Cengage.

Geurtzen, N., Keijsers, G. P. J., Karremans, J. C., Tiemens, B. G., & Hutschemaekers, G. J. M. (2020). Patients' perceived lack of goal clarity in psychological treatments: Scale development and negative correlates. *Clinical Psychology & Psychotherapy, 27*(6), 915–924. doi:10.1002/cpp.2479.

Gibson, D. M., Wolf, C. P., Kennedy, S. D., Gerlach, J., Degges-White, S., & Watson, J. (2021) Development of the counselor wellness competencies. *Journal of Counselor Leadership and Advocacy, 8*(2), 130–145. doi:10.1080/2326716X.2021.1925997

Gil, E., & Rubin, L. (2005). Countertransference play: Informing and enhancing therapist self-awareness through play. *International Journal of Play Therapy, 14*, 87–102. http://dx.doi.org/10.1037/h0088904

Glăveanu, V. P., Karwowski, M., Jankowska, D. M., & de Saint-Laurent, C. (2018). Creative imagination. In T. Zittoun & V. P. Glăveanu (Eds.), *Handbook of Imagination and Culture* (pp. 61–86). Oxford University Press.

Gold, S. H., Hilsenroth, M. J., Kuutmann, K., & Owen, J. J. (2015). Therapeutic alliance in the personal therapy of graduate clinicians: Relationship to the alliance and outcomes of their patients. *Clinical Psychology & Psychotherapy, 22*(4), 304–316. https://doi.org/10.1002/cpp.1888

Greenleaf, R. (1970). *The servant as leader.* www.greenleaf.org/products-page/the-servant-as-leader/

Hays, J. (2016). *People of the Caucasus.* Facts and Details. https://factsanddetails.com/russia/Minorities/sub9_3d/entry-5089.html

Hesse, H., & Rosner, H. (1956). *The journey to the East*. Noonday Press.

Holland, J. L. (1997). *Making vocational choices: A theory of vocation-personalities and work environments* (3rd ed.). Psychological Assessment Resources.

Holman, E. A., Jones, N. M., Garfin, D. R., & Silver, R. C. (2023). Distortions in time perception during collective trauma: Insights from a national longitudinal study during the COVID-19 pandemic. *Psychological trauma: Theory, research, practice and policy, 15*(5), 800–807. https://doi.org/10.1037/tra0001326

Homeyer, L. E., & Bennett, M. M. (2023). *The guide to play therapy documentation & parent consultation*. Routledge.

Internet Encyclopedia of Ukraine. (2023). *Caucasia*. www.encyclopediaofukraine. com/display.asp?linkpath=pages%5CC%5CA%5CCaucasia.htm

Jablensky, A. (2016). Psychiatric classifications: Validity and utility. *World Psychiatry, 15*(1), 26–31. doi:10.1002/wps.20284.

Jolley, A. (2023, September 19). *Forget Freud's couch: Does spiritual psychotherapy work?* John Templeton Foundation. www.templeton.org/news/forget-freuds-couch-does-spiritual-psychotherapy-work?utm_source=Receive+News+from+the+John+Templeton+Foundation&utm_campaign=575b2ddfee-EMAIL_CAMPAIGN_2023_therapy_prayer_20231004&utm_medium=email&utm_term=0_-79ff1ce380-%5BLIST_EMAIL_ID%5D

Jongsma, A. E. (Ed.). (2021). *The complete adult psychotherapy treatment planner* (6th ed.). Wiley.

Jongsma, A. E. (Ed.). (2023). *The adolescent psychotherapy treatment planner* (5th ed.). Wiley.

Jung, C. G. (1989). *Memories, dreams, reflections*. A. Jaffe (Ed.), C. Winston & R. Winston (Trans.). Vintage Books.

Jung, C. G. (2023). *The collected works of C. G. Jung: Revised and expanded complete digital edition*. (CW 1–20). G. Adler, W. McGuire, & H. Read (Eds.), R. F. C. Hull (Trans.). Princeton University Press. https://press.princeton.edu/books/ebook/9780691255194/the-collected-works-of-c-g-jungKalff, D. M. (2020). *Sandplay: A psychotherapeutic approach to the psyche*. B. L. Matthews (Trans.). Analytical Psychology Press, Sandplay Editions. (Original work published 1966).

Karwowski, M., & Kaufman, J. C. (2017). *The creative self: Effect of beliefs, self-efficacy, mindset, and identity*. Academic Press. doi:10.1016/C2015-0-07011-3.

Kelly, K. E. (2006). Relationship between the Five-Factor Model of Personality and the Scale of Creative Attributes and Behavior: A validational study. *Individual Differences Research, 4*(5), 299–305.

Kestly, T. A. (2014). *The interpersonal neurobiology of play: Brain-building interventions for emotional well-being*. Norton.

Keysers, C. (2011). *The empathic brain: How the discovery of mirror neurons changes our understanding of human nature.* Social Brain Press.

Kim, R. (2022, March 7). *Addressing the lack of diversity in the mental health field.* National Alliance on Mental Illness. www.nami.org/Blogs/NAMI-Blog/March-2022/Addressing-the-Lack-of-Diversity-in-the-Mental-Health-Field

Kottman, T. (2014). *Play therapy: Basics and beyond.* Wiley.

Lambert, M. J., & Barley, D. E. (2001). Research summary on the therapeutic relationship and psychotherapy outcome. *Psychotherapy: Theory, Research, Practice, and Training, 38,* 357–361. http://dx.doi.org/10.1037/0033-3204.38.4.357

Lammers, J. C., Atouba, Y. L., & Carlson, E. J. (2013). Which identities matter? A mixed-method study of group, organizational, and professional identities and their relationship to burnout. *Management Communication Quarterly, 27*(4), 503–536. doi:10.1177/0893318913498824.

Landreth, G. (2024). *Play therapy: The art of the relationship.* Routledge. (Original work published 1991).

Leader, C. (2015). Evil, imagination and the unrepressed unconscious: The value of William Blake satanic "error" for clinical practice. *British Journal of Psychotherapy, 31*(3), 311–332.

Lennie, C. (2007). The role of personal development groups in counsellor training: Understanding factors contributing to self-awareness in the personal development group. *British Journal of Guidance and Counselling, 35,* 115–129. http://dx.doi.org/10.1080/03069880601106849

Lewis, C. P. (2021). *The weaponization of mental health: A paradox.* LinkedIn. www.linkedin.com/pulse/weaponization-mental-health-paradox-dr-clif-p-lewis-

Lewis, J. A., Arnold, M. S., House, R., et al. (2018). *American Counseling Association advocacy competencies.* www.counseling.org/docs/default-source/competencies/aca-advocacy-competencies-updated-may-2020.pdf

Lilly, JP (2015). Jungian analytical play therapy. In D. A. Crenshaw & A. L. Stewart (Eds.), *Play therapy: A comprehensive guide to theory and practice* (pp. 48–65). Guilford Press.

Lilly, JP, & Gaskill, R. (2023, October 14). *Unifying Jungian Analytical Theory and neuroscience to build healing pathways with play therapy.* Annual APT International Conference. Palm Springs, CA.

Loue, S. (2015) Ethical issues in sandplay research. In S. Loue (eds.), *Ethical issues in sandplay therapy practice and research.* Springer. https://doi.org/10.1007/978-3-319-14118-3_5

Luke, M., & Kiweewa, J. M. (2010). Personal growth and awareness counseling trainees in an experiential group. *Journal for Specialists in Group Work, 35,* 365–388. http://dx.doi.org/10.1080/01933922.2010.514976

Malikiosi-Loizos, M. (2013). Personal therapy for future therapists: Reflections on a still debated issue. *The European Journal of Counselling Psychology, 2*(1). doi:10.5964/ejcop.v2i1.4.

Markos, P. A., Coker, J. K., & Jones, W. P. (2007). Play or supervision? Evaluating the effectiveness of sandtray with beginning practicum students. *Journal for Creativity in Mental Health, 2*(3), 3–15.

Markos, P. A., Coker, J. K., & Jones, W. P. (2008). Play in supervision. *Journal of Creativity in Mental Health, 2*(3), 3–15. doi:10.1300/J456v02n03_02

McCann, I. L., & Pearlman, L. A. (1990). Vicarious traumatization: A framework for understanding the psychological effects of working with victims. *Journal of Traumatic Stress, 3*, 131–149.

McCurdy, K. G., & Owen, J. J. (2008). Using sandtray in Adlerian-based clinical supervision: An initial empirical analysis. *The Journal of Individual Psychology, 64*(1), 96–112.

McRoberts, R. (2018). Informed consent: Addressing child autonomy. *Play Therapy Magazine, 13*(4), 8. www.modernpubsonline.com/Play-Therapy/PlayTherapyDec18/html/index.html

Metcalf, L. (2003). Countertransference among play therapists: Implications for therapist development and supervision. *International Journal of Play Therapy, 12*, 31–48. http://dx.doi.org/10.1037/h0088877

Meyer, O. L., & Zane, N. (2013). The influence of race and ethnicity in clients' experience of mental health treatment. *Journal of Community Psychology, 41*(7), 884–901. https://doi.org/10.1002/jcop. 21580

Myers, J. E., Witmer, J. M., & Sweeney, T. J. (1996). The Wheel of Wellness. *The WEL workbook: Wellness evaluation of lifestyle*. MindGarden.

National Museum of African History and Culture. (2024). *Talking about race*. https://nmaahc.si.edu/learn/talking-about-race/topics/whiteness

Nissen-Lie, H. A., Rønnestad, M. H., Høglend, P. A., Havik, O. E., Solbakken, O. A., Stiles, T. C., & Monsen, J. T. (2017). Love yourself as a person, doubt yourself as a therapist? *Clinical Psychology and Psychotherapy, 24*, 48–60. doi:10.1002/cpp. 1977.

O'Connor, K. J., & Ray, D. (2023, October 13). *What if we have more in common than we think? Core concepts that move play therapy forward*. Annual APT International Conference. Palm Springs, CA.

Ohrt, J. H., Clarke, P. B., & Conley, A. H. (2019). *Wellness counseling: A holistic approach to prevention and intervention*. American Counseling Association.

Online Etymology Dictionary. (2023). *Temple* (n. 1). www.etymonline.com/search?q=temenos

OpenNotes. (2023). *Federal rules mandating open notes.* www.opennotes.org/onc-federal-rule/

Painter, N. I. (2003, November 7–8). *Why white people are called "Caucasian".* Collective Degradation: Slavery and the Construction of Race. Proceedings of the Fifth Annual Gilder Lehrman Center International Conference at Yale University. https://glc.yale.edu/sites/default/files/files/events/race/Painter.pdf

Paone, T., Malott, K., Gao, J., & Kinda, G. (2015). Using sandplay to address students' reactions to multicultural counselor training. *International Journal of Play Therapy, 24*(4), 190–204. http://dx.doi.org/10.1037/a0039813

Pastner, B., Alexopoulos, J., Rohm, C., Preuche, I., & Loeffler-Stastka, H. (2014). Development of therapeutic attitudes: Attitudes of trainees in training. *European Journal of Educational Sciences, 1*(1), 110–123.

Pearlman, L. A., & MacIan, P. S. (1995). Vicarious traumatization: An empirical study of the effects of trauma work on trauma therapists. *Professional Psychology: Research and Practice, 26,* 558–565. https://doi.org/10.1037/0735-7028.26.6.558

Penner, F., Gambin, M., & Sharp, C. (2019). Childhood maltreatment and identity diffusion among inpatient adolescents: The role of reflective function. *Journal of Adolescence, 76,* 65–74. https://doi.org/10.1016/j.adolescence.2019.08.002

Perryman, K., Blisard, P., & Moss, R. (2019). Using creative arts in trauma therapy: The neuroscience of healing. *Journal of Mental Health Counseling, 41*(1), 80–94. https://doi.org/10.17744/mehc.41.1.07

Petchkovsky, L., Petchkovsky, M., Morris, P., Dickson, P., Montgomery, D., Dwyer, J., & Burnett, P. (2013). fMRI responses to Jung's Word Association Test: Implications for theory, treatment and research. *The Journal of Analytical Psychology, 58*(3), 409–431. https://doi.org/10.1111/1468-5922.12021

Phillips, L. (2021, November 22). Culture-centered counseling. *Counseling Today.* https://ct.counseling.org/2021/11/culture-centered-counseling/

Potapchuck, M. (2012). *White culture.* CAPD, MP Associates, World Trust Educational Services. www.seattle.gov/documents/Departments/RSJI/GRE/whiteculturehandout.pdf

Potash, J., & Chen, J. (2014). Art-mediated peer-to-peer learning of empathy. *The Clinical Teacher, 11,* 327–331. doi:10.1111/tct.12157

Ratts, M. J., Singh, A. A., Nassar-McMillan, S., Butler, S. K., & McCullough, J. R. (2016). Multicultural and social justice counseling competencies: Guidelines for the counseling profession. *Journal of Multicultural Counseling and Development, 44*(1), 28–48. https://doi.org/10.1002/jmcd.12035

Ray, D. (2011). *Advanced play therapy: Essential conditions, knowledge, and skills for child practice.* Routledge.

Robbins. S., & Jolkovski, M. (1987). Managing countertransference feelings: An intersectional model using awareness of feeling and theoretical framework. *Journal of Counseling Psychology, 34*, 276–282. http://dx.doi.org/10.1037/0022-0167.34.3.276

The Robert K. Greenleaf Center for Servant Leadership. (2021). *What is servant leadership?* www.greenleaf.org/what-is-servant-leadership/

Samuels, A. (1985). Countertransference, the "mundus imaginalis" and a research project. *The Journal of Analytical Psychology, 30*(1), 47–71. https://doi.org/10.1111/j.1465-5922.1985.00047.x

Sandplay Therapists of America (STA). (2024). *Guidelines for research in sandplay.* www.sandplay.org/wp-content/uploads/Guidelines-and-Procedures-for-Research-Using-Sandplay-Therapy.pdf

Searles, H. F. (1955). The informational value of the supervisor's emotional experience. *Psychiatry, 18*, 135–146.

Shamambo, L. J., & Henry, T. L. (2022). Rethinking the use of "Caucasian" in clinical language and curricula: A trainee's call to action. *Journal of General Internal Medicine, 37*(7), 1780–1782. https://doi.org/10.1007/s11606-022-07431-6

Shand-Lubbers, R. M. (2023). Becoming a white antiracist counselor: A framework of identity development. *Counselor Education and Supervision, 62*(3), 203–294. *https://doi.org/10.1002/ceas.12272*

Siegel, D. J. (2007). *The mindful brain: Reflection and attunement in the cultivation of well-being.* W. W. Norton.

Steinhardt, L. F. (2012). *On becoming a Jungian sandplay therapist.* Jessica Kingsley Publishers.

Stewart, A. L., Field, T. A., & Echterling, L. G. (2016). Neuroscience and the magic of play therapy. *International Journal of Play Therapy, 25*(1), 4–13. http://dx.doi.org/10.1037/pla0000016

Stillo, S. M. (2018). *Exploring supervisees' experiences of discussing personal issues in professional counselor supervision: An interpretive phenomenological analysis* (Doctoral dissertation). ProQuest Dissertations & Theses. (UMI No. 2086516161).

Tennessee Department of Mental Health and Substance Abuse Services. (2013). *TDMHSAS best practice guidelines: Obtaining informed consent for children and adolescents.* echappellTDMHSASResearchTeam, 363–366. www.tn.gov/content/dam/tn/mentalhealth/documents/Pages_from_CY_BPGs_363-366.pdf

Transcaucasian Trail. (2019). *About the Caucasus.* https://transcaucasiantrail.org/en/about/the-caucasus/#:~:text=The%20Caucasus%2C%20a%20mountainous%20isthmus,%2C%20Armenia%2C%20Turkey%20and%20Iran

Turner, B.A. (2005). *The handbook of sandplay therapy*. Temenos Press.

Urban, E. (1996). With healing in her wings: Integration and repair in a self-destructive adolescent. *Journal of Child Psychotherapy, 22*(1), 64–81.

Van Wagoner, S., Gelso, C., Hayes, J., & Diemer, R. (1991). Countertransference and the reputedly excellent therapist. *Psychotherapy, 28*(3), 411–421. http://dx.doi.org/10.1037/0033-3204.28.3.411

Viado, L. A. (2015). *Countertransference issues of wounded healers: A case study approach*. [Doctoral dissertation]. ProQuest Dissertations and Theses (UMI No. 3714348).

von Franz, M. L. (1980). *Projection and re-collection in Jungian psychology*. Open Court Publishing.

Wampold, B. E., & Imel, Z. E. (2015). *The great psychotherapy debate*. Routledge.

Wilkinson, M. (2005). Undoing dissociation: Affective neuroscience: A contemporary Jungian clinical perspective. *The Journal of Analytical Psychology, 50*(4), 483–501. https://doi.org/10.1111/j.0021-8774.2005.00550.x

Wilkinson, M. (2006). The dreaming mind-brain: A Jungian perspective. *The Journal of Analytical Psychology, 51*(1), 43–59. http://dx.doi.org/10.1111/j.0021-8774.2006.00571.x

Willemsen, H. (2014). Early trauma and affect: The importance of the body for the development of the capacity to symbolize. *Journal of Analytical Psychology, 59*(5), 695–712. doi:10.1111/1468-5922.12117.

Winnicott, D. W. (1971). *Playing and reality*. Basic Books.

World Population Review. (2023). *Age of consent for mental health treatment by state 2023*. https://worldpopulationreview.com/state-rankings/age-of-consent-for-mental-health-treatment-by-state

Yee, T., Ceballos, P., & Swan, A. (2019). Examining trends of play therapy articles: A 10-year content analysis. *International Journal of Play Therapy, 28*(4), 250–260. https://doi.org/10.1037/pla0000103

Yoo, H. (2011). *Supervisors' experience of empathetic understanding when using art-making in art therapy supervision*. [Doctoral dissertation]. ProQuest Dissertations & Theses (Order No. 3478778).

Ziff, K., Ivers, N., & Hutton, K. (2017). "There's beauty in brokenness": Teaching empathy through dialogue with art. *Journal of Creativity in Mental Health, 12*(2), 249–261. https://doi.org/10.1080/15401383.2016.1263587

7
Creative Techniques

Out of a playful movement of elements whose interrelations are not immediately apparent, patterns arise which an observant and critical intellect can only evaluate afterwards. The creation of something new is not accomplished by the intellect but by the play instinct acting from inner necessity. The creative mind plays with the objects it loves.

Jung, CW 6, p. 182, § 197

After learning a bit about Jung, students have told me they are often intrigued, but are left wondering what they might actually *do with* or *say to* clients if wanting to work from a Jungian framework. They're wanting *techniques*. I will admit that the word "techniques" makes me bristle a bit. Let me explain why.

The trick is, there is no trick.

No, the trick is that I titled this chapter "creative techniques" because I know counselors and play therapists want them so badly that I had to lure you through a little door in order to present you with this bigger idea. There are so many books filled with "creative techniques", and if you really want that, you are invited to go find and read them. No shade, but even after my proposal for this book was accepted, I was asked to put "techniques" in the title of this book. No. No, thank you. I know techniques sell. Techniques sell not just books but continuing education, inter/national conferences, expensive certification programs, and, I'm sorry, but they sell-out the relationship. To me, the word "techniques" has come to mean a kind of therapist designed, pre-fab lesson plan with a directive, goal-oriented activity, usually focusing on a problem, not the whole person. I can see how they can be tempting, even temporarily helpful, especially for insecure or new clinicians, or a seasoned clinician wanting to branch out with an original brand, but they're

DOI: 10.4324/9781003433736-7

tricks. They focus on the therapist, their goal, their sense of accomplishment, and what they want the client to do, which to me is dangerously close to not being client-centered, a foundational counselor value. Over-reliance on technique, especially without a strong professional identity and theoretical foundation, means the counselor is now "just a therapist" with a big ol' bag of tricks. Too much of that, and we've lost focus on who we are and how to be in relationship with both our-Selves and collaboratively with our clients. Being endlessly hungry for new techniques is, at its core, ego-focused, and a demonstration of a misalignment with the Self. I'm not about that; I don't think Jung was, either, and I certainly don't want to promote that to my students.

Several dictionary definitions of "techniques" and "skills", though, are almost interchangeable. I prefer "skills" for four good reasons. (1) We use the word "skills" in counselor education and supervision, to describe, teach, and measure competencies. I like to be consistent with language when it is more helpful to do so. (2) The subtext of the word "technique" as a marketing gimmick in our field is so obvious that I cannot conflate the two with good conscience. We need to be aware and wary of people trying to sell us the latest-and-the-greatest "techniques". (3) My teacher taught me that in Hindu mythology, *Kaushalya*, the name of the Queen Mother, means "skill" (Newell, 2021); it actually means the specific, spiritual, and (for our sake and purposes) psychologically skillful means of keeping the mind, body, and spirit focused on the Self. This concept is also known in Mahayana Buddhism (you know, where Westerners stole and re-packaged "mindfulness" from). That is my point, exactly. (4) Jung didn't like techniques and said in several places that they don't exist objectively.

Jung was intentionally elusive about his method, a sentiment that appears to be tattooed on the hearts of the Jungian community. In his writings, both personal and professional, he expressed a hesitation to concretize the process in favor of remaining open to new ideas and scientific findings as they emerge (Bulkeley & Weldon, 2011). Today, Jungian theory straddles across expressive arts, play, and mind-body therapies, aspects of which are validated by neuroscience and attachment theory. However, specific research on a single "Jungian" method remains rather elusive, in part because the community cannot agree on a single protocol, and many simply have no interest in attempting to manualize treatment. Sandplay therapy is a notable exception, though the research protocol currently outlined by the Sandplay Therapists of America (STA, n.d.) does not fully account for the further dialogue that may continue after the creation of the sand picture is made in silence, past that it should be client-centered (more about sandplay therapy below). For this reason, I often reinforce the integration of not only the basic

and advanced counseling skills, but those taught in child-centered play therapy (CCPT; Landreth, 2024). To me, there are many parallels between the
Jungian and person-centered theory, namely the view of human nature, trust
in the client, a spiritual core, the value of the person-of-the-therapist, facilitating creativity, and avoiding imposing our will. Landreth also really outlines some of those *non-quantifiable intangibles* about our biases that we tend
to dance around more in the counseling world. We might take it for granted
that our desire for our client to change or "perform" might actually get in the
way of their ability to feel safe and free to be themselves. While I am very
interested in what the symbols that emerge for the work might mean, I try
to do so with genuine curiosity and intentionally delayed interpretation. My
goal is to focus on the relationship and collaborating to understand.

Looking back, though, we can see glimpses of Jung's method as well as themes
that emerged, but he himself said there was no specific technique, especially
to working with Shadow material (Jung, 1973), a sentiment that is extended
to Jungian analytic play therapy today (Lilly, 2015). We want to encourage
creativity through mode-shifting (see Chapter 2), avoiding one-sidedness
(CW 8) in our thinking, and encouraging awareness and shifting within the
counseling relationship, but never imposing our will onto others, including
suggestions and interpretations.

But HOW, exactly, might we do that? There are innumerable ways to engage
both associative and analytic modes. However, it's been said that we need
to find a way to satisfy one side of the psyche without harming the other.
This is why consent and child assent are to be ongoing (ACA, 2014; APT,
2022). Interventions must always be invitations when working creatively
with whole Selves, including our clients. Our clients must feel safe, have
choices, and be free in our presence to act as they wish without overt pressure
from us to perform.

The sentiment stated by one of Jung's most beloved students, Marie-Loise
von Franz (1998), sets us up to begin to look at creative interventions, from
talking to art making, though she was speaking specifically about dreams. She
encourages us to attempt to understand every aspect of the creative process,
even the so-called "resistance", as drama. Much like in Indian mythology,
the Self is expressing itself through the divine play where it, and therefore
we, are symbolically everything in the story: from the writer to the characters
to the story to the ears hearing it. Dora Kalff, too, the mother of sandplay
therapy, stated in her book on the approach, which is traditionally a silent,
sand-focused process, that symbolic material may also appear verbally and
through art making (2020).

Some of the latest research in creative cognition suggests that we might help people feel more creative by expressing our value in creativity, believing that people are inherently creative, and making creative pursuits seem more do-able, or achievable (Karwowski et al., 2022). This takes a significant amount of creative knowledge and practice on our part. Our ultimate goal is to be present with ourselves and our clients, inviting the engagement of the symbolic, religious, and ultimately transformative function, acknowledging the needs of the drives (see Chapter 4), and listening to the symbolic language of the unconscious (Chapter 5). This might manifest through the body, mind, or spirit. Prepare for any and all of them to show up.

Clients who might be hesitant to engage in the creative process, for whatever reason, may be inspired by the counselor who embodies a sense of creative self-efficacy, and patience, and practice as a Wounded Healer turned Servant Leader. The therapeutic relationship may act not only as a container, but a ritualistic practice toward transformation. Psyche is often just as pleased with a symbolic, ritualistic act as a "real" one (Johnson, 1991). The safe and sacred space (temenos), the act of confession, the consistency of our therapeutic "liturgy", allowing clients to create their own, and transitioning through liminal space together, all has the potential for activating the religious function in clients. This is not to say that therapy is a substitute for organized religion – by no means! – but here we recognize and honor the interconnectedness of the psychospiritual, and the mystery of the transcendent function. We are to walk and work with clients humbly and reverently.

If we need an easy formula for inviting participation in creative, mode-shifting interventions, I like to borrow from the psychodynamic framework (Corey, 2021) but add a Jungian twist:

- maintaining a safe and protected space
- lowering consciousness through encouraging:
  - the associative process
  - free association, dreams, art making, play
- increasing conscious awareness of unconscious processes through:
  - the analytic process
  - discussion and interpretation – immediacy (here and now), resistance, the relationship
- encouraging transformative action.

We may get there by talking, co-interpreting dreams, making artwork, or even playing. We focus on being attuned, curious, and practicing mode-shifting. All of these involve being open and embody aspects of creativity. But what we must remember, from this Jungian discussion all the way to our counselor roots, is that what we are really creating is the therapeutic relationship IN COLLABORATION with our-Selves and our clients. Ancient wisdom, CCPT, and Jung all teach that the creative process is sacred and spontaneous.

Jung explains that people may naturally gravitate toward different methods for engaging the unconscious, which may be expressed verbally, by writing down details or by creating artwork (CW 8, pp. 118–119, § 170–171):

- Visual – more easily see images in their mind's-eye or may report having visions.
- Audio-verbal – may hear an internal voice, theirs or others, narrating, telling a story, or making suggestions.
- Movement – while rare, some adults will spontaneously gravitate toward creating images with their hands. Other types of physical expression may be encouraged, such as making wide gestures or even using a talking board to assist automatic writing.

Jung suggests that this process may not be fully known by the client (a phenomenon also known as *dissociative absorption* by Kuiken et al., 2018) so it is the creative counselor's duty to be on the lookout and help clarify the affect when appropriate (CW 8). Free, spontaneous speech, art, and play are considered the best start (von Franz, 1980), but Jung noted that it can be tough to fully experience and integrate unconscious material alone (CW 16). So, our roles as witness, container, and interpretive collaborator are all important as Jungian-oriented counselors.

This begs the question: should Jungian counseling be considered directive or non-directive?

TO BE OR NOT TO BE . . . DIRECTIVE

> Every form of communication with the split-off part of the psyche is therapeutically effective. This effect is also brought about by the real or merely supposed discovery of the causes. Even when the discovery is no more than an assumption or a fantasy, it has a healing effect at least by suggestion if the analyst himself believes in it and makes a serious attempt to understand.
>
> CW 13, p. 342, § 465

I tend to think about "being directive" on a continuum, especially about play therapy theory. This is where we're really having this conversation about *directives* (Gil, 2006). I don't hear about it much in the general counseling field, with the focus on talk therapy, but I think we should talk about it more. Directives include suggestions for others to think or do what the therapist would like. I know talk-therapists do this even without art materials and toys, with statements, suggestions, and questions: "Think about a time when . . .", "Tell me about . . .", "How about you . . .", "What would it look like it if . . .?". How about we start by owning that?

Sandplay therapy, which is a specific Jungian model, is non-directive, while Jungian Play Therapy might be more directive, so we will explore both below, in order of least to most directive. However, when integrated with other models, which we know is how most counselors practice, it can look very different. While Jungian counseling and play therapy are not symptom-focused, we might work in environments that require us to meet certain practice standards. Because of this, we might take a more non-directive stance. Many of the counseling skills listed on the CCS-R can also be considered non-directive interventions.

As a general rule, non-directive interventions tend to favor more:

- Facilitating an empathic, respectful, safe relationship and environment.
- Appearing relaxed and interested / leaning in.
- Intentional use of silence.
- Reflecting feelings/thoughts/content: Sometimes reflection is simply one word, repeating back something a client says (e.g., "that hurt!") but other times it is an interpretation of what we see (e.g., a child puts a toy down and we say, "You're done with that"). Reflecting content is also sometimes called "tracking" (e.g., "Now you're deciding to paint"). Paraphrasing (short restatements) and summarizing (longer restatements) are also considered reflecting on the CCS-R. An advanced reflection might be also called "enlarging meaning" (e.g., "You know a lot about . . .", "You trusted them . . ."). Reflecting what we notice about a client in the here and now is called "immediacy"; an example might be "That scowl lets me know you don't like that".
- Returning responsibility: e.g., "In here, you get to decide". "You're welcome to create whatever you like". "You get to name that miniature".
- Encouraging: Avoiding the use of judgments, either good or bad, encourages instead to invite continuation, such as non-verbals like "mmm-hmmm", nodding, etc. or acknowledgement of effort or unconditional positive regard, e.g., "You're working hard on that!", "Oh, I see!".

- Free play/exploration/association.
- Spontaneous drawings or artmaking, otherwise known as *art as therapy* (Kramer, 2000).

Interventions on the more suggestive/semi-directive/directive continuum include:

- "Strewing" – placing objects one thinks a person might "need" to communicate or learn. This is a term that I first heard in the Unschooling Community (Dodd, n.d.), which is a non-directive approach to learning. However, it also reflects practices of Ecosystemic Play Therapy (O'Connor, 1991) where therapists choose items for the child to play with based on various factors. I would also consider having items such as mandalas/round paper in a playroom (more on mandalas later), having books on therapeutic or mythic themes in the room, or obtaining items with a certain client in mind in the realm of strewing. An example of the latter might be collecting more natural materials, such as pine cones, leaves, sticks, and rocks for a client who commented that they wished there were more of these in the playroom.
- "Third hand interventions" – this is an art therapy term which refers to a variety of ways that a therapist might support and intervene a bit in someone else's creative process in an attuned way to assist the client. We act quite literally as their "third hand". It may be as subtle as squeezing more paint onto a pallet or as overt as making a mark on a sheet of paper at the client's request.
- Suggesting activities the therapist thinks the client might enjoy or be helpful. Less direct suggestions might be, "There are paints over there", or "You can show me in the sand if you like". More directive would be, "Would you show me a picture of your family in the sand?".
- Asking questions. Landreth (2024) gives the best explanation for how questions may disempower the most vulnerable and pull them from associative into analytic processes too soon. Often we ask questions when they could be reflective statements demonstrating greater understanding; for example, "You want to paint now?" and "You want to paint now!" are subtle differences, but to someone needing to be deeply heard, the latter may be more effective. In CCPT questions of any kind are practically forbidden. In the CCS-R, the use of questions should be "appropriate", and closed questions should be limited, with favor given to open-ended questions.
- "Soft interpretations" or "hunches" (dreams, symbol amplification, etc., see more below) – again, this is a question of authority vs collaboration.

Since the therapist is in a position of power over the client, their suggestions of what a symbol might mean could have an influential impact which might disrupt the natural healing process (JP Lilly, as cited in Kottman & Meany-Walen, 2018). Interpretations happen if our definition includes our very thoughts about what something might mean; I argue that we are always, especially as counselors, assessing and interpreting even micro-expressions and emotional tone, let alone a particularly chosen series of figures chosen and arranged in the sand. While we might keep these thoughts to ourselves, we may also cite them specifically in our progress and/or psychotherapy notes, even if they are only the determination of play themes, or assessing those themes as evidence of wounds or healing (Friedman & Mitchell, 1991; Yeh et al., 2015).

- Strongly suggesting or "assigning" homework, even if it is recording dreams, playing more, finishing a piece of artwork at home, or reading a story is directive.
- Psychoeducation / information sharing: sharing information in service of our clients can be a major component of many evidence-based integrative practices, such as CBT (Jongsma et al., 2021). Jungians might not disagree with CBT that feeling, thinking, and behaving are interconnected and that increased insight may be helpful in reducing symptoms; however, we might argue that they are not so easily identified and changed directly, as unconscious factors may influence them all.
- Putting together a guided imagery sequence or story; this directive might be changed to be based on information a client spontaneously presents.
- Pre-packaged "techniques", board games, worksheets, etc. are designed to be directive, though they might be used creatively.

For example, in sandplay therapy (discussed further below), there are no specific guidelines for how to respond to a person when they ask us something (such as a question, or for help), when we need to set a limit (such as throwing sand), or how to establish the therapeutic relationship, other than to be client-centered. For this reason, I often refer to the guidelines set forth by CCPT. Some credit Jung with influencing the development of person-centered counseling (Douglas, 2005), the initial basis for CCPT. Sandplay therapy and CCPT are similar in that they both:

- are evidence-based practices (Evidence Based Child Therapy, 2023; Wiersma et al., 2022)
- value creating sacred space and maintaining relational safety (Kalff, 2020; Landreth, 2024)

- are not simply a collection of techniques but are a philosophy or way of being
- acknowledge unconscious / sensory soothing / symbolic processing
- are client-led, therapist attuned
- focus on the present, not the past
- are non-pathologizing
- are accepting rather than correcting
- limit the use of questions
- trust the process, the wisdom of the psyche, and consider the play to be in and of itself therapeutic
- limit the use of verbal interventions
- highly suggest therapists do their own work
- delay interpretation but observe for themes

THE TALKING CURE

> "The psyche creates reality every day" through the creative process, bridging feeling and thinking, intuition and sensation, providing "answers to all answerable questions" from within.
>
> CW 6, p. 88, § 78

Freud is often credited with discovering the *talking cure*, or patients feeling better after free-associating on his couch while he wasn't looking at them. However, we really should go back and credit Anna O., the client herself, as inspiring the method, as Freud later did. See Breuer and Freud's *Studies in Hysteria* (2004) and an internet search of this amazing feminist pioneer. Jung's philosophical, spiritual, ethical, and practical differences led him to make great strides in changing the method Freud taught him, so much so that he's barely included in psychoanalytic or even psychodynamic textbooks.

Jung disagreed with Freud fervently in three major areas that impact how we might skillfully listen and utilize talking: the value and role of the unconscious, spirituality, and attachment. Freud thought of the unconscious like a garbage can, where we attempt to shove our unwanted thoughts and desires, and that dreams were like putrid clues for the doctor to convince their patients to capture so they might more fully examine and figure out what's infecting the client; Jung thought there was great wisdom in both the personal and collective unconscious, and that they spoke a symbolic language all their own, often unique to the dreamer, who was ultimately the one who could make meaning of them, which could enhance their life. While Freud was Jewish and integrated mythology into his theory and personal art collection, his position on religion, in general, is that he thought it quite feeble-minded to believe anything outside the realm of science; on the other hand, Jung took what is still considered quite a revolutionary and contemporary stance that religion is an ancient, global reality, which serves many essential psychological and social functions, and integrated both Eastern and Western thought into his work. Finally, while Freud highly sexualized even an infant's attachment to their parents, Jung saw our major drives to be working toward finding love, security, and expression in alignment with our true Self, which can still be seen throughout the development of attachment, humanistic, and I'd argue even Internal Family Systems theory.

In some ways we might say that Jung was more "anti-medical model" than "spiritual", but that would be too reductive. In a way, though, it reflects the spirit of the age he was living in. Until that point, other than confession or seeking guidance from a religious or other community elder, nothing else looked like what we now know as counseling. Jung was very interested in spirituality and sought a bridge to new scientific methods. To be truly free to say or do whatever we wish in the presence of someone who will be fully accepting of all of it is a rare occurrence in everyday life (sometimes even, or especially, in religious circles). However, it is the foundation of what it means to be a counselor, to be client-focused, especially a Jungian.

Be present and invite creative exploration.

I often say that Jung invites us to wonder with our clients, engaging the numinous with the knowledge and presence to *enrich associations* (CW 16). Jungianians all aim to honor the symbolic life. We actively work toward staying curious with our clients, suspending our analytic interpretations for some time while bathed in associative processes (see mode-shifting). However, we need first to be able to create an environment of safety in order for others to lower into their unconscious, or associative processes. We must listen to the unconscious material, verbal, emotional, or visual, that emerges as the map to Self-knowledge (von Franz, 1998). But we mustn't rush into that analytic thinking, or problem-solving mode, too quickly. This is a skill.

The skills I will discuss in this section under the "talking cure" aren't necessarily all about talking, but they do generally involve talking, or are the primary skills used by counselors who mostly rely on talking (as opposed to making art or playing). They may also be included in a play therapy relationship. They are also primarily skills reflected in The Counselor Competencies

Scale – Revised (CCS-R; Lambie et al., 2018), an assessment tool aligned with CACREP (2024) standards that is used as an assessment tool in counselor education training programs. I will also refer to many CCPT skills, especially where they integrate into Jungian theory, to help make the practice seem more concrete.

Basic Counseling Skills

Basic counseling skills are ones that aim to foster a sense of safety, freedom, and demonstrate that we are fully present with and curious about our clients. (We also say they're "basic" so as to not scare new students off, because they really involve a lot of complex philosophical underpinnings that we'll discuss in the Advanced section.) This includes non-verbal and verbal attending, reflecting feelings and thoughts, as well as sometimes, if necessary, asking questions.

We start with *non-verbal attending*, which can be challenging to describe, as it may vary depending on a variety of factors, including the size of the room, the arrangement of furniture, how comfortable each person is with the other, and if we're online. In general, we want to maintain a comfortable distance, a relaxed, open posture, and soft expression to communicate our sense of ease in the space. This cannot be faked. It's a skill we need to practice. Mindfulness, an *intentional use of silence*, and ongoing reflective practices are a must to be able to sit with our clients in non-verbal attending, and to truly see if and when we are, or aren't. Self-awareness, emotional stability, and openness are all considered aspects of our professional counselor disposition that can be observed non-verbally, and now assessed in many graduate counseling programs (Garner et al., 2020). I also would put what are sometimes called *non-verbal utterances*, or therapist sounds, like "hmm-hmm", "mmm . . .", or "aaah!" into this category. They are ideally used minimally, but with affective facial expressions, to let the client know we're listening and feeling with them. I am not a fan of keeping a neutral expression and don't encourage my students to "fix their face", either. I direct them to the now very famous Still Face Experiment (originally published as Tronick et al., 1975, but one of my favorite videos is by the Children's Institute, 2016, both of which I'll cite below). The Still Face Experiment shows us how quickly even securely attached babies can become distressed when their loving caregiver gives them a blank expression, but we still don't have a complete understanding of why. Remembering the difference between Freud and Jung on attachment, and our counseling values (ACA, 2014) we are not neutral; we are to communicate empathy, and that means emotion. Our capacity to emote comes from the symbolic function, and our connection to the Self.

Beginning with verbal attending, we start with typical "therapist speak", words or short phrases such as "Ok . . .", "yeah . . .", "wow!". Another major counseling skill, and one that will get a student high marks on the CCS-R (Lambie et al., 2018) is the PRIMARY use of reflecting in sessions. That means we want to hear the counselor reflect back to the client what they hear or otherwise perceive what they are FEELING, primarily, as well as thinking, saying, and meaning. That may sound like a feeling word (a feeling is one word), reflected back like "sad . . ." or a short phrase or summary like "That hurt you . . .". Verbal attending might also fall under the category of *immediacy* as well. Some consider immediacy to be an advanced skill, but I think that noticing what's literally going on in the room is pretty basic, though sometimes it takes courage to say so. This might sound like "You're really mad at me" based on the look on a child's face after we tell them it's almost time to go. We might also say, "I notice that your shoulders dropped just then . . . that looks like it was a relief!". However, there is a divide in the Jungian world about how much one should verbally interact at all with our clients, which we will discuss more below.

Questions are so common in everyday life, and in counselor training, and yet are so controversial in some circles, especially in play therapy, that I almost put them under advanced techniques, below. Well, I do discuss them below, but I want to mention them here first. Gary Landreth (2024), the developer of child-centered play therapy (CCPT) really taught me to always consider why we might ask questions at all, especially to children. He says that if we know enough to ask a question we can make a reflective statement. So, instead of asking "Do you want me to open that?" we can state "You want me to open that". He also says that when we ask a question we are making a demand on the client, imposing our desire to know, and not respecting where they are. With children, that is often in play, which is an associative process. In adults, that may be in silence, which is a sacred place of potentiality. A question is an analytic process, which pulls them out. Our question can both be an interruption and a powerful suggestion, which could be off base and lead a client down a path they were not planning to go down. That's not respecting their process. However, some questions can be encouraging, show interest, make the process seem more natural or conversational, put people at ease, and be quite open like, "Then what?", "What was that like?", or even, "Really?!". It's also a social norm in America to ask questions, and it makes some people really uncomfortable when we don't ask any. I've had clients, as young as five years old, express their annoyance at an over use of reflection and have asked to play "ask me about my day", so I might show interest in ways that they prefer. So the lesson is: use questions in a client-centered way, not to impose our own agenda.

Advanced Counseling Skills

Advanced counseling skills have more potential for the counselor to impose their own will. Though they might be seen as a little thing, they can lead to mis-attunement, so should be used with caution and intentionality. Advanced skills might be used because the counselor has an insight, thinks that what they know might be helpful to the client, or wants to hurry the process along, for whatever reason. They also might be truly helpful to the client, ethically warranted, and are considered some of the nuts-and-bolts realities of counseling.

Information sharing is the first one, and is something we do right from our first interactions with a client, be that online on our websites, or by presenting intake paperwork. Considering it starts at the beginning, I get that it seems like a basic skill, but there is so much nuance. Sometimes a client is in such a state when they first come in that we can sense right away that they don't know what they're reading and signing; they're so overwhelmed with emotion they aren't taking new information in. At times like that, we might need to get real basic, and just cover the informed consent forms, or other legal requirements, letting them know we're a professional listener, the limits of confidentiality, and that we'll revisit it all next time, and give them copies to take home. Information sharing time often happens in safety planning, crisis, or providing resources for people who may need a service we don't provide, such as food or shelter. In this way, we might need to *interpret* what we see or read between the lines of what a client is saying to be able to link them to appropriate resources. We also share information when we are providing psychoeducation, again, which should be presented conscientiously. We might engage in information sharing both indirectly or directly (Lilly & Heiko, 2019). For example, we might sing a lullaby to a babydoll when a child asks us to put them to bed. Or, a client might ask for something to do at bedtime to help quiet the mind. We might normalize the struggle by information sharing, as well as *self-disclose* what some of our favorites are, based on clinical experience. Appropriate self-disclosure might also be letting our clients know we're worried about them, which is why we're completing a safety plan, or reminding them of our ethical boundaries, such as "Thank you, but I don't accept gifts". More advanced self-disclosure might be letting a client know that you're comfortable praying with them, if they've been hinting that they'd like you to do so.

Telling stories may also fall under information sharing. The use of myth and metaphor as a descriptor of psychological functioning goes all the way back to Freud, but it is the Jungians who love to share stories with their clients and each other, from analysts to play therapists (Allan, 1988). A couple of my favorite books on the psychological implications of children's literature in general are *The Uses of Enchantment* (Bettelheim, 1975) and *Don't Tell the Grown-Ups* (Lurie, 1998). However, it is the work of Marie von Franz that is considered the gold standard for a Jungian examination of fairy tales; there are too many published titles to mention them all here but a few are: *Archetypal Patterns in Fairy Tales* (1997), *Animus & Anima in Fairy Tales* (2002), and *Shadow & Evil in Fairy Tales* (1974). While clients are often described as "telling their stories", we also want to listen for themes and stories-within-the-story, like a dream-within-a-dream. This may emerge as clients singing a bit of a favorite song, describing a new movie they saw, sharing memories of childhood bedtime stories, or reciting lines of scripture. To explore themes, we may seek out inspiration from looking at play-themes, as well as from literature.

Some of the research that we have about culturally sensitive practices suggests that clients often want counselors to invite them to talk about topics that might be particularly uncomfortable or taboo; this is called *broaching* (Day-Vines et al., 2020) and can also be considered somewhat confrontational, especially by counselors-in-training, because it makes them, not necessarily the client, uncomfortable. *Empathic confrontation* is a term I often use when supervising counselors-in-training because it just tends to come up. They generally tell me that they feel an urge, and are later told by their site-supervisors to "hold their clients accountable" for some inconsistency between what they are thinking/feeling, saying/doing, etc. I would argue that this is likely an example of the very thing that's brought them to counseling! It may likely be unconscious, so "directly confronting", yes, may be "mean" or "inappropriate" (what students often say they're afraid of being). Because we're there to help make the unconscious more conscious, we want to do so gently, with empathy, feeling with our clients, and letting the blow fall by degrees, so to speak. We may do this by gently bringing something up, or broaching a topic, as a statement, perhaps taking the responsibility for not yet quite understanding (because, honestly, we don't know for sure, right?). That might sound like: "I was wondering about that. It sounds different than . . .". Or, "Oh! I don't remember that being the plan . . .". It might also be restating a policy reviewed on intake, the treatment plan, or setting a limit (I prefer the ACT model of limit setting outlined in the Landreth text).

Now, a little rant about interpretation:

Interpretation is often said to be avoided in counseling, yet so much of what we do could not happen without it. That includes our *clinical judgment*. We need that, right? But that last little bit, "judgment", is also a big no-no word that we've pushed into Shadow. We interpret and judge the word "judgment", right? "It's BAAAAD". If we do it, it means we're "judgey". But how about this idea: any time we are perceiving, inferring, analyzing, or otherwise making meaning from any stimulus, we are engaging our symbolic function. This includes facial expressions, the way someone is dressed, scanning the environment to see if we're safe, and deciphering what someone says. All of that and more involves interpretation and judgment. We ask ourselves "what might this mean?" (interpretation) and "is this ok or not?" (judgment). I would argue that what makes these words dangerous for counselors is if we continue to deny, or are otherwise unaware that, we're interpreting and judging. We're more likely to do this if our culture (teachers, supervisors, peers, etc. in the profession) says it's wrong and represses this process, too. We risk these judgments turning inward, creating feelings of shame or superiority (as we sit in the position of power as Counselor), and unconsciously leeching our will out as fact; we call that *psychic discharge*. Ew.

Interpretation suggests we are an interpreter, translating, de-coding, say, symbolic, associative material to more analytic, verbal ones, making meaning. Even Jung's method is called "analytic psychology". However, verbalizing our interpretations, outside of a paraphrase or summary (see *reflection* above), is often discouraged, especially for new counselors. This isn't because it is wrong to interpret; it's because new counselors are often a bit too eager to prove themselves. They want to be seen as "good" at being a counselor, that they can figure things out, and have (good clinical) judgment. We do not want to interpret for our clients too soon, or get too far ahead. We need first to consider potential bias, personal and collective cultural considerations, and gauge where we are in the relationship. We might ask ourselves, "Might this be true for my client?" as well as "How might this comment land?"

We may present an interpretation of what we see, when the time is right, kind of like pulling a loose tooth for a child when they're showing us it's hanging by a thread. *Immediacy*, or commenting on the here-and-now, is an example of that: "You look tense right now". *Enlarging of meaning* or *facilitating understanding* (even promoted in CCPT that discourages "interpretation") I think also involves interpreting. We might hear a client say, "I hate him!" and we say what we've interpreted to be the meaning behind the message: "You trusted him and he really let you down. That hurts". Other interpretations might seem like something small, like a *hunch*, "And that's why you decided to leave . . .", or put together over several sessions, like, "There's the unicorn again . . .!", or packaged into a *core message* like, "Part of you thought you had to stay being mommy's baby . . .". These kinds of statements might be so clear to us that they seem to be fact, but they may really be intuitive clues from the unconscious, especially when presented in creative works. When presented at the wrong moment, or if we're misattuned, comments like this might slam into the client's consciousness, be rejected by the ego, and even damage the therapeutic relationship.

From my Jungian-oriented counseling perspective, there are two vital elements that we need to value and cultivate in order to ethically interpret and judge, because it is inevitable that we will be put in the position to do so: greater knowledge of and transparency about our own bias, and involvement of the client. By "bias" I mean bias in general. By objective definition, bias is our inclination, a preference, our response one way or the other; bias becomes "negative" when it is in Shadow, when we choose unjustly, usually in denial, and with distorted judgment. This includes some of the "non-quantifiable intangibles" proposed by Landreth (2024) in CCPT. We need to continuously deconstruct our assumptions that what we're doing as counselors is always "good" or "right" with our clients. We need to ask ourselves some tough questions that might hurt:

- Do we have an unspoken intention that our client should change? How does that sit with trust in the client, the psyche, and the process, as well as obligations by our site, the State, and other perceived professional commitments?
- Are we trying to be "tricky", or actually manipulative, by implementing techniques that the client doesn't understand, to try and get them somewhere, or "get better" faster?
- Do we hope that they will do or say something specific so they'll then be "acting right", and/or we can "win" in our pre-judged analysis (diagnosis, treatment plan, caregiver expectation, etc.)?
- Are we trying to rescue our client from themselves or others? Are we trying to solve their problem for them? How is this balanced with advocacy and respecting the client and their culture?

- Are we secretly judging their behavior? Are some of the things they say or do preferable, "good or bad"? "Realistic" or "distorted"? Why? Who set the standard? Based on what information or ideology?
- Are we trying to be liked by our client so that we can feel good about ourselves? Are we avoiding emphatically confronting our client or holding back out of a sense of false altruism or a duty to preserve the therapeutic relationship?

To do this work, we need to be real with ourselves, personally and collectively. We cannot make informed cognitive decisions without interpretation, therefore bias, and judgment; this includes our decision to abide by a code of ethics to guide us, which our clients should know about. For counselors, we have signed up to respect client autonomy as well as to be "aware of – and avoid imposing – [our] own values, attitudes, beliefs, and behaviors" on others (ACA, 2014, A.4.b.). This means that I need to let the client see who I really am so they can continue to make the informed decision to interact with me. If I'm silent, they might project too many of their old assumptions onto me, which, if they've come to counseling, might be part of the problem; if I say nothing, for the sake of saying nothing, and fail to interpret what I might notice as a client need, I'll likely be unhelpful. They might even leave and never come back. Suppose I think something is funny and I hide my expression. In that case, I might be missing an opportunity to *empathically confront* someone's unhelpful thoughts, feelings, or beliefs (that they've already told me they think are unhelpful and want to change). I might also be off base with a laugh and hurt their feelings; in this case I would want to take the opportunity to own my impact and try to build a repair. This type of "real" yet "symbolic" act is an example of the use of the counselor-as-instrument in the dance of the therapeutic relationship.

This is why we need continue to do our own work, whatever that might mean for us at this time (counseling, analysis, supervision, consultation group, or other reflective practices) and to be grounded in a primary theory that we can return to for a reality check. We need to know who we are and let our client truly see us. If we don't know ourselves, how can we trust ourselves, and expect others to trust us and our clinical judgment? While I don't believe we can be "neutral" (we want things for our clients, if even we say we only want what they want), we can work toward being open, attuned to others, and curious about various perspectives and paths to the Self.

I feel obligated to wonder aloud for my client so see if I might be off base so I can shift, because thoughts have power and can influence covertly if unspoken. This also means that if a client isn't ready to talk about something, I don't think I should try to "make" them. They have a right to their aesthetics of existence, their silence, or freedom to talk about what they wish. How do I know the path they're on won't lead to where they need to go? I also agree with the sentiment of CCPT, to avoid the use of questions, but to a degree. To me an *appropriate use of questions* is not just balancing open and closed ones, but presenting questions as invitations which are well timed and attuned to the client in the here-and-now. While I don't generally recommend asking a client to directly interpret their own work such as, "What does this figure represent?" or "Why did you paint the whole paper white?" I often do a lot of sincerely curious wondering aloud, like, "I wonder what that was like for you", "I wonder what that little bird is doing now", especially if I sense that a client is leaning that way. Not asking questions at all is pretty weird by American social norms, and can be considered disrespectful, negligent of our professional duties, and can cause us to appear disinterested. Clients have told me so, and I believe them.

DREAMS

> The symptom is like the shoot above ground, yet the main plant is an extended rhizome underground. The rhizome represents the content of a neurosis; it is the matrix of complexes, of symptoms, and of dreams. We have every reason to believe that dreams mirror exactly the underground processes of the psyche. And if we get there, we literally get at the "roots" of the disease.
>
> CW 11, p. 23, § 37

Remember our Tree of Psyche (Chapter 3)? Dreams get at the roots. In Jungian counseling, we take great interest in dreams, and assume they are the natural, spontaneous, symbolic messages from the unconscious, often embedded with wisdom. Jung said dreams are evidence of our symbolic function (CW 18). We consider them vital parts of the psyche's self-regulating system (CW 18); there is significant evidence now that dreams are vital to cognitive and emotional functioning, and that working with dreams can bring comfort and understanding (Hoss, 2018; Spangler & Sim, 2023; World Science Festival, 2022). Some clients, though, may not be interested in or may not remember their dreams. We want to be respectful of our client's preferences in their ways of working, which is why it's important to discuss dream analysis as an option in our intake paperwork.

Jungian dream interpretation should take the dreamer's context and personal associations deeply into account, both when looking at one dream, but also in a series, as in sandplay therapy. No matter what anyone assisting the dreamer might think the dream is saying, or "means", it's ultimately the dreamer who makes the meaning. However, Jung observed that many clients tend to take an overly analytic stance when recounting a dream, and might also assume the dream is trying to hide something (CW 16); the Freudian still runs deep in the culture, I'm afraid. Nightmares, particularly in children or those who've experienced trauma, notoriously try to capture our attention (Cromer et al., 2022). While Jung (CW 8) stated that he didn't put too much stock in the formal and concrete classification of dreams, psychologically or practically, and that there are no "rules" when it comes to interpretation (CW 18), he did indicate that dreams may be "little" or "big" (CW 16). Little dreams include recounts from the day, or other thoughts closer to consciousness; big dreams may be attempting to reveal something deeper.

It may be helpful, though, to refer to the types and stages of a dream that Jung (1974) roughly outlined:

Types of dreams:

1. Wish fulfillment dreams – These are often the stereotypical Freudian type-dreams that Jung criticized as being overly reductive and culturally insensitive (CW 16). They may present as overtly repressed sexual fantasies, claims to power, or prominent unfulfilled drives, which are most common in children (CW 16).
2. Reaction dreams – Reaction dreams, like reductive dreams, are more obvious reactions of the nervous system, often in direct response to an anxiety or trauma. Recurrent reaction-dreams may also be called "compensatory" (CW 16).
3. Prospective dreams – Prospective dreams look toward the future. They may be viewed as a kind of preparation of our deepest hopes or prayers, which, when powerful enough, can even seem prophetic.
4. Telepathic dreams – Telepathic dreams differ from prospective dreams in that they are not as personal. It may be so removed from the personal as to be confounding. Telepathic dreams may be speaking of collective disturbances, or even of another person outside of the dreamer's frame of reference.

Four stages of a dream:

1. stating the place or location of the dream
2. plot development
3. the culmination of events, where something changes or resolves
4. the final situation.

We can also refer to the Hero's Stages (Chapter 5) as a guide for us along the path of collaborative dream interpretation as well. Below are some of my thoughts using this method as presented by The Center for Applied Jungian Studies (n.d.), and the work of Max McDowell (McDowell et al., 2023).

1. Confession – Listening to and capturing the dream. This is often done by both writing it down, in as much detail as we can remember, and then presenting it. We might look at it ourselves, take a dream to a dream analysis group, or to an analyst or Jungian-oriented counselor. It is important that the confession be heard and accepted reverently, without judgment.

2. Illumination – In both reading and talking about the dream, identify any feelings, thoughts, or other associations with the dream material. Everything is still important at this point, including who the dreamer is, where they come from and are in relative space and time, their relationships, and the story itself, with all of its symbolic content. This is a time for associative process work (see mode-shifting). Don't edit yet. Just write down or say anything that comes to mind. We might make notes in the margins, either in our dream journal, on a piece of paper, or in a digital document.

3. Amplification – Identify any dream material that might be considered symbolic or archetypal to look for additional patterning or meaning. There may be a similar narrative to a myth, fairy tale, story, or movie. Or, conversely, what if we imagine the dream or dream-images were REAL? What would those implications be? What are the dream-objects' qualities in the "real world"? There may also be amplifications in the dream through something being bigger, shinier, faster, or otherwise MORE than other things in the dream. Also, repetition may be an amplification. Was something said multiple times? Are there many of one kind of object? Is there a situation that repeats, like on a loop? Take note of those things as well as the thoughts, feelings, and other associations that arise. Also, who and where is the dreamer in the dream? Is the dreamer watching passively or actively involved?

4. Education – In this phase we will actively and directly explore what the dream is trying to tell us . . . what does it want us to understand . . . how can we interpret it? We might educate ourselves about various aspects of the dream or our associations, including looking up the meaning of symbols, or asking characters in the dream directly what they want from us. Jung reminds us to also "stick as close as possible to the dream images" and describe them as if we have "no idea what the words" being used mean, nor the thing's history, function, associations, nor context (CW 16, p. 149, § 320). This may go for the most common of words such as "table", "bird", or "king". We might imagine each element of the dream as a part of the dreamer, which Jung called *interpretation on the subjective level* (Jung, 1974). This last exercise might be really weird or scary for folks. We might introduce it, again, as some psychoeducation with a wondering: "You know, some people say that one way of looking at a dream is by imagining that each aspect of the dream is a part of us. What about that?".

5. Transformation – With possible new information about unconscious material, how might we implement that back into our waking life? Sometimes simply knowing what the dream is saying is enough to bring about a shift. Sometimes it's an invitation to make a change, from something small like making a phone call, to something bigger like exploring a career change. Sometimes we might take a more symbolic approach to transformation, by spending more time with a dream image, writing a letter and burning it, or planting seeds for new ideas to grow.

We can also integrate active-imagination into dream interpretation, but it may transcend talking. While Jung first coined the term active imagination at the Tavistock Lectures in London in 1935, it wasn't published until 1968, in his work on analytical psychology (now in CW 18). For those who may want to delve deeper, Jung goes on to explain the method, without actually calling it by name in several places throughout the CW (. . . I can see why some people find Jung confusing and evasive . . .). Active-imagination can be helpful in activating the transcendent function (CW 7), or perhaps more plainly, riling up associative processes when people are stuck in analytic mode. Jung describes how a client who is over-intellectualizing may tell a story that feels "flat" or disconnected from them; he suggests this is because they are not actively engaged with their imagination (hence the term *active imagination*; CW 7, p. 293, § 344).

Jung explains that he tended to wait until a dream-image or an association spontaneously emerged from the unconscious, and he would then encourage them to take that theme and run with it through more focused interaction with the symbol. That might be through free-association (saying whatever comes to mind), talking to it, creating a dance, sculpture, painting, song, or the like (CW 8, p. 262, § 400). By consciously allowing unconscious material to "possess" us, we can become more unified (CW 7, p. 306, § 368).

I add Jung's use of the word *possession* here deliberately, because over the years clients have expressed such a soul-wrenching fear in many different ways. Some say they don't want to cry because they're afraid they'll never stop; or that they don't want to play because they sense additional memories will come up; or that the act of creating will bring up additional layers of disturbance that they're not ready for. This is why "interventions" should always be well-attuned invitations, where the client is empowered to say no to any suggestion.

Jung invited many of his clients to paint or draw their dreams as a way of liberation, both from the disturbance of the symbols that haunt them, and from over-reliance on him as the practitioner. While the images may be a bit "rough-and-ready" at first (CW 16, p. 49, §106), the process gets the client actively involved by physically engaging with materials and the symbols through active imagination. Once out of the imagination, they can then more easily be shared. Because people may have difficulty verbalizing a dream, or other unconscious content, the artwork, and the process of creating, can evoke additional layers of feeling and meaning. In fact, Jung says:

> Image and meaning are identical: and as the first takes shape, so the latter becomes clear. Actually, the pattern needs no interpretation: it portrays its own meaning.
>
> CW 8, p. 263, § 402

In this way, premature or over-interpretation is discouraged. We may observe and reflect more "objective" content from the work: aspects being near or far apart; colors or hues; line quality being straight, wavey, thick, or thin; repetition or orientation of elements. I will add here the CCPT suggestion, though, that we avoid naming objects or symbols and instead wait for the client to name them. Jung spoke quite harshly about pushing suggestions when they are "one-sided" or attempts at "convincing the patient or of achieving any therapeutic results" even when derived from theory (CW 16, p. 146, § 315). I think pushing suggestions can be even more dangerous without theory. In all instances in creative work it is important to remember that it is the creator's experience and meaning making that is important, not what the Jungian-oriented counselor may interpret or want.

ART & PLAY

> Seriousness comes from a profound inner necessity, but play is its outward expression, the face it turns to consciousness. It is not, of course, a matter of wanting to play, but of having to play; a playful manifestation of fantasy from inner necessity, without the compulsion of circumstance, without even the compulsion of the will. It is serious play . . . That is the ambiguous quality which clings to everything creative.
>
> CW 6, p. 182, § 196

Jung wrote extensively about his own formative experiences with play and art making, was an artist in his own right, encouraged creative expression with his own clients and students, and inspired the development of sand-play therapy. His contributions to the study of symbology and the language of the unconscious has influenced developmental theorists (Piaget, 1951), Hollywood screenplay writers (Vogler, 2020), and contemporary research on themes in mental health treatment (Lee & Jang, 2018; Sarah et al., 2021; Yeh et al., 2015).

While Jung never treated children, he worked with many adult survivors of childhood trauma as they revisited their dreams and experiential memories (Jung, 2008). Trauma affects both encoding and recall of memories; it is not uncommon for those who are traumatized, especially children, to adapt through dissociation as a primary defense, failing to retain, or quickly losing, at least partial memory of events to protect the mind from stress (Haley, 2011; van der Kolk, 2014; Wilkinson, 2005). While children's ability to conceptualize develops slowly, and therefore may limit cognitive ability to verbally express experiences, especially metaphorically, play is considered instrumental in assisting with the alchemical and assimilation process (Anderson, 2018; Landreth, 2024). Young children, especially, may have difficulty putting events into words, and may use play, art making, and other creative means as a primary way of working through their internal process.

Winnicott (1971) observed that a child's inability to play may be of greater concern than the vast array of initially witnessed symptoms of trauma, and may have more lasting negative consequences on future functioning; a child who does not feel the safe freedom to explore and be creative might be otherwise internally stifled, lack self-esteem, or capacity to interact with others. For this reason, early intervention with play-based therapy is considered best practice (APT, 2022; Evidence Based Child Therapy, 2023). When we invite thinking metaphorically, we encourage mode-shifting. From our knowledge of bottom-up-processing, we know that starting with latent, body-based material and applying it through and outside the body to an external object (play or art item) may not only seem less threatening, increasing the window-of-tolerance (Siegel, 2020) for processing the traumatic material, but can simply be more effective (Faranda, 2014; Freedle, 2019).

Overlap

The fields of art and play therapy are distinct, yet there is a great deal of overlap. Counselors may choose to train in one or many areas of the expressive arts through various organizations, but may find limited options for these expressive arts from a Jungian perspective, specifically. Of interest may be the International Expressive Arts Therapy Association (IEATA), the American Art Therapy Association (AATA), the Association for Play Therapy (APT) and the Sandplay Therapists of America (STA). Bear in mind that they all have their own codes of ethics, political musings, and community culture. We can only invest in so many areas. For example, while my master's is in art therapy, and I was a member of all of those organizations above at one time, I felt most at home at the APT, and became credentialed as a Registered Play Therapist-Supervisor, so that's where I hang out a lot, and how I publicly identify. Before we call ourselves an "art therapist" or a "play therapist", etc. we need to make sure we have the ethical right to do so. However, counselors with some specialized training and supervision may integrate aspects of art or play into their practice, and say so, without using another title. Being grounded in a theory of the mind is vitally important, though, and for our sake, here, that is Jungian. Suggestions presented here are only an overview and are not considered formal training. And for goodness sake, read Jung.

Perhaps due to Jung's influence, perhaps due to the mindfulness trend in mental health, appropriated from Eastern spiritual traditions, mandalas are a commonly "prescribed" first therapeutic art activity. There are even mandala coloring books. Jung's own artworks contained mandalas, and he wrote of the cultural and religious significance of them around the world. Mandala means "circle" in Sanskrit and refers to geometric patterning of shapes and symbols, often with a central point. They may appear like kaleidoscope images, a labyrinth, or even a clock. While Jung observed that mandalas may spontaneously appear in the dreams or artwork, indicating an encounter with the Self, he also noted that their appearance or fascination may indicate that the client is having trouble projecting internalized God-images and may be developing an inflated ego (as cited in Fordham, 1975). Some may refer to a centralized preoccupation as "navel gazing" or even narcissism. Others may fear closing their eyes in session or focusing on their breathing, as it brings attention to the center of the body that holds anxiety or isolation. More non-directive Jungian-oriented counselors may simply be on the lookout for mandalas, collect circular objects to have available, cut paper into circles, have printed mandalas available to color, or provide psychoeducation about them as appropriate. As I see it, a Jungian approach generally does not go for techniques, and is mindful not to exploit religious traditions as mental health techniques (Lilly, 2015; Loue, 2015).

To start, play is a human right, so that fits right into the counselor value of empowerment (Office of the United Nations High Commissioner for Human Rights, 1989). Play is spontaneous, self-motivated, and free; people don't need to be taught how to play and I don't have the right to coerce them to play . . . or to talk. Children have a right to play or not to play. They also have a right to silence. Questions can be coercive so they should be used mindfully and minimally. Children get questioned and told what to do all day long. Taking responsibility as the adult who creates space for wounded children to enter into means providing them with empowering, safe choices in the play materials I provide, and by holding the frame of the therapeutic relationship (see Chapter 6 for more information). It's been my experience that these precepts are most firmly held and best described in child-centered play therapy (Landreth, 2024). Yes, even though I'm a Jungian, I suggest you go read Landreth FIRST for the how-to of facilitating a non-directive play experience and being in relationship with a child. There's time to read Jung and philosophize more deeply with other Jungians later.

Jungians acknowledge that it is the *play itself* that has therapeutic power. While widely accepted as our universal first language as children, play is now also considered beneficial for people of all ages. As we've previously discussed in this book, play, as an activator of the symbolic function, provides direct access to the unconscious, promotes healthy relationship, and stimulates creativity and emotional regulation. Play has been found to have 20 core agents of change in four broad categories of communication, wellness, relationships, and personal strength (Schaefer & Drewes, 2014).

While we know that children need free time to play, it is disappearing from their lives. Play time is now marketed and sold in handheld, digital devices. Recess is one of the first "privileges" to be taken away from children who are having emotional and behavioral difficulties, even though educators, administrators, and school mental health teams know better. No . . . they're often called "behavioral health" teams and specialists, focused on the child's problematic behavior, not the child themselves. This is a larger problem which you may want to go back and read about again in Chapter 1. Children deserve to be seen, heard, develop deep connections so they can make healthy choices, and have lots of time to play. I look outside even in my small, rural town and rarely see kids outside playing anymore. This is harming our children's development in multiple ways: physically, cognitively, socially, emotionally, and creatively.

Most play therapists I know not only have toys in their room, but sandtrays, and art materials as well. However, some sandplay therapists don't consider themselves play therapists, so I will save them for a separate section. I've seen the integration of Jungian-oriented art and play therapy range from completely non-directive to very-directive, and we're a small community, so I can understand why folks may be confused about how it might look, and what makes it distinctive. My style tends to lean heavily toward being non-directive, which often looks quite a lot like CCPT, especially with younger children, but tends to be a bit more conversational as I work with older kids and adults. Preparing the environment with art supplies and play materials based on experience with them, as well as our clients' age range, is an important consideration.

Materials

If we see young children, a CCPT (Landreth, 2024) setup is nearly ideal for both play and art making. There is a great list in the Landreth text for both a fully stocked as well as a portable play kit. The idea, though, is that there are a variety of materials, carefully selected, in full view, at a child-friendly height, so they may choose and engage with whatever they wish. In general, we want a variety of objects from the real world (people, animals, food, structures, religious items, nature, etc.), fantasy (magical creatures, monsters, robots, characters from stories, miniature or play weapons, etc.) and means for personal expression (dress-up, building, drawing, painting, and sculpture materials). Toys which may inspire contained gross motor activities may also be considered to assist with dispelling physical energy (bop- or bean-bags, foam swords, exercise balls, hula hoops, and ribbon wands).

Especially because of my history with Waldorf and Montessori early childhood education, I have the added preference for the love of natural materials. This includes found objects like pebbles, shells, fallen branches, seed pods, feathers, leaves, collected and dried flowers, shed snakeskin, and even cleaned animal bones. Always check to see if it's ok to take things from sites. Choosing handmade cloth dolls, airy pieces of silk fabric, and wood over plastic whenever possible offers unique and varied sensory experiences. They're also REAL in a way that manufactured toys are not. They're both closer to the earth, and have a uniquely human feel, especially if we have collected or made the objects ourselves. The extra love and attention to the objects adds to the warmth of the space and extends into the relationship. When looking to purchase natural toys, I recommend supporting local artists when available; craft shows, church bazaars, and even yard sales are places to explore, but many larger companies have natural options, too. Bella Luna Toys (2023) and A Toy Garden (2023) are companies that have been around and share many values of our profession.

I also like having curtains on my shelves to "close" activities if I have to set a limit (such as if a child is having trouble keeping sand in the sandtray) or if certain toys or miniatures are triggering. Some children have hesitated coming into my playroom because they caught a glimpse of something scary. Because one of our first priorities is fostering a sense of safety I have no problem "hiding" scary items, especially if a child asks me to. Many children with attachment disruptions and relational trauma have delighted in asking me to hide items, and then, in later sessions, asking me to retrieve them. I also have a history of seeing adults in the playroom. Play therapy with adults is its own specialization (Schaefer, 2003) and is an integrative practice that may be offered in addition to traditional counseling; some adults are quite put off by the presence of any, or specific toys. In several of my counseling offices, I have had large closets where the majority of my toys and miniatures could be kept neatly tucked away.

Art supplies should, of course, be non-toxic and washable. While a large easel and tempera paints in pots are commonly seen in play therapy rooms, and are a time-tested choice, there are other materials to consider, again based on the early childhood models above. Chunky beeswax crayons stimulate multiple senses, are easy for small hands to hold, and can take the pressure that stressed out kids might draw with. Wet-on-wet watercolors also come to mind because the colors are clear, they flow together beautifully, and tend not to get "muddy" on the paper like tempras. Like the concept of knowing our own mind before tending to another in general, it is recommended that the counselor interested in incorporating art materials into their practice has explored the mediums extensively and been witnessed in this process.

PLAY THERAPY

Children are educated by what the grownup is and not by what he says.

CW 9i, p. 175, § 293

While it may be considered splitting hairs to some, others are quite particular about what they prefer to call themselves and their methods. The distinct terms Jungian play therapy and Jungian analytical play therapy are two examples. Some people consider sandplay therapy a form of play therapy, while others do not. I may be stirring the pot here, but I don't quite identify with any of the terms above: the title of this book is *Jungian Counseling and Play Therapy*. My professional identity today is rooted in my counselor values of empowering others by being client-centered, wellness-based, and culturally inclusive (ACA, 2014, 2023), but my theoretical framework for understanding the mind is based in Jungian theory.

Another area of splitting hairs is in defining what is "therapeutic-play", "play-based therapy", and "play therapy" (Hudspeth, 2021). One could argue that almost any free play where the child was in a safe environment might be considered therapeutic-play. Other play-based activities could also be considered therapeutic, such as teaching a psychoeducation lesson through the use of puppets, or playing a board game designed around mental health prompts. The definition of play therapy, though, widely advertised by the Association for Play Therapy (2023), focuses on the importance of the (1) theoretical foundation, (2) therapeutic relationship, (3) powers of play, and (4) specialized play therapy training and supervision of the provider. See the difference?

A big part of being a Counselor AND a Play Therapist, for me, is focusing on and advocating for my client. Did you notice all that talk of "power" up there? (See Chapter 1 for more discussion of biopower, post-modernism, and the ethics of existence.) That means I need to also know who I am, what that means in the positions of power which I sit in, and how I advocate for myself if I want to do that for others. *Healer heal thyself* is a tenet of transforming from a Wounded Healer to a Servant Leader in our professional identity.

One of the radical concepts that CCPT really reinforces for me is: it is the CHILD who is my client. Not the parents, not the state, not the insurance company, not the school. THE CHILD. I also must define my identity, my role, and hold the frame of the relationship, often for multiple caregivers. While I am a professional, I also embrace what a child called me once: the "weird adult" in their life – I'm not their parent, nor their teacher, nor a person who's there to tell them what to do. I don't give children "a talkin' to" about their behavior. I am not a "behavior specialist", and don't focus on "behavioral health". I don't talk about them behind their back or "tell on" them; if someone wants to talk to me about the child's progress, I talk to the child first, or am careful not to disclose anything about the child. My child clients get the same rights as anyone of any age does in my office: to say or do just about anything they want during our time together as long as they stay safe and aren't doing something else on their digital device.

Because I am very sensitive to children's rights to silence, choice, and emotional safety, I tend toward CCPT skills (how I respond), while rooted in my Jungian theoretical orientation. That often looks like "wondering" aloud a bit, a selective use of questions, telling stories, and sometimes providing suggestions or psychoeducation. I am often thinking, though, about various Jungian concepts such as the nature, structure, and function of the psyche, the language of the unconscious, and am on the lookout for mode-shifting in action.

While CCPT is focused primarily on the child and the relationship, Jungian/analytical play therapy has an additional theoretical focus on the value of the unconscious and inviting greater awareness and knowledge of it (Allan, 1988; Allan & Bertoia, 2003; Green, 2014; Lilly & Heiko, 2019). Jungian/analytical play therapists may use various levels and types of modeling, materials, directives, questions, conversations, and psychoeducation. Like analytic psychology, what that looks like in research and practice is notoriously resistant to being quantified. "Chief" JP Lilly (2015), (one of my most influential Jungian teachers) describes how Jungian analytical play therapy may easily be adapted to those who choose to utilize more CBT type language (but still don't like "techniques"); his model includes how disruptive incidents in a child's life can cause various types of dysregulation, including disequilibrium (cognitive), decompensation (emotional), deterioration (behavioral). He, incidentally, also participated in CCPT research (Scott et al., 2003) and is our active Jungian-oriented representative on the board of APT.

While we may still need more research on "Jungian art therapy" and "Jungian/analytical play therapy", we do have evidence of the effectiveness of psychodynamic psychotherapy with children and adolescents (Midgley et al., 2021), play therapy in general (Evidence Based Child Therapy, 2023), and sandplay therapy (Wiersma et al., 2022).

Let's get the "sandplay" vs "sandtray" conversation out of the way. Honestly, it's confusing to seasoned play therapists sometimes, not just noobs. Sand-PLAY therapy differs from sandTRAY therapy in that the former suggests a Jungian theoretical orientation. While some practitioners may shorten the practice to "sandplay", it is a part of Jungian legend that Dora Kalff herself preferred we use the whole phrase – "sandplay therapy" – in reference to her work. While there are many who integrate sand and miniatures in their work, or utilize "sandtray" as a modality, to sandplay therapists, "a sandtray" is an object in which sandworlds are created (Allan, 1988). Sandplay therapy tends to be governed by the Sandplay Therapists of America (STA), a "member society" of the International Society for Sandplay Therapy (ISST), and together they offer a training program with various levels of membership, from Associate to Certified Sandplay Therapist – Teaching Member (CST-T). Sandtray therapy is a much looser term, and is considered by many Jungians as potentially dangerous because it lacks a theoretical foundation; however, there are now organizations such as the International Association for Sandtray Therapy and World Association of Sand Therapy Professionals who are working to bridge the gap and find community. Trainings from all of these organizations may be co-sponsored by an Association for Play Therapy (APT) Approved Provider. I tend to hang out in those areas because it feeds my credential; each credential next to one's name tends to need specific continuing education.

Sandplay therapy was developed by Dora Kalff (1904–1990), under the guidance and direction of Carl Jung. She had trained as an analyst for many years, but because she did not have a formal graduate degree, was not credentialed by the Jung Institute (Kirsch, 2000). Kaff studied directly with Margaret Lowenfeld (1939) who had developed "the World Technique" after being inspired by H. G. Well's book *Floor Games* (1911). (We're going to excuse the use of the word "technique" here because it is foundational, a proper name, and it was 1911.) Buhler (1951) used the technique for research and diagnosis, in Jungian tradition of projective testing. Kalff combined the technique with Neumann's (1954) concepts of strengthening attachments and resolving trauma through expressing fantasies (Allan, 1988), to develop her own method and, eventually, the International Society for Sandplay Therapy in the 1980s (ISST, 2023; Kalff, 2020).

Sandplay therapy invites an externalized three-dimensional processing of internal regulation systems that may be less intimidating than talking, art making, or playing. The main components of sandplay include providing a safe and protected space in the therapy office, within the container of the sandtray, and with the therapist providing unconditional positive regard, minimal verbal interventions, so as to not interrupt the process, observation of symbolic patterning, in tandem with delayed interpretation (Allan, 1988; Friedman & Mitchell, 2008; Kalff, 2020). Observing sandtrays, or other expressive work, in a series over time is encouraged for greater insight into the client's internal working through common states of chaos, struggle, and resolution (Allan, 1988).

Sandplay therapy materials include trays of wet and dry sand, with blue bottoms and sides to suggest sky and water, access to water (at times), buckets, shovels, and rakes, and a variety of miniatures. The sandtray in sandplay therapy has traditional dimensions of 28 1/2" x 19 1/2" x 3", because it is said to just fill the field of vision, to be an immersive, but not consuming, confrontation with the unconscious. Examples of sandplay therapy rooms can be found on the ISST website. Themes include the content in the tray, the spatial relationships of objects to each other, the client, and the therapist, the movement of the figures and materials, and the affective responses before, during, and after the work, for both client and therapist (Turner, 2005). Wounding and healing themes, first identified by Mitchell and Friedman (1994), have been and continue to be observed and found to be meaningful in sandplay therapy practice and research (Mitchell & Friedman, 2017; Yeh et al., 2015).

Sandplay therapy may be utilized with children, teens, adults, couples, and groups to encourage more associative processing. However, sandplay therapy largely is a non-verbal modality. When integrating it into counseling, a client-centered approach is recommended (STA, n.d.). Sandplay therapy recognizes and honors that the practice may appear similar to the Japanese artistic tradition of creating miniature landscapes called *Hakoniwa* (Friedman & Mitchell, 1991) as well as Native American and Buddhist sand paintings (Weinrib, 2004). It has a very quiet, reverent, meditative feel. Some sandplay therapists even have designated areas for sandplay and for talking to keep them separate processes.

Because sandplay therapy has a distinct practice suitable for replication (STA, n.d.), we now have a good bit of research. Enough, actually, for two meta-analyses (Lee & Jang, 2015; Wiersma et al., 2022), as well as some firm theoretical footing. Dr. Freedle (2017, 2019) brought a neuro- and trauma-informed perspective to sandplay therapy and applied it to the trending neurosequential model of therapeutics (NPT; Perry, 2023; Perry & Hambrick, 2008). Sandplay therapy has been found to significantly reduce both internalizing and externalizing symptoms of emotional distress. We also have several studies which include neuroimaging. Sandplay therapy has been shown to improve brain function, namely the frontotemporal networks, responsible for memory and other cognitive functions (Akimoto et al., 2018), as well as the pre-frontal cortex and limbic system, thought to be involved in reducing anxiety (Foo et al., 2020; Foo & Pratiwi, 2021). While current data on American play therapists' knowledge and use of sandplay therapy is limited, in Japan, play therapists have reported they are more familiar with sandplay than even cognitive behavioral therapy; most play therapists integrate more than one theoretical orientation in their practice, with psychodynamic, person/child centered, and Jungian being the top three (Lambert et al., 2007; Sudo et al., 2023). A post-modern approach to sandplay therapy has been suggested elsewhere in the literature (Gallerani & Dybicz, 2011), which appeals to me both ethically and pragmatically. Critics of traditional sandplay therapy have said that the process does not seem to account for the client's preference to engage in an open dialogue during counseling sessions. A post-modern approach opens up the "free and protected space" to include freedom of dialogue, if the client chooses.

While it is assumed that in creating a picture in the sand, the client may be reimagining the projections of the past as well as future perceptions of the Self, we might consider the benefit of also adding in well-timed analytic processes to encourage mode-shifting. Traditionally, the sandplay therapist may photograph the work at the end of a session and keep them as part of the file, to be reviewed at the very end of "the process", as they call it, or what counselors call "termination", or the end of the therapeutic relationship. This may not only be developmentally inappropriate, as children may not remember sessions months or years past, triggering, as clients may not want to revisit certain images, but may also miss opportunities for deeper reflection in the moments around creation.

Though some may argue that such a post-modern approach to sandplay therapy is precariously close to devolving into "sandtray" territory, I find it even more Jungian, and honestly, Kalffian. Though I never trained with Dora Kalff, I have seen footage of her in session with clients, and frankly, she talks to them (Amman, 1972). While I'm not advocating for the therapist to mindlessly chatter away, I do see the benefit of incorporating verbalized reflections. By integrating CCPT skills of tracking, reflection of content, or even the Jungian concept of amplification, clients may go deeper, mode-shift with greater awareness and ability, and utilize their sessions more fully (Sedgwick, 2015). Clients of all ages, but especially teens and adults, might finish their sand picture in just a few minutes. To not talk about the content now sitting before us, as a counselor in the digital age, honestly feels like ignoring the elephant in the room. I often see clients start to deconstruct and verbalize what they think the tray means to them. This is a part of the aesthetics of existence. I think it is my ethical duty at that point to join with them as co-interpreter. Now, I've seen this taken too far, where the therapist takes the lead too quickly and starkly asks misattuned direct questions like "What does this mean?". But there is something to be said for observing and reflecting content: "There's that figure again!", "These are all together", "This one is right in the middle", or the active use of the attuned therapist such as, "I'm wondering . . . how it feels for you to look at this . . . what it is like for this [figure] . . .", etc. Clients might also directly introduce or evoke in the therapist existing stories (classically, just myths and fairy tales), which might be observed and shared.

Even if one argues that this approach is more "Jungian sandTRAY not sandPLAY", the Jungian theoretical orientation brings distinction. However, if we are re-defining the process to involve talking and well-attended suggestions by the therapist, then one might argue that an invitation by the therapist to create a picture in the sand at a particular time or regarding a particular salient topic might be a logical next step. How is this not unlike Jung inviting clients to create an image or write about a dream? In either case the client is in the lead, the artist of their experience. Jungian informed counselors are to assist clients in making their vision clearer, and perhaps acting at times as curator of their body of work to date.

YOGA & BODY-BASED THERAPIES

> People will do anything, no matter how absurd, in order to avoid facing their own souls. They will practice Indian yoga and all its exercises, observe a strict regimen of diet, learn the literature of the whole world – all because they cannot get on with themselves and have not the slightest faith that anything useful could ever come out of their own souls.
>
> CW 12, p. 99, § 126

One of the most transformative educational and therapeutic relationships in my life was with Zo Newell, the great yogi and spiritual scholar. When we met, I had been working with survivors of sexual trauma for some time, mostly utilizing art and play from a Jungian counseling framework. Body-based therapies and mindfulness practices were becoming increasingly popular. While I found them scientifically progressive, theoretically interesting, and even had a personal history of practicing yoga, they were (and are) often more directive than I prefer (see Levine, 1997; Linehan & Wilks, 2015; Somatic Experiencing, 2023; van der Kolk, 2014). At the time I was unfamiliar with what may have been the first contemporary trauma-informed somatic therapy based on interpersonal neurobiology and Jungian theory, by Dr. Sándor post World War 2; *Calatonia* is a technique designed to mobilize unconscious images through gentle activation of the limbic system (Calatonia International Training, n.d.).

I decided to deepen my own yoga and reflective practices first by attending Zo's therapeutic yoga classes, later training as a yoga teacher with her, and after, continued to seek spiritual guidance from her until her death in 2022. While teaching yoga was, of course, part of my training, it is a greater understanding of the Self, and our relationship to it, that is one of the biggest insights from our relationship. I have since studied with, and been inspired by her husband, James Newell (2023), who is a Jungian-oriented musician, theological scholar, and educator, active in the Depth Psychology Alliance (2023).

I am adding this section to this book not only because I believe that the integration of yoga- and other body-based therapies may be helpful in building bridges to the Self, and practicing mode-shifting, but to increase awareness that mental health has integrated many ancient spiritual practices without giving them proper consideration. This is an ethical concern for me on many levels, and an advocacy issue. Not only does appropriating other cultures' spiritual and religious practices and attempting to manualize and sell them as mental health treatment reek of colonialism, but it can be dangerous to our clients' spiritual, social, physical, and emotional health (Brewster, 2023). There are many different schools of thought about the practice of yoga in the West. Jung (CW 11) also had many thoughts about Westerner's incorporation of yoga and mindfulness, including our general appropriation, misunderstanding, and secularization of the entire practice; for this reason he encouraged caution. "Yoga as exercise" remains a popular, ego-focused practice, and is not my approach, especially in working therapeutically. While exercise's benefits on mental health are well established, that is not my area of expertise or professional focus. The person behind the inquiry about yoga seems to have been of greater interest to Jung, and is also to me.

In a general counseling practice, it is vital that we remain within our scope of practice (ACA, 2014). Incorporating touch, especially, into session requires specific training, supervision, ongoing consent, assent, and documentation (APT, 2012). For those without specialized body-based therapeutic training, it is not recommended that you integrate them until you are. However, we can provide psychoeducation and refer out. The International Association of Yoga Therapists (2023) and Yoga Alliance (2023) may be good places to start familiarizing oneself with various training programs and credentials to look for when seeking teachers and building a yoga referral list for clients. I also highly recommend both of Zo's books (Newell, 2007, 2021) for those practicing yoga, to deepen their reflection on the historical, cultural, and personal symbolic meaning and charge of the poses.

ADDITIONAL CULTURAL CONSIDERATIONS

> The externalization of culture may do away with a great many evils whose removal seems most desirable and beneficial, yet this step forward, as experience shows, is all too dearly paid for with a loss of spiritual culture. It is undeniably much more comfortable to live in a well-planned and hygienically equipped house, but this still does not answer the question of who is the dweller in this house and whether his soul rejoices in the same order and cleanliness as the house which ministers to his outer life.
>
> CW 11, § 962, p. 585

Creativity, like language, play, and art making is innately and deeply human. It is only natural that we would choose to mindfully integrate and invite these expressions into our counseling practices. However, we must also value, engage in, and process through our own creative experiences in order to hold the space and facilitate others in doing so. That means professional training and supervision, yes, but I think it extends all the way to the person, and our ongoing relationship with the Self, the very source of creation in the psyche. We must attempt to understand our own depths before we can begin to guide others in exploring theirs.

I am often saddened, but not surprised, when I learn that people don't think they're creative. I hear this from clients and counselors alike. While I believe that we're all creative, I can only be present, reflect, and invite. However, I think it is my ethical duty as counselor, educator, and mother to clearly state my position that it is both developmentally and culturally inappropriate to not allow children, especially, the space and opportunity to express themselves, learn, and grow through the free and ample use of creative expression. Children are a population and therefore a culture. In America, our Western culture tends to value and prioritize verbal processing and individual responsibility for behavior, even for the youngest and most vulnerable clients. In many cultures, speaking up and out against elders is taboo. It is therefore culturally insensitive for counselors to expect clients to talk about their troubles. Preparing ourselves and our spaces with tools for creative expression is more culturally informed and responsive, and therefore more ethical; this applies to all counselors (Ratts et al., 2016).

All of the functions of the psyche are interconnected: the symbolic, the religious, the reflective and the transformative functions (see Chapter 4). A block in one may impact another, and ultimately the latter, which can impede psychological, emotional, behavioral, and relational change. If a client has expressed interest in, or a history of spiritual or religious practices, I, like Jung, recommend that counselors explore the possibilities of clients engaging with, and building community outside of session, but remain open to clients' requests to process through and integrate them into sessions. This may be of particular relevance to those with a resistance to creative expression; they might need to develop routines and rituals in order to trust and access the Self. While counselors may be trained in and broach the subject of RSIP, they should remain wary of cultural appropriation, especially interventions that are directive and derivative of cultural practices, and the common pathologizing of numinous experiences (Morse & Lomay, 2021). Instead, we should stay within our wheelhouse, remain culturally alert, creating a space that is open, collaborative with, and adapted to our clients, so that they may integrate activities as they see fit (McAuliffe & Associates, 2013; Myers et al., 1996; Samuels, 2017). When in doubt, return to the basic counseling skills of reflection. We may choose to participate with them if they would like us to pray or meditate with them at the beginning or end of session, discuss their values, or prepare for a religious or spiritual event, perhaps in collaboration with elders in the community. Also, be aware that many of the things we take for granted in our practices may be considered offensive by religious or spiritual perspectives; this includes guided imagery, the use of pranayama (breathwork), hypnosis, or even representing or claiming ownership of certain items in our sandplay collections. Our aim as Jungian-oriented counselors is to remain curious and culturally responsive to the end.

Reflections

1. When do you feel most creative? What activities can you get lost in, and get into "flow", where you seem to lose time in the process?
2. How do you, or might you, schedule your time to prioritize these practices?
3. Notice any resistance you might have to identifying as "creative" or making time for creative activities. You might write down some of these thoughts or biases. Where might they come from?
4. How do you bring your creativity to your work? Do you have a preferred mode (associative or analytic)? Notice if there is an area that might need more attention.

REFERENCES

Akimoto, M., Furukawa, K., & Ito, J. (2018). Exploring the sandplayer's brain: A single case study. *Archives of Sandplay Therapy, 30*(3), 73–84.

Allan, J. (1988). *Inscapes of the child's world: Jungian counseling in schools and clinics.* Spring Publications.

Allan, J., & Bertoia, J. (2003). *Written paths to healing: Education and Jungian child counseling.* Spring Publications. (Original work published 1992).

American Counseling Association (ACA). (2014). *ACA code of ethics.* www.counseling.org/resources/aca-code-of-ethics.pdf

American Counseling Association (ACA). (2023). *What is a counselor?* www.counseling.org/about-us/what-is-a-counselor#:~:text=1%3A%20A%20Client%2DCentered%20Approach%20That%20Focuses%20on%20You&text=A%20professional%20counselor%20is%20likely,your%20relationships%20or%20self%2Desteem

Amman, P. (1972). *Sandplay: A method of psychotherapy.* [YouTube video]. Uploaded to Psychosmart Channel, September 30, 2013. https://youtu.be/aWd40dMH70c?feature=shared

Anderson, D. (2018). The alchemy of play. *Psychological Perspectives, 61*(2), 241–256. https://doi.org/10.1080/00332925.2018.1461506

Association for Play Therapy (APT). (2012). *Paper on touch: Clinical, professional & ethical issues.* https://cdn.ymaws.com/www.a4pt.org/resource/resmgr/Publications/Paper_On_Touch.pdf

Association for Play Therapy (APT). (2022). *Play therapy best practices: Clinical, professional & ethical issues.* https://cdn.ymaws.com/www.a4pt.org/resource/resmgr/publications/best_practices.pdf

Association for Play Therapy (APT). (2023). *What is play therapy?* www.a4pt.org/

Bella Luna Toys. (2023). *About Bella Luna Toys.* www.bellalunatoys.com/pages/about-us

Bettelheim, B. (1975). *The uses of enchantment: The meaning and importance of fairy tales.* Vintage Books.

Breuer, J., & Freud, S. (2004). *Studies in hysteria.* Penguin Classics. (Original work published 1895).

Brewster, F. (2023). *Race and the unconscious.* Routledge.

Buhler, C. (1951). The World Test, a projective technique. *Journal of Child Psychiatry, 2,* 4–23.

Bulkeley, K., & Weldon, C. (2011). *Teaching Jung.* Oxford Press.

Calatonia International Training. (n.d.). *Calatonia and subtle touch.* https://calatoniainternationaltraining.com/#calatonia-subtle-touch

The Center for Applied Jungian Studies. (n.d.). *The interpretation of dreams.* https://appliedjung.com/root/wp-content/uploads/2016/07/The-Interpretation-of-Dreams.pdf

Children's Institute. (2016). *Still face with dads.* [YouTube video]. https://youtu.be/7Pcr1Rmr1rM

Corey, G. (2021). *Theory and practice of counseling and psychotherapy.* Cengage.

Council for Accreditation of Counseling and Related Programs (CACREP). (2024). *2024 CACREP standards.* www.cacrep.org/wp-content/uploads/2023/06/2024-Standards-Combined-Version-6.27.23.pdf

Cromer, L. D., Stimson, J. R., Rischard, M. E., & Buck, T. R. (2022). Nightmare prevalence in an outpatient pediatric psychiatry population: A brief report. *Dreaming, 32*(4), 353–355. https://doi.org/10.1037/drm0000225

Day-Vines, N. L., Cluxton-Keller, F., Agorsor, C., Gubara, S., & Otabil, N. A. A. (2020). The multidimensional model of broaching behavior. *Journal of Counseling & Development, 98,* 107–118. doi:10.1002/jcad.12304.

Depth Psychology Alliance. (2023). Home page. https://depthpsychologyalliance.com/

Dodd, S. (n.d.). *Strewing our children's paths.* https://sandradodd.com/strewing.html

Douglas, C. (2005). Analytical psychotherapy. In R. J. Corsini & Q. Wedding (Eds.), *Current psychotherapies* (pp. 96–129). Thomson Learning.

Evidence Based Child Therapy. (2023). Home page. http://evidencebasedchildtherapy.com

Faranda, F. (2014). Working with images in psychotherapy: An embodied experience of play and metaphor. *Journal of Psychotherapy Integration, 24*(1), 65–77. https://doi.org/10.1037/a0035967

Foo, M., Freedle, L. R., Sani, R., & Fonda, G. (2020). The effect of sandplay therapy on the thalamus in the treatment of generalized anxiety disorder: A case report. *International Journal of Play Therapy, 29*(4), 191–200. https://doi: 10.1037/pla0000137

Foo, M., & Pratiwi, A. (2021). The effectiveness of sandplay therapy in treating patients with generalized anxiety disorder and childhood trauma using magnetic resonance spectroscopy to examine choline level in the dorsolateral prefrontal cortex and centrum semiovale. *International Journal of Play Therapy, 30*(3), 177–186. https://doi.org/10.1037/pla0000162

Fordham, F. (1975). *An introduction to Jung's psychology.* Penguin Books. (Original work published 1953).

Freedle, L. R. (2017). Healing trauma through sandplay therapy: A neuropsychological perspective. In B. Turner, (Ed.), *The Routledge international handbook of sandplay therapy* (pp. 190–206). Routledge.

Freedle, L. R. (2019). Making connections: Sandplay therapy and the Neurosequential Model of Therapeutics. *Journal of Sandplay Therapy, 28*(1), 91–109. www.sandplay.org/journal/abstracts/

Friedman, H. S., & Mitchell, R. R. (1991). Dora Maria Kalff: Connections between life and work. *Journal of Sandplay Therapy, 1*(1), 17–23.

Friedman, H. S., & Mitchell, R. R. (Eds.) (2008). *Supervision of sandplay therapy.* Routledge.

Gallerani, T., & Dybicz, P. (2011, May 2). Postmodern sandplay: An introduction for play therapists. *International Journal of Play Therapy, 20*(3), 165–177. https://doi.org/10.1037/a0023440

Garner, C., Freeman, B., Stewart, R., & Coll, K. (2020). Assessment of dispositions in program admissions: The Professional Disposition Competence Assessment – Revised Admission (PDCA-RA). *The Professional Counselor, 10*(3), 337–350. https://doi.org/10.15241/cg.10.3.337

Gil, E. (2006). *Helping abused and traumatized children: Integrating directive and nondirective approaches.* Guilford Press.

Green, E. (2014). *The handbook of Jungian play therapy with children & adolescents.* Johns Hopkins University Press.

Haley, D. W. (2011). Relationship disruption stress in human infants: A validation study with experimental and control groups. *Stress: The International Journal on the Biology of Stress, 14*(5), 530–536. https://doi.org/10.3109/10253890.2011.56 0308

Hoss, R. J. (2018). *Learning in dreams: Psychological growth.* The International Association for the Study of Dreams: Brain Awareness Week. www.asdreams.org/baw-learningindreams/

Hudspeth, E. F. (2021). Play therapy versus play-based therapy. *Play Therapy Magazine.* https://cdn.ymaws.com/www.a4pt.org/resource/resmgr/magazine_articles/Play_Therapy_vs_Play-Based_T.pdf

International Association of Yoga Therapists. (2023). *Accredited programs.* www.iayt.org/page/AccrdPrgms

International Society for Sandplay Therapy. (2023). *Home page.* www.isst-society.com/

Johnson, R. A. (1991). *Owning your own shadow: Understanding the dark side of the psyche.* HarperOne.

Jongsma, A. E., Peterson, L. M., & Bruce, T. J. (2021). *The complete adult psychotherapy treatment planner.* Wiley.

Jung, C. G. (1973). *C. G. Jung Letters: Volume 1, 1906–1950.* G. Adler, A. Jaffe, et al. (Eds.), R. F. C. Hull (Trans.). Routledge.

Jung, C. G. (1974). *Dreams.* R. F. C. Hull (Trans.). Princeton University Press.

Jung, C. G. (2008). *Children's dreams: Notes from the seminar given 1936–1940.* L. Jung & M. Meyer-Grass (Eds.), E. Faizeder & T. Woolfson (Trans.). Princeton University Press.

Jung, C. G. (2023). *The collected works of C. G. Jung: Revised and expanded complete digital edition.* (CW 1–20). G. Adler, W. McGuire, & H. Read (Eds.), R. F. C. Hull (Trans.). Princeton University Press. https://press.princeton.edu/books/ebook/9780691255194/the-collected-works-of-c-g-jung

Kalff, D. M. (2020). *Sandplay: A psychotherapeutic approach to the psyche.* B. L. Matthews (Trans). Analytical Psychology Press, Sandplay Editions. (Original work published 1966).

Karwowski, M., Zielińska, A., & Jankowska, D. M. (2022). Democratizing creativity by enhancing imagery and agency: A review and meta-analysis. *Review of Research in Education, 46*(1), 229–263. https://doi.org/10.3102/0091732X221084337

Kirsch, T. B. (2000). *The Jungians: A comparative and historical perspective.* Routledge.

Kottman, T., & Meany-Walen, K. K. (2018). *Doing play therapy: From building the relationship to facilitating change.* The Guilford Press.

Kramer, E. (2000). *Art as therapy: Collected papers.* L. A. Gerity (Ed.). Jessica Kingsley Publishers.

Kuiken, D., Porthukaran, A., Albrecht, K.-A., Douglas, S., & Cook, M. (2018). Metaphoric and associative aftereffects of impactful dreams. *Dreaming, 28*(1), 59–83. https://doi.org/10.1037/drm0000067

Lambert, S. F., LeBlanc, M., Mullen, J. A., Ray, D., Baggerly, J., White, J., & Kaplan, D. (2007). Learning more about those who plays in session: The national play therapy in counseling practices project (phase I). *Journal of Counseling & Development, 85,* 42–46. http://dx.doi.org/10.1002/j.1556-6678.2007.tb00442.x

Lambie, G. W., Mullen, P. R., Swank, J. M., & Blount, A. (2018). The Counseling Competencies Scale: Validation and refinement. *Measurement and Evaluation in Counseling and Development, 51*(1), 1–15. doi:10.1080/07481756.2017.135 8964.

Landreth, G. (2024). *Play therapy: The art of the relationship* (4th ed.). Routledge. (Original work published 1991).

Lee, J.-S., & Jang, D.-H. (2015). The effectiveness of sand play treatment meta-analysis. *Korean Journal of Child Psychological Therapy, 10*(1), 1–26.

Lee, S. H., & Jang, M. (2018). A study of themes and symbols in group sandplay therapy of Rohingya refugee children in Malaysia. *Journal of Symbols & Sandplay Therapy, 9*(1), 63–82. https://doi.org/10.12964/jsst.18004

Levine, P. (1997). *Waking the tiger: Healing trauma.* North Atlantic Books.

Lilly, JP (2015). Jungian analytical play therapy. In D. A. Crenshaw & A. L. Stewart (Eds.), *Play therapy: A comprehensive guide to theory and practice* (pp. 48–65). Guilford Press.

Lilly, JP, & Heiko, R. H. (2019). Jungian analytical play therapy. *Play Therapy, 14*(3), 40–42. https://cdn.ymaws.com/www.a4pt.org/resource/resmgr/publications/pt_theories/Jungian_Sept2019_FINAL.pdf

Linehan, M. M., & Wilks, C. R. (2015). The course and evolution of Dialectical Behavior Therapy. *American Journal of Psychotherapy, 69*(2), 91–239. https://doi.org/10.1176/appi.psychotherapy.2015.69.2.97

Loue, S. (Ed.). (2015). *Ethical issues in sandplay therapy practice and research.* Springer. https://doi.org/10.1007/978-3-319-14118-3_5

Lurie, A. (1998). *Don't tell the grown-ups: The subversive power of children's literature.* Bay Back Books.

McAuliffe, G. J., & Associates (Ed.) (2013). *Culturally alert counseling: A comprehensive introduction.* Sage Publications.

McDowell, M. J., Roberts, J. E., & McRoberts, R. (2023). *The dream of the six-legged dog: An experimental system that tests a dream's interpretation.* [Unpublished manuscript].

Midgley, N., Mortimer, R., Cirasola, A., Batra, P., & Kennedy, E. (2021). The evidence-base for psychodynamic psychotherapy with children and adolescents: A narrative synthesis. *Frontiers in Psychology, 12,* 662671. doi:10.3389/fpsyg.2021.662671.

Mitchell, R. R., & Friedman, H. S. (1994). *Sandplay past, present & future.* Routledge Press.

Mitchell, R. R., & Friedman, H. S. (2017). Archetypal themes in the sandplay process. *Journal of Sandplay Therapy, 26*(1), 7–22. www.sandplay.org/journal/abstracts/volume-26-number-1/rogers-mitchell-rie-and-friedman-harriet-s-archetypal-themes-in-the-sandplay-process/

Morse, G. S., & Lomay, V. T. (2021). *Understanding indigenous perspectives: Visions, dreams, and hallucinations.* Cognella.

Myers, J. E., Witmer, J. M., & Sweeney, T. J. (1996). The Wheel of Wellness. *The WEL workbook: Wellness evaluation of lifestyle.* MindGarden.

Neumann, E. (1954). *The origins and history of consciousness.* Routledge & Kegan Paul.

Newell, J. R. (2023). *Symbols of transformation.* www.symbolsoftransformation.com/index.htm

Newell, Z. (2007). *Downward dogs & warriors: Wisdom tales for modern yogis.* Himalayan Institute Press.

Newell, Z. (2021). *Flying monkeys, floating stones: Wisdom tales from the Ramayana for modern yogis.* Himalayan Institute Press.

O'Connor, K. J. (1991). *The play therapy primer: An integration of theories and techniques.* Wiley.

Office of the United Nations High Commissioner for Human Rights. (1989). *Convention on the rights of the child.* (General Assembly Resolution No. 44/25). www.ohchr.org/en/instruments-mechanisms/instruments/convention-rights-child

Perry, B. D. (2023). *NMT.* www.bdperry.com/clincal-work#:~:text=The%20Neurosequential%20Model%20of%20Therapeutics&text=It%20is%20an%20approach%20that,communities%20in%20which%20they%20live

Perry, B. D., & Hambrick, E. (2008). The neurosequential model of therapeutics. *Reclaiming Children and Youth, 17*(3), 38–43.

Piaget, J. (1951). *Play, dreams, and imitation in childhood.* Norton.

Ratts, M. J., Singh, A. A., Nassar-McMillan, S., Butler, S. K., & McCullough, J. R. (2016). Multicultural and social justice counseling competencies: Guidelines for the counseling profession. *Journal of Multicultural Counseling and Development, 44,* 28–48. https://doi.org/10.1002/jmcd.12035

Samuels, A. (2017). The future of Jungian analysis: Strengths, weaknesses, opportunities, threats ("SWOT"). *The Journal of Analytical Psychology, 62*(5), 636–649. https://doi.org/10.1111/1468-5922.12351

Sandplay Therapists of America. (n.d.). *Procedure manual for research using sandplay therapy as origionated by Dora Kalff.* www.sandplay.org/wp-content/uploads/2012/11/Procedure-Manual-for-Sandplay-Research.pdf

Sarah, B., Parson, J., Renshaw, K., & Stagnitti, K. (2021). Can children's play themes be assessed to inform play therapy practice? *Clinical Child Psychology and Psychiatry, 26*(1), 257–267. https://doi.org/10.1177/1359104520964510

Schaefer, C. E. (Ed.). (2003). *Play therapy with adults.* John Wiley & Sons.

Schaefer, C. E., & Drewes, A. A. (Eds.). (2014). *The therapeutic powers of play: 20 core agents of change* (2nd ed.). https://cdn.ymaws.com/www.a4pt.org/resource/resmgr/education_&_training/therapeutic_powers_of_play_2.pdf

Scott, T. A., Burlingame, G., Starling, M., Porter, C., & Lilly, JP (2003). Effects of individual client-centered play therapy on sexually abused children's mood, self-concept, and social competence. *International Journal of Play Therapy, 12*(1), 7–30. https://doi.org/10.1037/h0088869

Sedgwick, D. (2015). On integrating Jungian and other theories. *The Journal of Analytical Psychology, 60*(4), 540–558. https://doi.org/10.1111/1468-5922.12169

Siegel, D. J. (2020). *The developing mind: How relationships and the brain interact to shape who we are.* (3rd ed.). The Guilford Press. (Original work published 1999).

Somatic Experiencing. (2023). *Somatic Experiencing International.* https://traumahealing.org/

Spangler, P. T., & Sim, W. (2023). Working with dreams and nightmares: A review of the research evidence. *Psychotherapy, 60*(3), 383–395. doi:10.1037/pst0000484.

Sudo, H., Shelby, J., Kuniyoshi, T., Ishitani, S., Tsuruta, H., & Kobayashi, T. (2023). Play therapists in Japan: Training, methods, practices, and perceptions. *International Journal of Play Therapy, 32*(4), 218–229. https://doi.org/10.1037/pla0000205

A Toy Garden. (2023). About us. https://atoygarden.com/pages/about-us

Tronick, E., Adamson, L. B., Als, H., & Brazelton, T. B. (1975, April 10–13). Infant emotions in normal and pertubated interactions. In *Proceedings of the Biennial Meeting of the Society for Research in Child Development, Denver, CO, USA*. Vol. 28, pp. 66–104.

Turner, B.A. (2005). *The handbook of sandplay therapy*. Temenos Press.

van der Kolk, V. (2014). *The body keeps the score*. Penguin Books.

Vogler, C. (2020). *The writer's journey: Mythic structure for writers*. Michael Wiese Productions. (Original work published 1998).

von Franz, M. L. (1974). *Shadow and evil in fairy tales*. Shambhala.

von Franz, M. L. (1980). *Projection and re-collection in Jungian psychology*. Open Court Publishing.

von Franz, M. L. (1997). *Archetypal patterns in fairy tales: Studies in Jungian psychology by Jungian analysts #76*. Inner City Books.

von Franz, M. L. (1998). *Dreams: A study of the dreams of Jung, Descartes, Socrates, and other historical figures*. Shambhala.

von Franz, M. L. (2002). *Animus and anima in fairy tales: Studies in Jungian psychology by Jungian analysts #100*. Inner City Books. (Original work published 1991).

Weinrib, E. (2004). *Images of the self: The sandplay therapy process* (2nd ed.). Temenos Press. (Original work published 1983).

Wiersma, J. K., Freedle, L. R., McRoberts, R., & Solberg, K. B. (2022). A meta-analysis of sandplay therapy treatment outcomes. *International Journal of Play Therapy, 31*(4), 197–215. https://doi.org/10.1037/pla0000180

Wilkinson, M. (2005). Undoing dissociation: Affective neuroscience: A contemporary Jungian clinical perspective. *The Journal of Analytical Psychology, 50*(4), 483–501. https://doi.org/10.1111/j.0021-8774.2005.00550.x

Winnicott, D. W. (1971). *Playing and reality*. Basic Books.

World Science Festival. (2022, November 17). *The dreaming mind: Waking the mysteries of sleep*. Big Ideas Series, John Templeton Foundation. https://youtu.be/wvvovktKKa4

Yeh, C. J., Aslan, S. M., Mendoza, V. E., & Tsukamoto, M. (2015). The use of sandplay therapy in urban elementary schools as a crisis response to the World Trade Center attacks. *Psychology Research, 5*(7), 413–427. doi:10.17265/2159-5542/2015.07.004.

Yoga Alliance. (2023). *Teachers*. www.yogaalliance.org/Credentialing/Credentials_for_Teachers

8
When We Reach the End

The afternoon of life is just as full of meaning as the morning; only, its meaning and purpose are different . . .

Jung, CW 7, p. 112, § 114

How do we know when we reach the end of counseling, or really any relationship? Who gets to determine when it's time to go and how? This brings us back to our examination of power (Chapter 1). While counseling ideally begins with the end in mind, there may be other extenuating circumstances including additional life events, interactions with other systems, or financial concerns that may interrupt the process. Some people simply do not find any type of psychotherapy to be helpful, and for some, it can actually do harm (Cuijpers et al., 2021; Roesler, 2013; Wampold & Owen, 2021). While Jungians and other psychoanalytically oriented counselors may be accused of "keeping" their clients longer in therapy than others, I argue that managed care and various systems that limit accessibility to services force clients to "break up" with their therapists prematurely which can do harm as well. I include here suggestions from various "evidence-based practices" that proclaim that clinical results can be obtained in a limited number of sessions. While I have participated in such research in order to bring legitimacy to the competition in the field for what is considered "evidence-based", it is certainly not the be-all, end-all of when to end the process (Wiersma et al., 2022). In all cases, for me, it comes down to the counselor value of client empowerment and our commitment to ethical care. There are so many things to consider.

How do we know when our client is "done"? How are we supportive of our most vulnerable clients including children, those who can no longer afford services, or those who simply want to leave with our blessing? How do we prepare for the inevitable goodbye? How might we provide closure? Failing

DOI: 10.4324/9781003433736-8

to do so can leave a residual sense of incompleteness at best, and at worst, abandonment and resentment. Ending well is important. Anyone who has experienced a death, any type of attachment disruption, a breakup, or has been *ghosted* knows this. We need to be ready to go. We want closure. Even after we think we're done, we still may have questions or want to check in on holidays, after a life change, or just because.

From a Jungian perspective, the individuation process, or becoming fully who we are, is a lifelong journey. If that is the ultimate goal of counseling, we may never "arrive" unless we specialize in end-of-life care. Mental health maintenance is also a value in our profession, and an ethical obligation (ACA, 2014). As counselors, we may want to stay in counseling ourselves to manage the stress and trauma of what we do, keep addictions at bay, or navigate life as it comes. The same goes for our clients. What about the Jungian tradition of being required to stay in analysis or "process" for an undetermined length of time, or while in training, which can take innumerable years? Where are we going? How might we know when to change course?

There has recently been debate in the play therapy community about if there is a difference between the *therapeutic relationship* and the *working alliance*, and if so, what those differences are (O'Connor & Ray, 2023). Counseling itself is a relationship (ACA, 2014). Yes, it's a professional relationship, but it's a real one, which should be genuine, heartfelt, and empowering. One might argue that they're the same, which could be backed up by references in the literature. However, I think, especially from a person-centered, trauma- and neuro-informed, attachment, post-modern perspective that we could consider the "relationship" to be something that might remain in our hearts, minds, bodies, and souls even after the active session "work" is done.

There is much discourse about "the end" in counseling, and the surrounding power dynamics. Here we will discuss how we might plan for the end, and our vision for the future, individually, didactically, and collectively. We will also reach the end of this book.

THERAPEUTIC ENDS

Creation is as much destruction as construction . . .

CW 8, p. 163, § 245

Ideally, *termination*, or the end of counseling or play therapy, is a process that is planned at the beginning and when ready, happens naturally and gradually. The very choice to be in or out of the therapeutic relationship is one of informed consent, which should be both a formal document, signed at intake, and an ongoing process, broached by the counselor. I advocate for even the youngest of clients to be involved in the consent process, also referred to as *assent* (McRoberts, 2018). My general sense of client-centeredness conflicts with some of the specifics of child-centered theory (Landreth, 2024) here; I think it is important for children to know some of why they are invited into relationship with me, and have some say in why and how our time together will end. While a child client may say, like an adult, that they don't think they need to come to sessions anymore, we also want to be on the lookout for signs that this might be on the horizon.

Treatment Plans

While counselors-in-training are taught that the treatment plan, and the resolution of goals, determine the end of treatment, this is more symptom- and therapist-focused than many Jungians like. Clients, as well, may not be interested in a formal treatment plan, even though we must write one up for various governing reasons, and may even "forget" that they have them. The explorative nature of the process may lead us "off track" of the plan, which can be expected in this method. More open, creative, and psychodynamically oriented practitioners may also have a higher tolerance of ambiguity (Kornilova & Kornilov, 2010; Qian & Yarnal, 2011; Weiss, 1973). For this reason, though, we might review the treatment plan peri- odically, as an intervention itself, to reorient the client to where they said they wanted to go when they first came in. Starting with the end in mind, when co-developing a treatment plan, we may also anticipate what the termination summary might look like. Clients may have a goal to even- tually be more open with friends and family, to attend group, school, or engage in more recreational activities that take up the time, and some- times function, that counseling does. Other clients may be welcome to return whenever they think they need to. It is important to know what our boundaries around this are so we can help hold the frame. When working with children, especially as play therapists, I recommend one of the latest and greatest sources available in documentation and community collabo- ration (Homeyer & Bennett, 2023).

Some practices have written policies to conduct a treatment plan review every three to six months or once a year for chart audits. We might take this opportunity to ask our clients if they think they've resolved their goals, or give formal assessments to quantify levels of reported symptoms. Other clients may come to us with a certain number of "required" or "allowed" hours. Some examples may be those who have been court ordered to six months of counseling, or those whose insurance policies only pay for eight sessions. Initial treatment plans ideally have these conditions built in, and we'd then review the plan at that time to determine if they'd like to continue with the process. I encourage counselors to build into their practice an allotment for a certain number of clients to receive services at a reduced rate or pro bono (free) especially when an established client's circumstances change so that clients aren't abandoned (ACA, 2014, A.12, C.6.e.). If this is not possible at the agency where the counselor works, it is important to have a list of trustworthy and accessible referral sources.

Breaks

Counselors need to take breaks. There are many reasons for this, both planned and unplanned. Either way, we have a responsibility to our clients' continuation of care. We want to make arrangements in advance so they may be tended to in times of crisis if and when we can't be there. We might need a vacation, attend a conference, or take extended time off due to injury or illness, a death or birth in the family. Ideally, even breaks are discussed at the start of treatment planning (see Chapter 6). As discussed in Chapter 1, having a network of like-minded colleagues is invaluable. In agency settings, there may be another counselor who could step in for a time; a release of information could be prepared in advance in case of an emergency. Another option may be providing a list of local Jungian discussion, dream, or process groups. While Jungian seminars may be primarily training centers, they also may provide these services. Of course, local and national crisis line numbers should also be presented for clients to contact during a break.

Phasing-Out

Sometimes, in very active therapeutic relationships, the treatment process is observed by the counselor and the client to be "slowing down" or "wrapping up". I've had many clients who come in several weeks in a row and actually apologize for not having anything "negative", "bad", or distressing to talk about. I think these times are important opportunities to dig deeper into what is going well, to celebrate life, and to reinforce accomplishments and gratitude. While we may have a natural negativity bias (Norris, 2021), that propensity may change over time, which may even be a goal for some clients. We have evidence that continued positive experience, including mindful engagement on positive emotions and ongoing healthy interactions, can also have healing effects, mentally and physically (Ford et al., 2021; Wright, 2015). Taken in tandem with the importance of the counselor's role as a resource, I am hesitant to initiate ending the relationship abruptly or too soon, especially if I know that a client may be likely to experience other life stressors in the near future. While it may take more of a balancing act with our schedules, I recommend phasing-out whenever possible. That is, when a client, who has been seen weekly, has been doing well for several weeks, a discussion and co-decision to step down to every other week, with the option to schedule if needed, is begun. When that goes well, the step-down may look like every three weeks, or once a month, again, with the option to schedule more frequently if needed. This way, the end of counseling is more gradual, and the heart of the relationship can go with the client.

Symptoms Vs Enhancement

Though psychodynamically oriented therapies typically include more sessions than CBT (for various reasons) response rates for symptom reduction are initially similar; however results from psychodynamic treatment tend to last longer, reducing the chance of remission, and results may continue to improve over time (Cuijpers et al., 2021; Midgley et al., 2021; Roesler, 2013; Shedler, 2010). Research on sandplay therapy indicated that while symptom reduction may occur in fewer than ten sessions, further sessions may be life-enchanting (Wiersma et al., 2022). This does not mean, though, that Jungian-oriented counselors and play therapists should "hold" their clients and prevent them from "graduating", being "released", or leaving counseling of their own free will. (It also doesn't mean clients are more likely to be "done" sooner with CBT.)

If a client has noticeably reduced symptoms, that should be documented in their progress notes and the treatment plan. If a symptom is completely gone, we might consider it being in a "maintenance" phase, and add an objective to, or reword an existing goal. However, we may choose to mark that goal as "achieved" or "completed", and add a life-enhancing goal. For some, this is a paradigm shift; moving from pathology, or medical model, to one based in wellness, can be tough, even though counseling is based on a wellness model (CSI, 2023; Myers et al., 1996). How much counseling is "too much", though?

While there is limited research on the concept, dependency on the therapist is a conversation long had among practitioners, and a dynamic that might be avoided if we have clear, collaborative working goals (Geurtzen et al., 2018). Counselors have a responsibility to hold the frame of their practice and encourage clients to develop skills and relationships that will ultimately work us out of a job. If a client seems to lack personal, spiritual, or community resources, we might encourage that as a goal. We don't want to be the only person in a client's life that they can talk to. We often say we're trying to work ourselves out of a job. It is important to approach this concept early on in the relationship, and revisit it often, so that clients don't end up feeling shamed and rejected by our negligence.

This leads us to further discussion of therapeutic relationships, or working alliances, that are established to work us into, rather than out of, a job: doing our own work to become a Jungian-oriented counselor or play therapist.

PROCESS AS A TRAINING REQUIREMENT

> A hostile opposition takes place only when consciousness obstinately clings to its one-sidedness and insists on its arbitrary standpoint, as always happens when there is a repression and, in consequence, a partial dissociation of consciousness.
>
> CW 18, p. 621, § 1418

Back when Jung was first developing his theory, in the early 1900s, the field of psychology was new and lacked many professional and ethical standards we now hold dear. Until Jung's time, mental health treatment was conducted by medical doctors, mainly in hospitals and "lunatic asylums", reserved for those with severe symptoms, or whom those in power wanted to lock away (Foucault, 1965).

Jung helped change things by suggesting that those who wanted to learn his method had to experience their own process first, regardless of their mental health (Kirsch, 2000). Dora Kalff (2020) also made this a requirement for sandplay therapists. However, the accreditation process, or receiving Jung or Kalff's "blessing", was highly subjective to how much analysis or further education they personally thought a trainee might need, and other various, often mysterious, extenuating circumstances (Kirsch, 2000, p. 5). While Jungian analytic and sandplay therapy training is now governed by organizations, (which Jung was notoriously suspicious of), these requirements of personal process continue to be highly subjective, as well as increasingly expensive, lengthy, and inaccessible to most. This perpetuates the stigma of Jungians being elitist, cultish, unprofessional, and even racist (Brewster, 2023; Noll, 1994).

While it is inarguable that a deep understanding, appreciation, and culti-vation of the language of the unconscious, and ongoing reflective practices, is vital to practicing from a Jungian orientation, assessing what a trainee's personal process "should" look like was, and still is, controversial. Back in the day, possible trainees often had to travel great distances for sessions with Jung or Kalff in Switzerland, so the process was often much shorter, and sometimes, the blessing was bestowed without it. Sometimes, analysands (Jungian analysts-in-training) requested and were granted permission to receive analysis from someone untrained, and if Jung thought they could do it, he granted permission (Kirsch, 2000). There are also living, circulat-ing myths of Kalff inviting American sandplay therapists-in-training to her home, but then refusing to see them.

Gatekeeping in Jungian circles, because they tend to be small, has always involved a good deal of navigating the dual relationship of one's therapist also being one's teacher. It wasn't until the 1950s, with the development of the IAAP (International Association for Analytical Psychology) that any authority other than Jung himself could provide authorized accreditation as a Jungian analyst (Kirsch, 2000). Only then did standards include a graduate degree, though in any field, as well as additional training in analytic psychol-ogy, and extensive personal analysis. While organizations have power, indi-viduals do, too. Counselors, specifically, aim to support the empowerment of others. How are we advocating for ourselves through the organizations we choose to fund and allow them to "speak" us through our training and credentialing?

While "personal process" is considered a cornerstone of Jungian therapies, the number of required hours is not based upon Jung's teachings, nor sci-ence, but institutional policies and the official "blessing" of the one in the therapist role. Currently, to become a Jungian analyst in the US through the Inter-Regional Society of Jungian Analysts (IRSJA, 2023) requires 100 hours of personal analysis before even applying and continued analysis through the training. To become a Certified Sandplay Therapist through the Sandplay Therapists of America (STA, 2022) requires a minimum of 30–40 sessions. I've been told personally that they don't budge on the min-imum suggestion, and most require the sessions to be in-person. This is a real barrier for many potential trainees who don't have teaching members in their area, who tend to cluster in cities, as well as those who can't afford to pay out of pocket indefinitely. It may be of interest that the Association for Play Therapy (APT, 2023) does not have such requirements, though there are a few of us who identify as Jungian/Analytic Play Therapists (APT, n.d.).

Though reportedly growing, STA had only 381 members in 2020 (McRoberts, 2022). Current training and ethical guidelines do not fully encapsulate and prepare potential trainees for the very real likelihood of dual relationships within STA, such as one's sandplay therapist becoming their teacher, and vice versa (STA, 2018, 2022). While this tends to be common in small communities, additional, specific measures should be taken, including open and ongoing conversations about boundaries and specific, written confidentiality agreements (Bernard & Goodyear, 2014). There are few studies to empirically illustrate how these and other potential ethical boundary crossings affect the supervisory relationship or professional identity (Kozlowski et al., 2014), but it may impact counselors pursuing their own work in sandplay therapy, certification through STA, or ultimately, the quality of their personal and professional identity.

While often suggested, requiring therapists to pursue their own therapy, whether in training, supervision, as part of gatekeeping, or for a previously disclosed ongoing mental health maintenance process, is still debated due to mixed and inconclusive outcomes of the effectiveness of such a requirement on job performance, as well as various ethical considerations. Global studies suggest that psychodynamic- and humanistic-oriented therapists are more likely than cognitive behavioral therapists to independently pursue their own therapy by approximately 30%; in addition, psychodynamic approaches are pursued by therapists of various theoretical orientations by up to 40–60% (Norcross et al., 2009, as cited in Malikiosi-Loizos, 2013). Perhaps not surprisingly, American counselors seem to be attending counseling as part of their training at significantly lower rates than in the rest of the world (Egunjobi, 2020). Attending counseling for treatment, though, is not the same as attending to meet a requirement, so goals and expectations should be different, but also clear and held to the same ethical standards of practice (Edwards, 2018).

Some Jungian analysts and sandplay therapy teachers have admitted to me that requiring a certain number of process hours may be for job security or unspoken gatekeeping practices (like to keep an eye on trainees). It has also been disclosed to me that most Jungian trainees stop their personal processes after completing requirements, but why, we can only speculate, given the mythos that Jungians are to keep doing the work for their whole lives. Perhaps it is because by that point they have spent thousands of dollars out of pocket, as many analysts and sandplay therapists are private-pay only. Perhaps, too, they no longer feel that the process is empowering, since they were required to attend, disclose their most private fantasies, sometimes to their therapist who is also a teacher, and continue to pay for the privilege.

So when do we reach the end? If the individuation process takes our whole lives, how do we know when we're done? When do we "meet requirements"? When our analyst or sandplay therapist declares it so and releases us? By what assessment? What if we don't want the governing organization to know our personal business? What if our therapist moves away and there isn't another in the area that meets those standards? Well, I can tell you from experience that it happens, and puts the credentialing process on hold, sometimes indefinitely. I can understand why people don't want to invest in a long, expensive, emotional credentialing process only to have it cut short. This is part of our Jungian heritage and our reputation.

I pose these questions of "we" not only because traditionally Jungian students first go through their own process, but to encourage this "we" mentality as humans in general, as we're working with clients, and within our communities. There is a power dynamic at play when someone comes to us for help, and we must wield that power with great respect, giving it back to the individual whenever possible. I believe in the aesthetics of existence: that our life is a work of art for the sake of the Self. Our journey and interactions with others along the way shape that process. We each have the power to choose where we want to invest our time and resources. Even the tiniest babies know when their bellies are full. And like Jung said, the individuation process is lifelong. None of us here have "arrived" yet, so how about we not act like it?

FUTURE VISION

> Through the new ethic, the ego-consciousness is ousted from its central position in a psyche organized on the lines of a monarchy or totalitarian state, its place being taken by wholeness or the self, which is now recognized as central. The self was of course always at the centre, and always acted as the hidden director.
>
> CW 18, p. 621, § 1419

Identification with a theory of practice is a developmental process that takes time, experience, supervision, peer support, and reflection (Fitzpatrick et al., 2010; Muro et al., 2015; Werries, 2015). Though integrative or eclectic styles are increasingly popular in today's post-modern world, a strong theoretical foundation with intentionality as well as appropriate supervision and mentorship is nonetheless recommended, as it can impact client care outcomes, and our sense of professional identity (Aguilera, 2010; APT, 2023; Arthur, 2001; Bernard & Goodyear, 2014; O'Connor & Ray, 2023). While even Jung knew that "there is no single theory . . . that cannot on occasion prove basically wrong" (CW 16, p. 116, § 237), it is still prudent to make a valiant effort to really dig in. We need to be able to see ourselves pictured and reflected in the world (CW 16).

Because of the reputation of being elusive and complex, and competition in the market, the depth practitioners, including Jungians, are recognizing the need for a bit of rebranding in order to carry on the tradition into the digital age; this requires constructing a more user friendly conceptual framework, including scaffolding of basic skills in a developmental sequence and measurable competencies (Friedman & Anderson, 2019; Poston & Bland, 2020). Contemporary education in general is, hopefully, realizing it's in need of a paradigm shift, waking up to the notion that technology's rapid fire pace is here to stay for its ease in accessibility and affordability, but not at the expense of the search for, and solace found in, depth of meaning and human interaction (Darden, 2014; Lee et al., 2020; Murthy, 2020; National Center for Education Statistics, 2018). Heutagogy offers a post-modern approach, identifying the "spirals of reflection" (Canning & Callan, 2010) involved in learning when empowered and connected through collaboration, and therefore aligned with the Jungian aesthetic. Collaborative mentoring fosters solidarity, work satisfaction, self-efficacy, creativity, and intrinsic motivation for individual and collective advocacy (Chong & Ma, 2010; Deci, 1972; Grant & Berry, 2011; Reynolds, 2011; Zellars et al., 2002).

Jungian scholars have observed ongoing resistance to scientific pursuits openly acknowledging or building upon the psychodynamic and analytic foundation, often by Jungians themselves, which is being critiqued and challenged in the literature (Brown et al., 2013; Cochrane et al., 2014; Roesler, 2018; Schmidt, 2014; Wakefield, 2014; Wilkinson, 2005; Winborn, 2016). Due to Jung's foundational influence on the counseling field and the rising popularity in play therapy and sandplay therapy, greater focus and further investigation into Jungian study and depth psychology is necessary in order to ultimately ensure that quality services are provided to particularly vulnerable populations, including traumatized and marginalized clients, especially children, as well as the mental health professionals who care for them (CACREP, 2024; Malikiosi-Loizos, 2013; McRoberts, 2018).

What are we going to do as counselors? Many of us have lost touch with our identities of being client-focused, wellness-based, culturally alert, and sell out to the latest and the greatest thing. While yes, let's look to the future, also, please READ THE CLASSICS. Yes, read Jung, but also Rogers, Landreth, Sweeney, Adler, and more. I recommend ALL COUNSELORS read the *Art of the Relationship* (Landreth, 2024) whether they are interested in play therapy or not. We have a lot to learn about our Selves. As Servant Leaders (Greenleaf, 1970), our collective values, and how we influence the shaping of society, personally and professionally, will be shaped by our creative cognition and action.

Advocacy

This is a book about my perspectives on being a Jungian-oriented counselor and play therapist, but it is also an act of advocacy. Clients have not been, and still are not consistently empowered in the mental health field, including in counseling and research; and to be clear, the result of true empowerment is not supposed to be crippling, isolating independence. Counselors are so creative, and want to be helpful, yet struggle with their personal and professional identity, resilience, and self-efficacy, too (McRoberts & Epstein, 2023). We're interconnected. For me, Jung provides the metaphorical language necessary for a deeper understanding of these dynamics, our psyches, both conscious and unconscious processes, personally and collectively, with that spiritual core that is being neglected. I understand that this is not a popularly held view, but it makes intuitive sense to me. While much of the research here is new, the broad Jungian concepts have always guided my practice. It's kind of creepy sometimes. That's the numinous at work.

Jung also keeps me humble. He was a prolific writer and deep thinker; I must forever be a student if I want to remain curious and seek understanding, especially of the subjective. It is counterproductive to hold and wield the power of expertise over our clients' heads if our aim is to assist them in being more empowered. To regard people as objects, or otherwise overly focus on "objective content" (I'm looking at you, SOAP notes) devalues the person, the process, and ultimately the Self. I'd like to see more of these ideas come together in Jungian counseling and play therapy. I'd wager that there are more folks out there that have read Jung, or are Jung-curious, but are too afraid to hang their shingle out saying so. Even if we are brave enough to say so, sometimes "Jung" or "Jungian" doesn't show up on a provider database search so clients who might like a Jungian perspective can't even find us. This is its own advocacy issue which I encourage anyone else who cares to join me in. However, I'd also like to encourage anyone who knows who they are and what they believe in to be braver and say so. There's a heap of evidence that it's ultimately good for us and our clients. I've said it before and I'll say it again: I may not be everyone's cup of tea, but I'm still a fine cup of tea. You're welcome to adopt that saying yourself.

There's an undeniable tension between the "legitimate" Jungians (credentialed analysts, sandplay therapists, and invested trainees) and "others" (including academics and the average soul hungry mental health practitioner) which needs to be directly addressed before it can be transcended. While it has been said that the Jungian fear of research interfering with "the process" is unfounded (Roesler, 2013), I do hear some legitimate concerns. Beyond simply more pre- and post-test quantitative research on specific pathologies, which could "get us our numbers" needed to compete in this over-analytic field, but be an ethical dilemma, it would require us to explore and agree on additional terminology, and at least a few minimal factors, more clearly defining our method. Jungians often don't want to pathologize. What measures, then, "should" they use? How might we begin to manualize a relationship that is attempting to be receptive to the numinous? While we do have the STA (2012) Research Manual for sandplay therapy, Jungian counselors might look to the CCPT protocol for further non-verbal interventions, adding in our own Jungian twist. CCPT has nailed it on the integration of philosophy, standards of practice, the person of the client and the therapist, and they have the numbers to back it up.

I came to research nearly 20 years into my career. Jung (CW 17) postulated that midlife is a metamorphic time on the path to individuation, which inspired me to take a deeper look (McRoberts, 2023). Academic writing became an act of Self-awareness, preservation, and advocacy. Theoretical integration of the personal and the professional takes time but can be propelled by our curiosity, commitment to lifelong learning, and engagement in the spiritual and expressive arts, especially with well-attuned mentoring (Leader, 2015; Mullen et al., 2007; Roesler, 2019; Rønnestad & Skovholt, 2003). As I continue to read Jungian journals, I see some research, but a lot of creative writing. That's not a bad thing. I think I've made a case for the creative already here. What I'm saying is, I get it, but: with a bit more intentional and transparent methodology we could elevate our qualitative research presence and span the creative and scientific, as we've been raised to do. There are a lot of great stories being told, but I fear that they'll be lost in a generation, as our Jungian elders die out. Many articles are nearly legitimate case studies and autoethnographies but lack the rigor and structure that the general market demands. I would love to see Jungians doing more "real" research and publishing in counseling and other mental health journals. This work is about our experiences and insights, yes, but isn't it ultimately about something bigger than ourselves? How might we get more Jungian research into the hands of more counselors and mental health practitioners in general? What are we doing to see that our research practices, from design to dissemination, are anti-racist (Belser et al., 2023; Rowe, 2023)?

I am both personally and professionally interested in the discourse of creativity, spirituality, trauma, and professional identity in counselors and play therapists. I do this because there has long been, and continues to be, a focus on pathologizing marginalized, vulnerable people, and oppressing them with our colonialist ideals under the guise of "reformation" or "healing"; Foucault said this is more cruel than prison (Wade, 2019). For example, Jung called it years ago that substance use disorders were spiritual problems (McCabe, 2015), a sentiment that continues in treatment today. There is wonderful, grassroots work being done in the field of addiction and the homeless, especially here in the South. Yet we, as a mental health field, continue to bow down to the for-profit prison-industrial complex, complicit in the legal enslavement of our own people, and making a living at it. That's a problem I don't hear us addressing directly. While I believe mental health care, like all healthcare, is a human right, I would like to see more counselors speaking up and out about how they manage confidentiality within oppressive systems, and how we can do better. As a counselor, educator, and supervisor, I have seen too many counselors bullied by the education and legal system, not to mention insurance companies, to engage in ethically questionable behavior. I've said it before and I'll say it again: In order to advocate for others, we have to first advocate for ourselves. We have our own psychological and spiritual growth to do.

Psychological & Spiritual Growth

Therapy has been called the "new religion" of Generation Me (Twenge, 2014; Vernoy, 2023). Funny . . . wasn't Jung falsely accused of trying to start a new religion with his spiritually integrated theory over a century ago? In all seriousness, as counselors, we need to be vigilant that our egos don't become inflated, or that we start practicing outside our scope. Our communities are so divided, even within denominations and non-denominations of Christianity, which still makes up more than half of our population in America. About 25% of us identify as "spiritual but not religious", and about the same number consider ourselves neither spiritual nor religious, with an increasing number of "nones" (Pew Research Center, 2018, 2022). Where does that leave our spiritual center, the heart of counseling? What of our God-image? What of our personal and collective sense of Self?

I am not surprised that counselors are not more "multiculturally competent" let alone culturally alert, humble, or responsive. Where are we? Who are we? If the majority of us can't reconcile this amongst ourselves, what are we doing in the face of our vulnerable clients belonging to minority religious and spiritual traditions including Buddhism, Hinduism, Judaism, Islam, Native American Life-Ways, and Paganism (National Geographic, 2023; the Pluralism Project, 2023; Sonnex et al., 2022)? How are we not "othering" them? How do we come to truly empathize with each other on a deep, spiritual level?

I thought we were having a creativity crisis (McRoberts, 2022), which was bad enough, but this spiritual crisis may be worse and at the root of it all. We're lost, isolating, and think our individual egos can figure it all out. While we are leaving our spiritual communities and families of origin in favor of greater independence and happiness, we are flocking to individual counseling, with our mental health worse off than ever before (Gallup, 2022). The mental health field continuously steals from religions, East and West, rebranding it "secular" in favor of being "scientific". This needs to stop. It's leaving a God-shaped hole in our psyches that Jung saw coming (Hagedorn & Moorhead, 2010). Spiritual integration is considered an important aspect of mental health care in general, is central to our identity and competency as counselors, and research says clients value it (Rogers et al., 2023). Trying to be in control all the time is exhausting . . . and futile. I invite us to all get more comfortable talking about the religious function, and all of the functions of the psyche, really, as a starting point. They are all interconnected. WE are all interconnected.

I would also like to see a greater bridge between the mental health and spiritual professions. Jung was one of the first to call out the largely semantic and power-dynamic shift from the spiritual to the scientific as a thin veil of illusion (Main, 2007). This shift, while reflective of a value of knowledge and facts, also contributed to the ongoing colonialist, individualistic mindset that may be contributing to the mental health crisis. There is a strong link between spiritual maturity and mental health, and it's just on the other side of virtuous humanism (Choi et al., 2020). Again, I think we need to read more about cultures and subcultures around the world, but also to get out, get curious, and get to know people. One of the criticisms of the digital age is that we are immersed in echo chambers and have forgotten our manners, let alone our ability to mode-shift or be person-centered in our daily life. By engaging in a spiritual discipline, we build community. Historically, communities often disagreed with one another but took care of each other out of respect for themselves, their heritage, and their elders.

That takes hard work, commitment, and Self-respect. We can't throw out culture for ideology; I'm with Jordan Peterson on that one.

Aesthetics of Existence

To hold the ethical view that our life is a work of art requires us to value and sacredly engage with the unconscious. After a career relatively well balanced between life and work, with a few years of doing the most, I am hearing the call to return to a simpler life. Jung valued large swaths of time alone, writing, and making artwork (Jung, 1989). I remember, too, the time Edith Kramer, the great art therapist, told me, when I was visiting her New York City flat, to see that I made art as much as I saw clients. That was in the 90s. I'm still working toward that goal. See, I wrote a whole book on this stuff and I will still admit that I haven't arrived. That's what doing our own work looks like, with a dollop of 12-Step lingo.

I have been in several heated debates about the seemingly arbitrary training requirements that do not account for the limited number, and aging-out, of Certified Sandplay Therapist Teaching Members (CST-Ts) and Jungian Analysts. What does it mean, collectively, to be a Jungian in the digital age? Is there evidence that the next generation of counselors will invest in the 5–20 years that it takes post-master's to become credentialed? Would they be more interested if we made it more accessible? More personable? What do they need and how might we adapt?

More intentional examination of ongoing training and supervision practices in Jungian-oriented counseling, play therapy, and sandplay therapy is needed. Providers want specific support, including a greater sense of community (Felton, 2016; Friedman & Mitchell, 2008; McRoberts, 2022; Penn & Post, 2012). APT members obtain continuing education, specifically in play therapy training and supervision, at a higher rate than ACA members overall; in addition, over half of surveyed sandplay therapists report obtaining training through APT (Lambert et al., 2007), making APT an identified leader in the field to collaborate with universities to develop quality Jungian play therapy graduate programming. However, the Jungian tradition of formal analysis training post-graduate remains the gold standard. Therefore, it seems that collaboration between APA, CACREP, IRSJA, IAAP, STA, and APT would be ideal for a well-rounded graduate course of study in Jungian analytical play therapy. Because such programs do not yet exist, a century after Jung first postulated his theory, and predicted it would take more than a lifetime to complete, the work of Jungian scholars and leaders remains, even as science projects the field forward. And many Jungian elders don't even want this level or type of growth. They want to hold Jung tight to their chests and if people seek them out, so be it. That's fine if that's the way they want to work, but I'm here to tell you that they don't own Jung. Jung's teachings, like all works of art and scientific discoveries, are accomplishments of the individual but belong to the collective. I agree with the nearly 50-year-old sentiment that more servants should only seek guidance from Servant Leaders and follow the Self to trust their emergence and path (Greenleaf, 1970). Like Jung and Kalff, we might need to forge our own.

I would like to see bolder discourse around how our field continues to be complicit in an exploitative, medicalized system resonant with dystopian science fiction. If you haven't, please read or re-read *Brave New World* (Huxley, 2006). There are forces in this digital age that are over-sexualizing, numbing, and pathologizing our humanity, our collective unconscious, and selling personae as a mental health treatment. We've been uprooted, stripped of our religions, forced off the land, imprisoned, and homogenized. Jung saw it coming and I don't believe I'm the only one who sees that it's here. I am not proposing that we band together and drop out of society like the cult we've been accused of being (Noll, 1994), but I do think that this will involve a movement. Counselors in general have a lot of power because the People are suffering and are asking for our help. We have that power due to our privilege and responsibility, a combination of our hard work, the systems we work for, and the power our clients give us when they look to us for answers. We have the ethical duty not to be an exclusive club of woke saviors selling ego-focused snake oil. We must continue to challenge ourselves, our clients, loved ones, and the systems we work in to answer: given the situation we're in, what is empowerment, really? What then, is the right thing to do with that power? What are the World and the Self asking of us? What kind of balance are we aiming to strike? What is mental health? Is it attainable under these conditions? What are we willing to do to get it? What are we actively doing to truly protect the privacy and integrity of ourselves and our clients? How do we help support the empowerment of people in building healthy, collaborative communities? We are part of this discourse. There are already some pretty clear answers out there, and we ignore them. I think we need to step up and own that, holding ourselves and others accountable. To paraphrase Chalmers (1995), we can't explain consciousness, or the unconscious, on the cheap. There's always a price.

I'll admit it: I would like to see more counselors read Jung and come to identify as Jungians. I think many will find a home there, even if we're often alone. Jung said we all have to spend time alone in order to reflect, have creative thoughts, come home to the Self, and see those visions come to life (CW 12). This might "just" be my bias, but research, including my own, indicates that creatives might really enjoy this way of working, this theory, this worldview (see McRoberts, 2022). But it needs to be more accessible; we need teachers. The Tao Te Ching says when the time is right they'll arrive. I got called to be one, but I'm just one. Challenging dualistic thinking requires the practice of mode-shifting. As we become more aware of our ability to shift between associative and analytic processes, we might not only become better counselors, but also find greater meaning, peace, and fulfillment in our lives.

Ultimately, I'd like to see us all come home to the Self.

SAYING GOODBYE

> Therefore we stand with our soul suspended between formidable influences from within and from without, and somehow we must be fair to both. This we can do only after the measure of our individual capacities. Hence we must bethink ourselves not so much of what we "ought" to do as of what we can and must do.
>
> CW 7, p. 324, § 397

All right y'all. As we reach the end of our time here together, I hope that you have found some things useful, or at least thought provoking. I've worked my whole life, let alone my career, to get to this point, and I thank you for joining me on this little leg of the journey.

When I know it's time to say goodbye, I want to make it a good one. If it's a big deal for my client, student, or loved one, I let it be a big deal. Routines and rituals are important (because of attachment, symbols, and all those functions of the psyche we talked about). If I know someone is fixin' to leave, especially if they're tore up about it, especially a kid, or an adult who's moving, we're gonna celebrate. I like us to plan together. Is it a graduation? We might have a procession, inspirational speeches, a diploma, cake, and pictures. Is it some other kind of big transition? If the person's favorite defense mechanism is humor, we might have a "roast" full of funny stories from several people, a "year in review" of trials, tribulations, and growth. We might both share our highlight reels and photo albums of our time together (like the sandplay therapists do), with talk of periodic postcards. I think this can be done with ethical grace. It takes time, Self-knowledge and ongoing support. And I'm always down for cake. Honestly, a lot of clients just stop coming, and I don't really like the "reach out three times" policy of a lot of places I've worked at; it seems invasive and is more about "the policy" than the client or the counselor. Many of us have a sense of when a client "forgot" their session, and when they're trying to peace out. I think it's gracious to let them save face. In between these two extremes are those clients who are ready to let go of the work, but not the relationship. In these cases, we do a "see you later", or "call me when you need me". I've had the honor of working with a child who then tells their parent they want to make an appointment when they're a teenager, and then call me themselves when they're an adult. The relationship is a professional one, but it's real. We don't always need to start from square one.

Part of my future vision for Jungian-oriented counseling and play therapy is that it is more prevalent, integrated, flexible, and accessible. I think Hermes, who may be our psychopomp for the digital age, laughs at our attempts to cage Jungian thought; it walks between the Worlds, speaking with the personal and collective. Just as sandplay therapy is more researched and practiced in Asia (Lee & Jang, 2015; Wiersma et al., 2022), Jungian academics are also more common (Kawai as cited in Casement, 2018). Brazil also has several universities that integrate Jung into graduate and undergraduate courses in medicine, psychology, human development, philosophy, education, art, and Jungian certificate programs, thanks to the revolutionary pioneer who got to know Jung personally, Dr. Nose da Silvera (Ramos, as cited in Casement, 2018). Like Knox says in the book *Who Owns Jung* (Casement, 2018), "own" might mean we think we have the rights to claim something or it might mean that we acknowledge it. I propose we all start owning Jung.

In the US it seems that we not only remain willfully ignorant of the developments in Jungian thought, but we're gun-shy when it comes to discussing even the basic concepts Jung presented through his introduction to the nature, structure, and functions of the psyche, even with mounting evidence. That's a lot of unaligned ego. While we pay more lip service to words like "multiculturalism" in the field and are putting more people from marginalized communities into positions of power, the transformative axiologies leading the charge are tragically secular (Tracey as cited in Casement, 2018). We are still attempting to create rigid, analytic models around forever transforming, associative processes while ignoring our universally human elements. Our culture is crying for nourishing depth, yet we continue to produce, distribute, and feed thin, homogenized theory. I'm convinced that Jung's the bridge to a more holistic way. The digital age has made us all over-reliant on the analytic process, maybe with the best of intentions. But make no mistake, we all function within systems of power that would like nothing more than for us to continue to be complicit. We have a responsibility to awaken, live mindfully, creatively, and co-exist ethically. This calls for more exploration, internally and externally, listening to the Self, and practicing mode-shifting. Yes, there's risk involved. Feathers will definitely be ruffled. But there is so much numinosity to be experienced. Let's fly. I hope to see you on the other side.

Reflections

1. What is one of your main takeaways from this book?
2. How might you apply Jungian theory or practice to your life and/or work?
3. Recalling a time when you have ended a relationship or event well. What elements did it include? How might you adapt them into your policies and procedures with clients?
4. Do you have any visions for the future of *Jungian Counseling and Play Therapy*? If so, please feel free to reach out!

REFERENCES

Aguilera, M. E. (2010). *An exploratory study of the developmental experience of novice play therapists*. [Doctoral dissertation]. Dissertation Abstracts International; Section A, 70, 3352.

American Counseling Association (ACA). (2014). *ACA code of ethics*. www.counseling.org/resources/aca-code-of-ethics.pdf

Arthur, A. R. (2001). Personality, epistemology and psychotherapists' choice of theoretical model: A review and analysis. *European Journal of Psychotherapy, Counselling and Health*, 4(1), 45–64.

Association for Play Therapy (APT). (n.d.). *Find a play therapist*. www.a4pt.org/search/custom.asp?id=3571

Association for Play Therapy (APT). (2023). *Play therapy credentials: Program overview*. www.a4pt.org/page/CredentialsInfo

Belser, C., Dillman Taylor, D., McRoberts, R., & Sami, W. (2023). Introduction to the special issue on outcome and evidenced-based research with children and adolescents. *Journal of Child and Adolescent Counseling*, 9(2), 67–71. doi:10.1080/23727810.2023.2229218.

Bernard, J. M., & Goodyear, R. K. (2014). *Fundamentals of clinical supervision* (5th ed.). Pearson Allyn & Bacon.

Brewster, F. (2023). *Race and the unconscious.* Routledge.

Brown, M. L., McDonald, S., & Smith, F. (2013). Jungian archetypes and dreams of social enterprise. *Journal of Organizational Change Management, 26*(4), 670–688. https://doi.org/10.1108/JOCM-Sep-2012-0146

Canning, N., & Callan, S. (2010). Heutagogy: Spirals of reflection to empower learners in higher education. *Reflective Practice, 11*(1), 71–82.

Casement, A. (Ed.). (2018). *Who owns Jung?* Routledge.

Chalmers, D. J. (1995). Facing up to the problem of consciousness. *Journal of Consciousness Studies, 2*(3), 200–219.Chi Sigma Iota (CSI). (2023). *Wellness in counseling.* www.csi-net.org/group/wellness

Choi, S., Hoi-Yun McClintock, C., Lau, E., & Miller, L. (2020). The dynamic universal profiles of spiritual awareness: A latent profile analysis. *Religions, 11*(6), 288. doi:10.3390/rel11060288. www.researchgate.net/publication/342357407_The_Dynamic_Universal_Profiles_of_Spiritual_Awareness_A_Latent_Profile_Analysis

Chong, E., & Ma, X. (2010). The influence of individual factors, supervision and work environment on creative self-efficacy. *Creativity and Innovation Management, 19*(3), 233–247. https://doi.org/10.1111/j.1467-8691.2010.00557.x

Cochrane, M., Flower, S., Mackenna, C., & Morgan, H. (2014). A Jungian approach to analytic work in the twenty-first century. *British Journal of Psychotherapy, 30*(1), 33–50. https://doi.org/10.1111/bjp.12060

Council for Accreditation of Counseling and Related Programs (CACREP). (2024). *2024 CACREP standards.* www.cacrep.org/wp-content/uploads/2023/06/2024-Standards-Combined-Version-6.27.23.pdf

Cuijpers, P., Karyotaki, E., Ciharova, M., Miguel, C., Noma, H., & Furukawa, T. A. (2021). The effects of psychotherapies for depression on response, remission, reliable change, and deterioration: A meta-analysis. *Acta Psychiatrica Scandinavica, 144*(3), 288–299. https://doi.org/10.1111/acps.13335

Darden, D. (2014). Relevance of the Knowles theory in distance education. *Creative Education, 5,* 809–812. doi:10.4236/ce.2014.510094.

Deci, E. L. (1972). Intrinsic motivation, extrinsic reinforcement, and inequity. *Journal of Personality and Social Psychology, 22*(1), 113–120. https://doi.org/10.1037/h0032355

Edwards, J. (2018). Counseling and psychology student experiences of personal therapy: A critical interpretive synthesis. *Frontiers in Psychology, 9*(1732), 1–13. https://doi.org/10.3389/fpsyg.2018.01732

Egunjobi, J. P. (2020). Prevalence of personal therapy for therapists-in-training across the world. [Self-published manuscript]. doi:10.13140/RG.2.2.32958.43840/1

Felton, A. D. (2016). *Identity in the sand: The exploration of counselor educators'-in-training professional identity development through sandtray.* [Doctoral dissertation]. University of Wyoming.

Fitzpatrick, M. R., Kovalak, A. L., & Weaver, A. (2010). How trainees develop an initial theory of practice: A process model of tentative identifications. *Counselling and Psychotherapy Research, 10*(2), 93–102. doi:10.1080/14733141003773790.

Ford, C. G., Kiken, L. G., Haliwa, I., & Shook, N. J. (2021). Negatively biased cognition as a mechanism of mindfulness: A review of the literature. *Current Psychology.* https://doi.org/10.1007/s12144-021-02147-y

Foucault, M. (1965). *Madness & civilization: A history of insanity in the age of reason.* Vintage Books.

Friedman, H. S., & Anderson, M. (2019). Embracing the past: Moving into the future. *Journal of Sandplay Therapy, 28*(1). www.sandplay.org/journal/abstracts/volume-28-number-1/friedman-harriet-anderson-marion-embracing-the-past-moving-into-the-future/

Friedman, H. S., & Mitchell, R. R. (Eds.). (2008). *Supervision of sandplay therapy.* Routledge.

Gallup. (2022). *America's reported mental health at new low; more seek help.* https://news.gallup.com/poll/467303/americans-reported-mental-health-new-low-seek-help.aspx

Geurtzen, N., Keijsers, G. P. J., Karremans, J. C., & Hutschemaekers, G. J. M. (2018). Patients' care dependency in mental health care: Development of a self-report questionnaire and preliminary correlates. *Journal of Clinical Psychology, 74*(7), 1189–1206. doi:10.1002/jclp. 22574.

Grant, A. M., & Berry, J. W. (2011). The necessity of others is the mother of invention: Intrinsic and prosocial motivations, perspective taking, and creativity. *Academy of Management Journal, 54*(1), 73–96. https://doi.org/10.5465/AMJ.2011.59215085

Greenleaf, R. (1970). *The servant as leader.* www.greenleaf.org/products-page/the-servant-as-leader/

Hagedorn, W. B., & Moorhead, H. J. H. (2010). The God-shaped hole: Addictive disorders and the search for perfection. *Counseling and Values, 55*(1), 63–78. https://doi.org/10.1002/j.2161-007X.2010.tb00022.x

Homeyer, L. E., & Bennett, M. M. (2023). *The guide to play therapy documentation & parent consultation.* Routledge.

Huxley, A. (2006). *Brave new world.* Harper Perennial. (Original work published 1932).

Inter-Regional Society of Jungian Analysts (IRSJA). (2023). *Training.* https://irsja. org/become-an-analyst/analyst-training-program/

Jung, C. G. (1989). *Memories, dreams, reflections.* A. Jaffe (Ed.), C. Winston & R. Winston (Trans.). Vintage Books.

Jung, C. G. (2023). *The collected works of C. G. Jung: Revised and expanded complete digital edition.* (CW 1–20). G. Adler, W. McGuire, & H. Read (Eds.), R. F. C. Hull (Trans.). Princeton University Press. https://press.princeton.edu/books/ ebook/9780691255194/the-collected-works-of-c-g-jung

Kalff, D. M. (2020). *Sandplay: A psychotherapeutic approach to the psyche.* B. L. Matthews (Trans). Analytical Psychology Press, Sandplay Editions. (Original work published 1966).

Kirsch, T. B. (2000). *The Jungians: A comparative and historical perspective.* Routledge.

Kornilova, T. V., & Kornilov, S. A. (2010). Intelligence and tolerance/intolerance for uncertainty as predictors of creativity. *Psychology in Russia: State of the Art, 3,* 240–256. https://doi.org/10.11621/pir.2010.0012

Kozlowski, J. M., Pruitt, N. T., DeWalt, T. A., & Knox, S. (2014). Can boundary crossings in clinical supervision be beneficial? *Counseling Psychology Quarterly, 27*(2), 109–126. http://dx.doi.org/10.1080/09515070.2013.870123

Lambert, S. F., LeBlanc, M., Mullen, J. A., Ray, D., Baggerly, J., White, J., & Kaplan, D. (2007). Learning more about those who plays in session: The national play therapy in counseling practices project (phase I). *Journal of Counseling & Development, 85,* 42–46. http://dx.doi.org/10.1002/j.1556-6678.2007.tb00442.x

Landreth, G. (2024). *Play therapy: The art of the relationship* (4th ed.). Routledge. (Original work published 1991).

Leader, C. (2015). Supervising the uncanny: The play within the play. *Journal of Analytical Psychology, 60*(5), 657–678. doi:10.1111/1468-5922.12178.

Lee, H. K., Chang, H., & Bryan, L. (2020). Doctoral students' learning success in online-based leadership programs: Intersection with technological and relational factors. *International Review of Research in Open and Distributed Learning, 21*(1), 61–81. https://doi.org/10.19173/irrodl.v20i5.4462

Lee, J.-S., & Jang, D.-H. (2015). The effectiveness of sand play treatment meta-analysis. *Korean Journal of Child Psychological Therapy, 10*(1), 1–26.

Main, R. (2007). *Revelations of chance: Synchronicity as spiritual experience.* The State University of New York Press.

Malikiosi-Loizos, M. (2013). Personal therapy for future therapists: Reflections on a still debated issue. *The European Journal of Counselling Psychology, 2*(1). doi:10.5964/ejcop.v2i1.4

McCabe, I. (2015). *Carl Jung and Alcoholics Anonymous: The Twelve Steps as a spiritual journey of individuation.* Routledge.

McRoberts, R. (2018). Informed consent: Addressing child autonomy. *Play Therapy Magazine, 13*(4), 8. www.modernpubsonline.com/Play-Therapy/PlayTherapy Dec18/html/index.html

McRoberts, R. (2022). Addressing the creativity crisis: Sandplay therapists' mode-shifting and professional identity development. *Journal of Sandplay Therapy, 31*(2), 129–142. www.sandplay.org/journal/research-articles/addressing-the-creativity-crisis-sandplay-therapists-mode-shifting-and-professional-identity-development/

McRoberts, R. (2023). The white rabbit: Sacred & subversive. The Archive for Research in Archetypal Symbolism. *ARAS Connections: Image and Archetype, 2*, 1–32. https://aras.org/newsletters/aras-connections-image-and-archetype-2023-issue-2

McRoberts, R., & Epstein, J. (2023). Creative self-concept, post-traumatic growth, and professional identity resilience in counselors with traumatic experiences: A canonical correlation analysis. *Journal of Creativity in Mental Health*, 1–15. doi :10.1080/15401383.2023.2232730.

Midgley, N., Mortimer, R., Cirasola, A., Batra, P., & Kennedy, E. (2021). The evidence-base for psychodynamic psychotherapy with children and adolescents: A narrative synthesis. *Frontiers in Psychology, 12*(662671), 1–18. doi:10.3389/ fpsyg.2021.662671.

Mullen, J. A., Luke, M., & Drewes, A. A. (2007). Supervision can be playful, too: Play therapy techniques that enhance supervision. *International Journal of Play Therapy, 16*, 69–85. http://dx.doi.org/10.1037/1555-6824.16.1.69

Muro, J. H., Holliman, R. P., Blanco, P. J., & Stickley, V. K. (2015). Exploring play therapy training: An investigation on the impact of practice on attitudes, knowledge, and skills with master's level students. *International Journal of Play Therapy, 24*(4), 234–247. http://dx.doi.org/10.1037/a0039811

Murthy, K. (2020). Paradigm shift: A need of the hour in the techno era. *Borneo Journal of Medical Sciences.* https://jurcon.ums.edu.my/ojums/index.php/bjms/ article/view/2224

Myers, J. E., Witmer, J. M., & Sweeney, T. J. (1996). The Wheel of Wellness. *The WEL workbook: Wellness evaluation of lifestyle.* MindGarden.

National Center for Education Statistics. (2018). *Integrated postsecondary education data system (IPEDS): Table 311.15.* [Data file]. https://nces.ed.gov/programs/ digest/d17/tables/dt17_311.15.asp

National Geographic. (2023, March 22). *Paganism is on the rise.* www.nationalgeo graphic.com/culture/article/where-to-go-to-explore-pagan-culture#

Noll, R. (1994). *The Jung cult: Origins of a charismatic movement*. Free Press Paperbacks.

Norris, C. (2021). The negativity bias, revisited: Evidence from neuroscience measures and an individual differences approach. *Social Neuroscience*, *16*. doi:10.108 0/17470919.2019.1696225

O'Connor, K., & Ray, D. (2023, October 13). *What if we have more in common than we think? Core concepts that move play therapy forward*. Keynote. Association for Play Therapy International Conference. Palm Springs, CA.

Penn, S. L., & Post, P. B. (2012). Investigating various dimensions of play therapists' self-reported multicultural counseling competence. *International Journal of Play Therapy*, *21*, 14–29. http://dx.doi.org/10.1037/a0026894

Pew Research Center. (2018). *Categorizing Americans' religious typology groups*. www. pewresearch.org/religion/2018/08/29/religious-and-spiritual-practices-and-beliefs-2/

Pew Research Center. (2022). *How US religious composition has changed in recent decades*. www.pewresearch.org/religion/2022/09/13/how-u-s-religious-composi tion-has-changed-in-recent-decades/

The Pluralism Project. (2023). *Native American traditions*. Harvard University. https://pluralism.org/native-american-traditions

Poston, J. M., & Bland, E. D. (2020). Not just anything goes: Psychoanalytic psychotherapy competencies in psychology doctoral programs. *Psychoanalytic Psychology*, *37*(1), 62–73. http://dx.doi.org/10.1037/pap0000209

Qian, X., & Yarnal, C. (2011). The role of playfulness in the leisure stress-coping process among emerging adults: An SEM analysis. *Leisure/Loisir: Journal of the Canadian Association for Leisure Studies*, *35*(2), 191–209.

Reynolds, V. (2011). Supervision of solidarity practices: Solidarity teams and people-ing-the-room. *Context*, *116*, 4–6. https://vikkireynoldsdotca.files.word press.com/2017/12/reynolds2011solidarityteamscontextuk.pdf

Roesler, C. (2013). Evidence for the effectiveness of Jungian psychotherapy: A review of empirical studies. *Behavioral Science*, *3*(4), 562–575. doi:10.3390/bs3040562.

Roesler, C. (2018). *Research in analytical psychology: Empirical research*. Routledge.

Roesler, C. (2019). Sandplay therapy: An overview of theory, applications and evidence base. *The Arts in Psychotherapy*, *64*, 84–94. https://doi.org/10.1016/j. aip.2019.04.001

Rogers, M., Wattis, J., Stephenson, J., Khan, W., Curran, S., & Walters, P. (2023). A questionnaire-based study of attitudes to spirituality in people using mental health services and their perceptions of the relevance of the concept of spiritually

competent practice. *Journal of Spirituality in Mental Health.* https://doi.org/10.10
80/19349637.2023.2205036

Rønnestad, M. H., & Skovholt, T. M. (2003). The journey of the counselor and
therapist: Research findings and perspectives on professional development.
Journal of Career Development, 30(1), 5–44. doi:10.1023/A:1025173508081.

Rowe, D. A. (2023). *Disseminating research with an equity-focused lens.* Method-
space. Sage. www.methodspace.com/blog/disseminating-research-with-an-equity-
focused-lens

Sandplay Therapists of America (STA). (2012). *Procedure manual for research
using sandplay therapy as originated by Dora Kalff.* www.sandplay.org/wp-content/
uploads/2012/11/Procedure-Manual-for-Sandplay-Research.pdf

Sandplay Therapists of America (STA). (2018). *STA standards for professional
conduct.* www.sandplay.org/wp-content/uploads/STA-Standards-of-Professional-
Conduct-Sept2018.pdf

Sandplay Therapists of America (STA). (2022). *STA handbook.* www.sandplay.org/
membership/sta-handbook/

Schmidt, M. (2014). Influences on my clinical practice and identity Jungian analysis on the couch – What and where is the truth of it? *The Journal of Analytical
Psychology, 59*(5), 661–679. http://dx.doi.org/10.1111/1468-5922.12116

Shedler, J. (2010). The efficacy of psychodynamic psychotherapy. *American
Psychology, 65*(2), 98–109. doi:10.1037/a0018378. PMID: 20141265.

Sonnex, C., Roe, C. A., & Roxburgh, E. C. (2022). Flow, liminality, and eudaimonia:
Pagan ritual practice as a gateway to a life with meaning. *Journal of Humanistic
Psychology, 62*(2), 233–256. https://doi.org/10.1177/0022167820927577

Twenge, J. M. (2014). *Generation me – revised and updated: Why today's young
Americans are more confident, assertive, entitled – and more miserable than ever
before.* Atria.

Vernoy, K. (2023, March 6). Has therapy become the new religion? Therapy
Reimagined. [Podcast episode]. https://therapyreimagined.com/modern-therapist-
podcast/has-therapy-become-the-new-religion/

Wade, S. (2019). *Foucault in California [A true story – wherein the great French philosopher drops acid in the Valley of Death].* Heyday.

Wakefield, C. (2014). In search of Aphrodite: Working with archetypes and an
inner cast of characters in women with low sexual desire. *Sexual and Relationship
Therapy, 29*(1), 31–41. http://dx.doi.org/10.1080/14681994.2013.861594

Wampold, B. E., & Owen, J. (2021). Therapist effects: History, methods, magni-
tude, and characteristics of effective therapists. In M. Barkham, W. Lutz, &

L. G. Castonguay (Eds.), *Bergin and Garfield's handbook of psychotherapy and behavior change: 50th anniversary edition* (pp. 297–326). John Wiley & Sons.

Weiss, S. L. (1973). Differences in goals, interests, and personalities between students with analytic and behavior therapy orientations. *Professional Psychology, 4*, 145–150.

Werries, J. R. (2015). *Factors associated with the choice of a theoretical orientation for master's level counselors-in-training.* [Doctoral dissertation]. University of the Cumberlands. ProQuest: 10629202.

Wiersma, J. K., Freedle, L. R., McRoberts, R., & Solberg, K. B. (2022). A meta-analysis of sandplay therapy treatment outcomes. *International Journal of Play Therapy, 31*(4), 197–215. https://doi.org/10.1037/pla0000180

Wilkinson, M. (2005). Undoing dissociation: Affective neuroscience: A contemporary Jungian clinical perspective. *The Journal of Analytical Psychology, 50*(4), 483–501. https://doi.org/10.1111/j.0021-8774.2005.00550.x

Winborn, M. (2016). Analytical psychology and science: Adversaries or allies? *Psychological Perspectives, 59*(4), 490–508. doi:10.1080/00332925.2016.1240536.

Wright, L. M. (2015). Brain science and illness beliefs: An unexpected explanation of the healing power of therapeutic conversations and the family interventions that matter. *Journal of Family Nursing, 21*(2), 179–185. https://doi.org/10.1177/107484071557582

Zellars, K. L., Tepper, B. J., & Duffy, M. K. (2002). Abusive supervision and subordinates' organizational citizenship behavior. *Journal of Applied Psychology, 86*, 1068–1076. http://dx.doi.org/10.1037/0021-9010.87.6.1068

Index

Note: Locators in *italic* indicate figures and in **bold** tables.

assessments, tests 36; Counselor
Competencies Scale – Revised (CCS-R)
96, 189, 190, 193–194, 195; counselor
training 48, 49, 153; creativity evaluation
(Mode-Shifting Index) 38–39; delay
131; formal, informal 39, 131, 165–166,
230; SOAP (subjective, objective,
assessment, progress) notes 171; spiritual
168; therapy alliance, documentation 39,
131, 165–166, 230; treatment plan review
230–231
Association for Creativity in Counseling
(ACC) 39
Association for Play Therapy (APT) 22,
23, 163, 207, 211, 212, 213, 234,
242
Association for Spiritual, Ethical, and
Religious Values in Counseling
(ASERVIC) 86, 88
associations: archetype material 117;
as complex expressions 111; dream
interpretation 202; enriching 193; free
195, 205; and memory 74; positive,
negative 122; poverty of 111–112;
sensory 38; symbolic charge 111; Word
Association Test (WAT) 38, 121
associative mode 40, 64
associative process 41, 46, 193, 195, 214;
see also mode-shifting
atman 70, 87
attachment / attachment theory 38, 88–89,
122, 193, 210, 213, 229
Attachment Regulation & Competency
Framework (ARC) 88
attitudes: analytic 36; negative 127;
reflective 95; religious 88, 89, 92;
symbolic 111, 113
attunement, mis-attunement 39, 94,
159, 196; see also co-regulation;
co-transference
autonomy 6, 167, 200
awe; see numinous

beginning with the end in mind 154
behavior, ethical; see ethics
behavioral health 7, 208, 212
behavioral management 168
behavioral therapies: cognitive behavioral
therapy (CBT) 11, 17, 40, 74, 83, 132,

191, 232, 235; dialectical behavioral
therapy (DBT) 11, 16–17
behaviorism 10
behaviors, professional dispositional 153
best practices 6, 164, 166, 168, 206
bias 38, 74, 92, 113, 158, 162, 186, 198–199,
241
biopower 3, 6, 22, 23
The Body Keeps the Score (Van der Kolk) 75
body-based therapies 217, 218
bracketing 19, 91
brain: archetypal symbolic knowledge
absorption 106–107; circuit activation
38; function improvement, sandplay 215;
hemispheres (left, right) 37–38, 40, 64;
imaging 35, 38; structural development
42
Brave New World (Huxley) 5–6, 243
breath / breathing / breathwork 87, 105,
208, 219
broaching 155, 197
Buhler, C. 213

Campbell, Joseph 110
Carroll, Lewis 3
catharsis 131
CBT; see Cognitive Behavioral Therapy
(CBT)
CCPT (Child Centered Play Therapy); see
Child Centered Play Therapy (CCPT)
The Center for Applied Jungian Studies
203
Certified Sandplay Therapist Teaching
Members (CST-Ts) 213, 234, 242
chaos stage 117, 130, *130*, 214
Child-Centered Play Therapy (CCPT)
45–46; characteristics 191–192; child
(vs parents) as client 211–212;
development, approach (Landreth) 12,
45, 237–238; vs Jungian play therapy 36,
45, 186; materials 209; naming objects/
symbols 205; non-directive 209; *Play
Therapy: The Art of the Relationship*
(Landreth) 12; questions, verbal
intervention 190, 191, 195, 201, 208; vs
sandplay therapy 191–192; verbal /
non-verbal 192, 215–216, 239
circumambulating/tion 11, 13–14, 40, 94,
161

Milton Keynes UK
Ingram Content Group UK Ltd.
UKHW020845270824
447372UK00003B/27